Biosensors

IEEE Press
445 Hoes Lane
Piscataway, NJ 08854

Biosensors

Nanomaterials, Approaches, and Performance-Enhancement Strategies

Baljinder Kaur
Department of Physics, Madhav Institute of Technology & Science
Gwalior, Madhya Pradesh, India

Santosh Kumar
Department of Electronics and Communication Engineering, Koneru Lakshmaiah Education Foundation Deemed to be University, Vaddeswaram, Guntur, India

Brajesh Kumar Kaushik
Department of Electronics and Communication Engineering
Indian Institute of Technology Roorkee, Roorkee, India

IEEE Press Series on Sensors
Vladimir Lumelsky, Series Editor

IEEE Press

WILEY

Published by John Wiley & Sons, Inc., Hoboken, New Jersey.
Published simultaneously in Canada.

Library of Congress Cataloging-in-Publication Data Applied for:

Hardback ISBN: 9781394268207

Cover Design: Wiley
Cover Image: © zf L/Getty Images

Set in 9.5/12.5pt STIXTwoText by Straive, Pondicherry, India

Contents

About the Authors

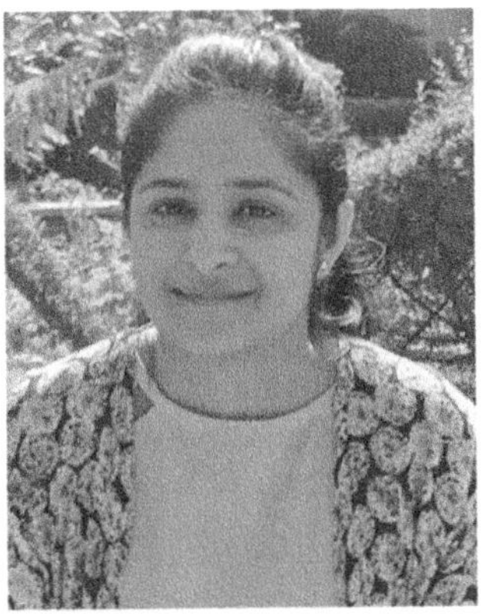

Baljinder Kaur received her Doctorate of Philosophy (PhD) in 2020 from the National Institute of Technology, Delhi, India. She completed her Post-Doctoral Fellowship in 2023 at the Indian Institute of Technology, Roorkee, India. She is currently an assistant professor in the Department of Physics at Madhav Institute of Technology & Science, Gwalior, Madhya Pradesh, India. She has published more than 30 research articles in national and international SCI journals. Her research interests include plasmonic sensors, optical device modelling, fiber optics, and 2D materials.

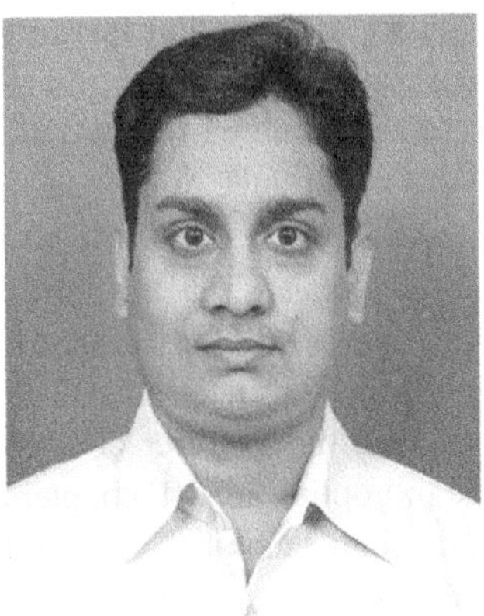

Santosh Kumar (Fellow of SPIE) received his PhD degree from IIT (ISM) Dhanbad, Dhanbad, India, in 2014. He was with Liaocheng University, Liaocheng, China, from 2018 to 2023. He is currently a professor in the Department of Electronics and Communication Engineering at Koneru Lakshmaiah Education Foundation, Vaddeswaram, India. He has been recognized as one of the worlds's top 2% scientists by Stanford University during the last three consecutive years. With extensive research experience, he has supervised 20 MTech dissertations and 7 PhD candidates. His contributions to the field include the publication of over 400 research articles in prestigious SCI journals and conferences, with more than 8000 citations and an H-index of 55. His work has been featured in renowned journals such as *Biosensors and Bioelectronics, Journal of Lightwave Technology, Optics Express, Optics Letters, Applied Physics Letters, ACS Applied Nano Materials*, and *Biosensors*, and various IEEE Transactions. He has presented his research at conferences across in India, China, Belgium, and the USA, demonstrating his global reach. He is the author of four scholarly books published under CRC Press (Taylor & Francis) and Springer Nature. He was recently granted a patent application for his groundbreaking optical fiber-sensing technology. As a highly regarded expert, he has reviewed over 2200 manuscripts for esteemed SCI journals published by IEEE, Elsevier, Springer, OPTICA, SPIE, and Nature. With expertise in electronics, communications engineering, and physics, his research focuses on WaveFlex biosensors, fiberoptic sensors, photonics and plasmonic devices, nano- and biophotonics, waveguides, interferometers, and the Internet of Things. Through fruitful collaborations with renowned universities in India, China, Portugal, Brazil, and Italy, he conducts cutting-edge scientific research.

Dr. Kumar is a Fellow of SPIE, a Life Fellow member of the Optical Society of India (OSI), and a senior member of IEEE, OPTICA, and SPIE. He also serves as an OPTICA traveling lecturer. Recognizing his contributions, he has been appointed as the Chair of the Optica Optical Biosensor Technical Group and as an associate editor for *IEEE Sensors Journal, IEEE Internet of Things Journal*, and *Biomedical Optics Express.*

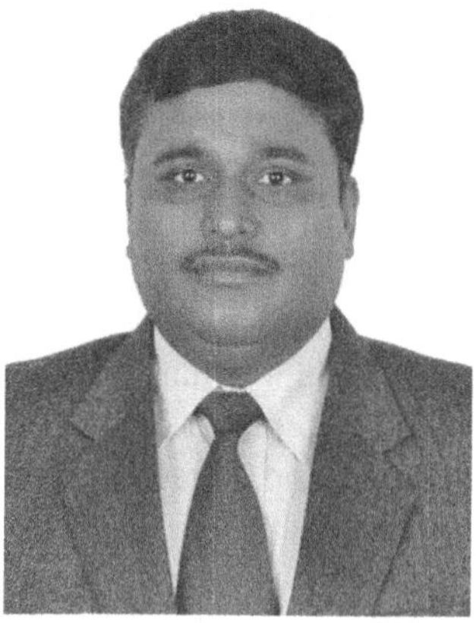

Brajesh Kumar Kaushik received his Doctorate of Philosophy (PhD) in 2007 from the Indian Institute of Technology, Roorkee, India. He joined the Department of Electronics and Communication Engineering, Indian Institute of Technology, Roorkee, as an assistant professor in December 2009; promoted to associate professor in April 2014; and since August 2020, he has been serving as a full professor. He had been a visiting professor at TU-Dortmund, Germany, in 2017; McGill University, Canada, in 2018; and Liaocheng University, China, in 2018. He served as a visiting lecturer of SPIE Society to deliver lectures in the area of spintronics and optics to SPIE chapters located across the world. He regularly serves as general chair, technical chair, and keynote speaker at reputed international and national conferences. He also served as the chairman and vice chairman of IEEE Roorkee Sub-section. Dr. Kaushik is a senior member of IEEE and a member of many expert committees constituted by government and nongovernment organizations. He is currently serving as a distinguished lecturer (DL) for the IEEE Electron Devices Society (EDS) to offer EDS chapters with quality lectures in his research domain. He is editor-in-chief of the *Elsevier Journal, Memories – Materials, Devices, Circuits and Systems*; an editor for *IEEE Transactions on Electron Devices*; an associate editor for the *IEEE Sensors Journal* and *IET Circuits, Devices & Systems*; an editor for *Microelectronics Journal*, Elsevier; and an editorial board member for *Circuit World*, Emerald. He is among the top 2% scientists in world as per Stanford University reports in 2019 and 2021. He is currently serving as a member of two technical committees – namely, Spintronics (TC-5) and Quantum Computing, Neuromorphic Computing and Unconventional Computing (TC-16) of IEEE Nanotechnology Council. He is also the regional coordinator (R10) for IEEE Nanotechnology Council chapters. He has 12 books to his credit, published by reputed publishers such as CRC Press, Springer, Artech, and Elsevier. One his books, titled *Nanoscale Devices: Physics, Modeling, and Their Application*, CRC Press, won the 2018 Outstanding Book and Digital Product Award in the Reference/Monograph Category from the Taylor and Francis Group. He has attained fellowships and awards from DAAD, Shastri Indo-Canadian Institute (SICI), ASEM Duo, and the United States–India Educational Foundation (Fulbright-Nehru Academic and Professional Excellence). His research interests are in the areas of high-speed interconnects, optics- and photonics-based devices, image processing, spintronics-based devices, circuits, and computing.

Preface

Due to advancement of new technologies in synthesis methods, the biosensing field has emerged as a promising tool in diverse fields that include healthcare, environmental monitoring, food, and agriculture industry. The need of early diagnosis of globally spread deadly diseases, such as cancer, tuberculosis, and cardiovascular disease, has increased the demand for rapid, cost-effective, highly sensitive, and accurate methods and devices.

This book embarks on a journey through the captivating progress made in biosensors to detect various diseases on the basis of bio-recognition elements. Nucleic acid, enzyme, aptamer, antibodies, bacteriophages, peptides, and synthetic molecular imprinted polymer-based sensor design in optical, electrochemical, and mass-based biosensors are discussed for different biomedical applications. More precisely, sensing techniques include plasmonic surface plasmon resonance (SPR)/localized (L) SPR sensors, surface-enhanced Raman scattering (SERS), colorimetric, fluorescence, electrochemical, magneto, and piezoelectric biosensors to detect the different biosamples will be discussed in detail.

The chapters are divided on the basis of bioreceptors and new nanomaterials that cover recent advances in diseased detection using various biosensor design that are not summarized in a single book in the previously published reviews. This book also focuses on advancements in nanostructured materials synthesis, signal enhancement strategies, and biomarker detection the diseases such as cancer, pathogenic bacterial infection, and tuberculosis. It also includes the main challenges, limitations, and future prospects to develop the biosensor for point-of-care and clinical applications. The cons and pros of each technique and bioreceptors are discussed in a summary section.

This book will be of interest to researchers in the fields of physics, chemistry, and biomedical science and a broad audience of researchers and experts in the diagnostic and analytical industry. We envisage that people working in medical diagnostics, biosensors, environmental and food safety monitoring, electronics and material engineers, defense/homeland security, and professors/postgraduate students in these sectors will benefit greatly by reading this book. Therefore, this book will attract the attention of various industries and researchers that will help to improve the performance of sensors. The new technologies include gene editing known as clustered regularly interspaced short palindromic repeat (CRISPR), quorum sensing that utilizes inter- and intra-cell signal, two-dimensional (2D) materials, and aptamer-mediated sensor designs with high performance and low detection limits required in case of bio-samples; these are discussed in detail.

Outline of This Book

This book provides a comprehensive overview of recent advancements in biomedical sensors. It includes advanced materials and various enhancement strategies to improve the performance of different biosensing platforms. It presents an exploration of ECL, mass-based biosensors, and optical biosensor technologies grounded in resonance, absorption, interference, fluorescence, and scattering. This book provides an overview of the innovations and their applications, as well as future perspectives and insights to ensure reader's confidence and enhance knowledge in the biosensing field. It also covers the immobilization methods used in industry and the lab to fabricate different bioreceptor-based biosensor structures.

The book provides readers with deep knowledge regarding nanomaterial-based biosensors to detect biomarkers and pathogens associated with diseases that spread throughout the world. This book will be of interest to researchers in the fields of physics, chemistry, and biomedical science, and to people working in medical diagnostics, biosensors, environmental and food safety monitoring, electronics and material engineers, defense, and homeland security. Professors and postgraduate students in these sectors will greatly benefit from reading it. Examples are usually pulled from everyday life and recent advancements in plasmonic biosensing devices to pique the readers' interest and make them eager to learn more. Following are descriptions of the book's outline.

Chapter 1 introduces biosensors, constituents, and operating principles. This chapter will give insight on bioreceptor types and their role in the detection process of various sensing schemes. Various biosamples, including cancer cells, tuberculosis, and infectious pathogens, are discussed, as well as various signal enhancement strategies and nanomaterials.

Thereafter, **Chapter 2** introduces the currently and previously used immobilization techniques used to immobilize antibodies, aptamers, cells, nucleic acids, bacteriophages, enzymes, and imprinted polymers. It focuses on adsorption or electrostatic interaction, covalent binding, entrapment, cross-linking-based immobilization techniques, and the battle among them toward the selection of a method to immobilize a specific bioreceptor. It also demonstrates the details and properties of different materials used as supports, such as glass, polymers, hydrogels, self-assembled monolayers (SAM), metals, nanoparticles, and membranes. It also summarizes the recently reported ECL, optical, and mass-based biosensors that use different immobilized methods for each receptor in the different biosensing applications.

Chapter 3 discusses recent developments in biosensors for detecting various diseases in food, beverages, and clinical samples using nucleic acid-based sensor technology. It provides a summary of the different types of aptamer-based biosensors (e.g. optical, ECL, piezoelectrical, and SERS) for the detection of microorganisms, toxins, and diseases.

Chapter 4 discusses the development of antibody-based optical sensor designs for detecting cancerous cell lines, highlighting the various sensor types. The possibilities of integration of these biosensors, point-of-care testing, and the emergence of new materials that include black phosphorus, phosphorene, silicene, Mxenes, immobilization methods, synthesis methods, and gene editing technologies are addressed. Additionally, the disadvantages of antibodies and the benefits of aptamers over antibodies are discussed.

Chapter 5 discusses the development of biosensor technologies based on small and 3D-shaped aptamers as compared to bulky antibodies that can surpass conventional *in vitro* diagnostics for disease detection and health monitoring. It explores the criteria to choose the target-specific aptamer and design strategies from the pool of aptamers through the SELEX method. It also discusses section-wise details of various types of SELEX and non-SELEX methods and steps involved in aptamer synthesis.

Chapter 6 discusses the bacteriophage-based biosensor designs, structure, family of phages used to specifically detect viruses, bacteria, and microorganisms related to various diseases. The chapter presents a comparative study of bacteriophage-based and traditional bacterial detection methods. It includes the details of reporter, stained, lytic, capturing, and receptor-binding protein-based probes. As this technology is still limited to the detection of microorganisms, its possibilities to explore other analytes have been discussed.

Chapter 7 discusses a peptide-based biosensor to detect analytes. It also provides an overview of the operating principle, the synthesis of peptides, and their use in the fabrication of sensors. This chapter examines the function of peptides as specific sequence cleavers, hydroxyl group phosphorylation catalysts, and antifouling agents in biosensors.

Chapter 8 discusses synthetic BRE, such as molecule imprinted polymers, and several nanomaterials-based biosensor designs for detecting various diseases, biomolecules, and other infected biosamples. It is concerned with the advantages and disadvantages of carbon, polymers, metals, metal oxides, and quantum dot-based nanomaterials in medical biosensing applications. A section also discusses the challenges and developments in the field of wearable biosensors to detect diseases.

Chapter 9 discusses the role of novel nanomaterials and advancements in optical biosensors for cancer detection due to the increased incidence of cancer-related diseases. It also illustrates various types of nanoparticles, including organic and inorganic, with different optical platforms to detect cancer-related diseases. Table 9.1 summarizes various biosensors designed to detect cancer. In addition, the chapter presents future development directions and characteristics of the next generation of paper-based devices.

Baljinder Kaur
Santosh Kumar
Brajesh Kumar Kaushik

Acknowledgments

The authors wish to extend their heartfelt appreciation to IEEE-Wiley Press, especially the editor, who diligently polished the book for its publication. Apart from the contributions of a solitary individual, the accomplishment of research work is dependent on the motivation, support, effective input, discussion, and guidance provided by the experts, and colleagues. It has been a great pleasure working with them, and we trust they feel the same, too.

Baljinder Kaur extends her wholehearted and deep gratitude to Prof. B. K. Kaushik and Prof. Santosh Kumar for their priceless mentorship, motivation, guidance, and unwavering backing during the write-up of this book. Dr. Kaur would also like to express her deep sense of appreciation to her family and friends for their constant support, encouragement, and cooperation.

Santosh Kumar would like to express his sincere gratitude to Shri Koneru Satyanarayana Garu, honorable president of the Koneru Lakshmaiah Education Foundation (deemed to be University), Vaddeswaram, Andhra Pradesh, India, for his immense encouragement and support throughout the writing of this book. Dr. Kumar would also like to express his heartfelt gratitude to his wife, Dr. Ragini Singh, and son, Ayaansh Singh, for their unwavering support, encouragement, and cooperation, as well as to his loving parents.

Brajesh Kumar Kaushik acknowledges the relentless efforts made by the co-authors in bringing this book to the final stage. The support provided by the Indian Institute of Technology-Roorkee is also highly acknowledged. This book is dedicated to all the friends and family members – especially to my mother, Mrs. Karuna Kaushik; wife, Dr. Supriya Kaushik; and son, Partha Kaushik for their unwavering support and understanding.

We hope that this book serves as a foundation for future advancements in the field and serves as a valuable reference for engineers, researchers, and students working in the fields of nano-optics, nano-photonics, plasmonics, and optical fiber biosensors in general.

List of Abbreviations

2D	Two-dimensional
AEM	Absorption enhancement material
Al_2O_3	Aluminum oxide
BRE	Bio-recognition element
BSA	Bovine serum albumin
CaF_2	Calcium fluoride
CRISPR	Clustered regularly interspaced short palindromic repeats
D.A.	Detection accuracy
DNA	Deoxyribonucleic acid
E. Coli	*Escherichia Coli*
ECL	Electrochemical
ELISA	Enzyme-linked immunosorbent assays
EW	Evanescent wave
FRET	Förster resonance energy transfer
FPI	Fabry–Perot
FOM	Figure of merit
FWHM	Full width at half maximum
HRP	Horseradish peroxidase
IR	Infrared
LSPR	Localized surface plasmon resonance
LOD	Limit of detection
MIP	Molecular imprinted polymer
MoS_2	Molybdenum disulfide
$MoSe_2$	Molybdenum diselenide
MZI	Mach–Zehnder interferometer
NIR	Near infrared
NA	Nucleic acids
NP	Nanoparticle
ORD	Optimum radiation damping

PathoBact	Pathogenic bacteria
PCF	Photonic crystal-fiber
PF	Perfluorinated
PT	Polythiophene
RI	Refractive index
RIU	Refractive index unit
RNA	Ribonucleic acid
S	Sensitivity
SAM	Self-assembled monolayers
SELEX	Systematic evolution of ligands by exponential enrichment
SERS	Surface-enhanced Raman scattering
SP	Surface plasmon
SPP	Surface plasmon polariton
SPR	Surface plasmon resonance
TE	Transverse electric
TIR	Total internal reflection
TM	Transverse magnetic
TMDCs	Transition metal dichalcogenides
TMM	Transfer matrix method
UV	Ultraviolet light
WS_2	Tungsten disulfide

About the Companion Website

This book is accompanied by a companion website:

www.wiley.com/go/kaur

The website includes sample programs with MATLAB and Simulation data files.

1

Fundamentals of Biomedical Sensors

1.1 Introduction

The use of sensors, education, communication, computers in daily routines, and development of technology over the years has played a significant part in simplifying the human lifestyle [1–3]. Figure 1.1 shows the schematic of a sensor that involve input signal, sensing unit, and output signal. A sensing unit transforms the input signal to an output signal that can be measured using diverse principles, structures, and geometry. Consequently, a sensor converts a physical parameter (temperature, humidity, index of refraction) into a signal that may be processed (e.g. optical, electrochemical (ECL), electrical, and mechanical) [4–7]. Fluorescence, absorbance, scattering, polarization, interference, color change, and luminescence are among the phenomena utilized in the development of sensors.

Sensors have been explored in the numerous sectors that include biomedicine, electronics, military applications, biochemical sensing, and environmental monitoring [8]. A wide variety of research articles on diverse sensing applications has been published in the recent few years due to advancement in various technologies. A biosensor structure is designed using a transducer, light source, and bioreceptor to detect an analyte. Clark reported a glucose oxidase solution encased in a semipermeable membrane as an electrode sensor for measuring the oxygen level in the blood in 1962 [9]. Updike and Hicks reported a sensor that entraps glucose oxidase solution within polyacrylamide gel in 1967 [10]. Guilbault and Montalvo reported a potentiometric sensor to detect the urease [11]. Then in 1972, 1975, 1976, and 1984, the ion-selective field effect transistor, immunosensor utilizing a potentiometric transducer, ECL glucose sensor, and fiberoptic sensor utilizing polymerization techniques were reported [12–15].

Biosensors: Nanomaterials, Approaches, and Performance-Enhancement Strategies,
First Edition. Baljinder Kaur, Santosh Kumar, and Brajesh Kumar Kaushik.

Published 2025 by John Wiley & Sons, Inc.
Companion website: www.wiley.com/go/kaur

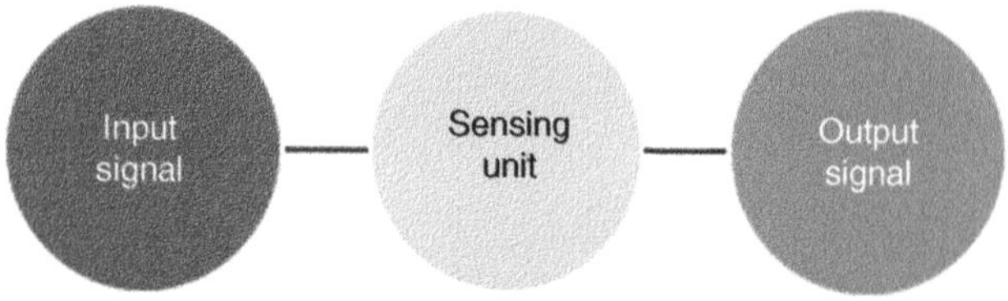

Figure 1.1 An illustration of components of a sensor structure.

Optical biosensors have been explored to detect the neurotransmitters that convey intercellular chemical messages within the nervous system [16, 17]. These neurotransmitters are generated by nerve cells that move to another part of the body and convey information in the form of chemicals such as acetylcholine, dopamine, serotonin, norepinephrine, gamma-aminobutyric acid, glutamate, endorphins, histamine, oxytocin, serotonin, and melatonin. Imbalances of these neurotransmitters are responsible for various neurological disorders such as Parkinson's disease, Alzheimer's, schizophrenia, depression, acetylcholine dysfunction, and altered levels of dopamine serotonin, and norepinephrine [18–25].

The emergence of the surface plasmon resonance (SPR) phenomenon advanced this research even more. Wood observed that reflected spectrum of light is associated with bright and dark bands as light passes through diffraction grating and become polarized [26]. Rayleigh and Fano explained this effect on the basis of the wave scattering from the diffraction grating [27]. Zenneck confirmed the existence of radio frequency waves at the metal-dielectric interface and presented the corresponding Maxwell's equation solution [28]. Otto offered a comprehensive and exact comprehension of the SPR phenomenon using experimental methods in 1968 [29]. Liedberg et al. demonstrated the first SPR-based sensor for measuring bimolecular interactions in 1983 [30]. In 1993, Jorgenson and Yee described a silver plasmonic metal-based fiberoptic sensor, in which the prism is replaced with fiber core to detect the sucrose solution [31]. Later, numerous biosensor designs, including an ECL glucose sensor, the utilization of various enzymes, antibodies, and aptamers for glucose and other biochemical detection, were reported [32, 33]. Technological advances have led to a diversity of biosensor designs [34, 35]. Before they may be used, enzymes must undergo a number of processes, including isolation and purification [36].

Figure 1.2 is a timeline of the development of various biosensor design and milestones. Researchers have studied transducer systems to detect air, soil, and water pollution, as well as numerous infections, toxins, and diseases [37–40]. Identifying ultrasensitive biosensors with sensitivities in the nano, femto, and Pico range is vital to detect diseases at the initial stages – including cancer, tuberculosis infection, cardiovascular disease, and Alzheimer's disease, which are responsible for so many deaths worldwide.

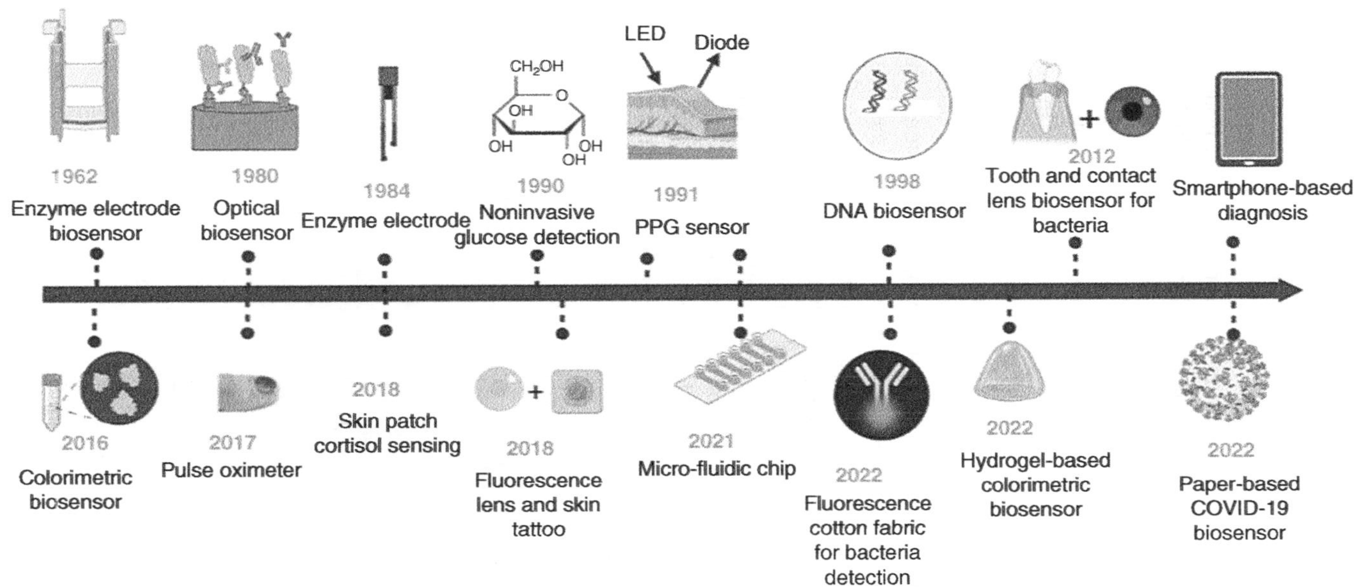

Figure 1.2 A schematic illustration of year-wise progress made in the field of biosensors.

In order to investigate plasmonic, ECL, surface-enhanced Raman scattering (SERS), chemiluminescence, and mass-based biosensors, researchers have investigated numerous methodologies [41–44]. The biosensors market, which includes thermal, ECL, piezoelectric, and optical sensors with applications in medical, food toxicity, bioreactors, agriculture, environment, home healthcare diagnostics, and point-of-care testing, was valued at US$24.9 billion in 2021 globally. It will reach up to US$49.6 billion through 2030 – an indication of an annual growth rate of 8.0% in the years 2022–2030 [45, 46].

Diabetes and cancer-related diseases have increased due to several factors, including environment, food habits, and daily lifestyle. In recent years, the demand for biosensors has rapidly increased due to their wide medical applications, their potential for early diagnosis, and the number of patients affected by diabetes [47]. Of all types of optical sensor designs, ECL glucose biosensors and lateral flow assay-based test for pregnancy have been commercialized most successfully in the global market. Fluorescence-based polymerase chain reactions (PCR) are used in nucleic acid-based tests due to its high specificity and sensitivity. Colorimetric biosensors are commonly used in serological tests that include lateral flow assays and enzyme-linked immunosorbent assays (ELISA) to detect different type of antibodies. Colorimetric methods have the drawback of low sensitivity values. Most plasmonic and refractive-index-based biosensors are still limited to lab research use only [48]. Figure 1.3 illustrates the market demand of different types of biosensors; the sizes of slices indicate the estimated share for each type of biosensor.

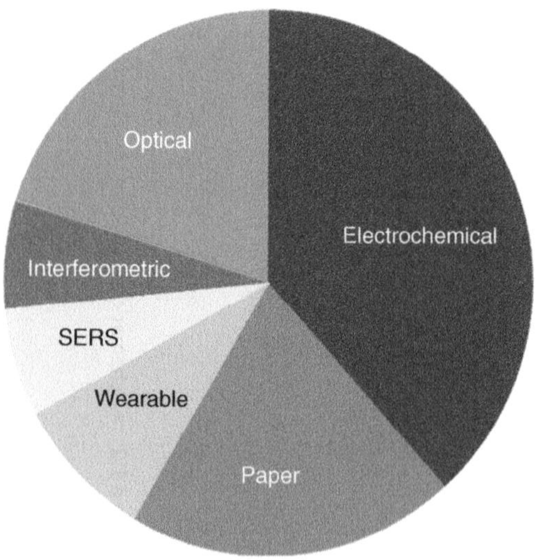

Figure 1.3 Commercialization and market pull of different types of biosensor platforms.

1.2 Classification of Biosensors

Biosensors can be classified on the basis of bio-recognition elements (BREs), different types of transducers, and physical phenomenon. The enzymes, molecular imprinted polymers (MIP), antibodies, nucleic acids, cells, and aptamers have been explored as a biological recognition element to detect numerous analytes [49]. Types of transducers include ECL, optical, piezoelectric, thermal, and magnetic transducers that changes the form of signal. Various optical sensing techniques, such as the evanescent wave (EW) technique [50], fiber grating, SPR-based sensing, and SERS spectroscopy, are available for different applications [51]. ECL biosensors operate in potentiometric, amperometric, and conductometric mode while mass-based sensors can be magnetoelectric and piezoelectric.

1.3 Elements of Biosensors

Figures 1.4a and b show the necessary components of a biosensor, including BRE and transducers to process the signal and output display [52].

1.4 Bio-recognition Elements

BREs consist of nucleic acid (NA), lectins, enzymes, entire cells, antibodies, aptamers, bacteriophages, peptides, and molecularly imprinted polymers, as illustrated in Figure 1.4c [53]. Figure 1.4d depicts the many types of transducers. Bacteriophages are a type of pathogen that infects and replicates within bacteria by selectively attaching to tail-spike proteins. Peptides consist of a short segment of 12–15 amino acid residues that are stable in harsh environments, inexpensive, and simple to produce on a large scale. NA utilize genetic materials such as deoxyribonucleic acid (DNA) and ribonucleic acid (RNA) as bioreceptors and aptamers are single-stranded DNA or RNA molecules [54]. Aptamers have a lower molecular weight, are readily produced at a low cost, and have excellent chemical stability [55]. Whole cells include microorganisms or cultivated tissues of multicellular organisms used in numerous biosensing applications due to its lower expenditures [56]. MIPs are artificial bioreceptors that are synthesized in the laboratory with binding sites designed corresponding to the target molecule [57].

1.4.1 Nucleic Acids

NAs are chains of linear polymers that consist of five nucleotides called bases: guanine, adenine, cytosine, uracil, and thymine. DNA is made up of a thymine base, while RNA uses uracil as a base. DNA is a unique genetic component of each

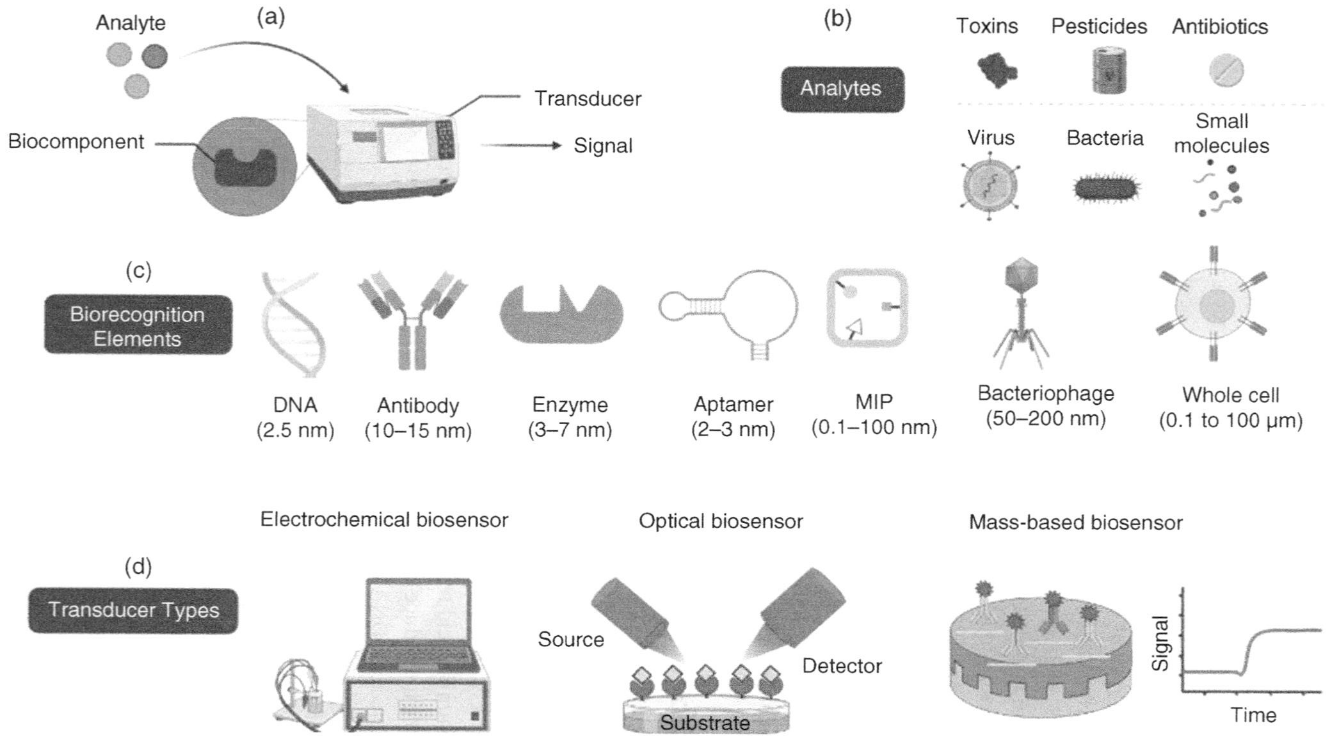

Figure 1.4 Schematic design of the (a) biosensor components (b) different analytes for sensing (c) bio-recognition elements (d) biosensor classification based on types of transducers.

individual organism. Due to its unique sequence and properties, NAs are used to design bioreceptors that match the complementary DNA of the concerned individual. The matching strand can be detected with different transducing mechanisms [54]. NA-based biosensor designs are simple, easy, fast, and low-cost, and they have high specificity to detect an analyte. Various NA biosensors have been reported to detect viruses, cancer cells, microorganisms, and biochemicals [58].

1.4.2 Aptamers

Aptamers are short sequences of oligonucleotides that form a three-dimensional structure that is very specific to the target molecules [55]. To synthesize the aptamers, various chemical or enzymatic procedures or a combination of chemical and enzymatic methods are used [59, 60]. Aptamers are chosen from the systematic evolution of ligands by exponential enrichment (SELEX) techniques using several repeatable steps. The production steps for a single-stranded DNA and its incubation are shown in Figure 1.5. Aptamers are selected using the repletion of various cycles, as these cycles increase the specificity toward the target [39].

1.4.3 Enzymes

Enzymes are target-specific, another type of BRE combined with an appropriate substrate that generates electrons and transfers them to a transducer. Proteins are widely explored enzymes, except RNA enzymes [62]. Enzymes are preferred as labels compared to other BRE, as they can be conjugated with antibodies or aptamers for bioreceptor purposes. Horseradish peroxidase (HRP) and beta-galactosidase are two examples of enzymes used in biosensor designing. Various enzymatic biosensors are also developed based on mass, plasmonic, ECL, thermistor, and piezoelectric techniques for different applications [63]. Enzyme immobilization in the biosensor design is advantageous as it can be used repetitively due to catalytic activity to detect the analyte as compared to the mobile enzyme [63]. Glucose and urease-based biosensors are well-known enzymatic biosensors, of which glucose biosensors are commercialized on different platforms due to their small detection limits and lifetimes.

1.4.4 Antibodies

Antibodies are another class of bioreceptors. They can be polyclonal and monoclonal depending on their production method [64]. Antibodies are proteins generated by plasma cells and classified into five groups that depend on their structure of heavy chain constant region sequences. Their structure is Y-shaped, formed from heavy and light chains, as shown in Figure 1.6. Binding sites specific to

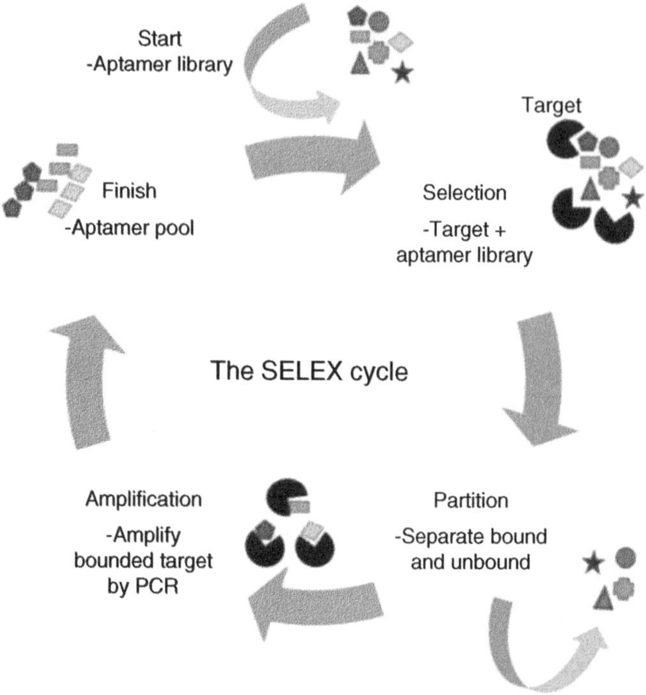

Figure 1.5 Stepwise diagram of the SELEX technique to choose the specific aptamers from the library that includes the separation of bound and unbound targets, target amplification, and generation of a specific aptamer. *Source:* [61]/with permission of Elsevier.

antigens, known as epitopes, can be classified as monoclonal or polyclonal. Monoclonal antibodies can bind to a single epitope while polyclonal antibodies target different epitopes. The production cost and time for making monoclonal antibodies are both higher than for polyclonal antibodies. As compared to other bioreceptors, antibodies involve high costs and stability challenges requiring low-temperature storage. Monoclonal antibodies act as the primary bio-recognition element and polyclonal antibodies act as the secondary bio-recognition element.

Most antibodies are produced by living organisms. Antibodies contain different numbers of epitopes that can be single or multiple [65]. Recombinant antibodies can also be synthesized in the lab with the help of synthetic genes; they are monoclonal in nature. Polyclonal antibodies suffer from high cross-reactivity as compared to monoclonal antibodies due to multiple epitopes. Instead of polyclonal antibodies, monoclonal antibodies are used to design highly specific biosensors because they bind only one epitope. The most important steps during the use of

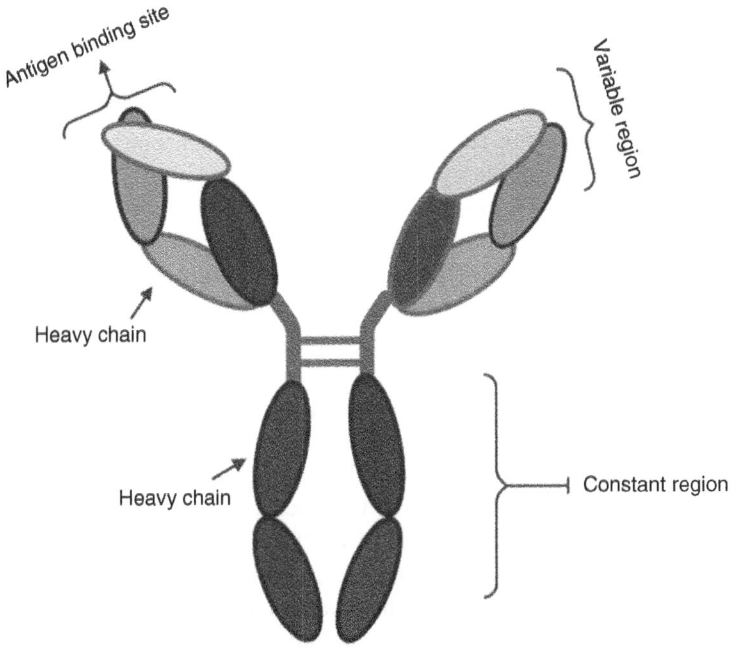

Figure 1.6 Structure of a Y-shaped antibody.

antibodies as a BRE are their immobilization and control of orientation on the surface without damaging their activity and specificity, as this affects the various performance factors, including the limit of detection (LOD), sensitivity, and figure of merit (FOM) [66].

1.4.5 Bacteriophages

A bacteriophage belongs to a family of viruses that contaminate bacteria and are used as BREs to detect the pathogen, cancer biomarkers, tuberculosis, and other pathogenic diseases. Phages are very specific in nature and can affect a single bacterial species. T4, M2, Φ29, and MS2 are a few examples of commonly used phages. A polyhedral head, collar of short length, and a helical tail are the basic components of a phage. Bacteriophages are found in nature and can be used at high pressure, temperature, and pH values. Several biosensor designs have been reported that consider the bacteriophage as a BRE for various types of bacteria detection [67–70]. Pathogenic bacteria (PathoBact) cause infection that consists of single cells with diameter and length in the range of a few μm [71]. PathoBacts have different shapes and can survive in a harsh environment. Bacteria are prokaryotic microorganisms, without membrane-bound organelles such as a nucleus or mitochondria [72]. The five PathoBacts *Pseudomonas Aeruginosa, Klebsiella Pneumoniae, Staphylococcus Aureus, Escherichia Coli,* and *Streptococcus Pneumonia* were responsible for 13.7 million global deaths in 2019 among 33 investigated PathoBacts [73]. The main structure components of bacteria are DNA, cell wall, ribosomes, capsule, cytoplasm, flagellum, and pili.

Gram-positive and Gram-negative bacteria are classified based on response of bacteria to Gram staining. Gram-positive bacteria don't change from crystal violet color and thus remain purple while Gram-negative bacteria turn red due to different thickness of outermost peptidoglycan cell wall that are made from glucose molecules and connected three short peptide chains [74]. In Gram-positive bacteria, the peptidoglycan layer is 30–100 nm thick; this layer is 1–3 nm thick for Gram-negative bacteria surrounded by extra lipopolysaccharides layer [75]. Microscopy, culture, cytological, biochemical test methods, Gram staining, hemagglutination assays, ELISA, and western blotting (serological tests) are conventional; and polymerase chain reaction, fluorescence in situ hybridization, next-generation sequencing, spectroscopic, CRISPR technology, loop-mediated isothermal amplification, microarray technology, and biosensors are advanced method to detect the PathoBacts [76, 77]. The advanced methods are highly sensitive, can select specific target stable, and have short detection time, low cost, simple structures, and less sample preparation. These advantages overcome the drawbacks of conventional methods [78]. Biosensors are advanced emerging and competitive techniques for detecting pathogens and other analytes [79–82]. They involve ECL, piezoelectric, and optical platforms to detect various microorganisms. However, it is important to mention that each technique suffers from several challenges to commercialize it for various applications as it is in the developing stage.

Bacteriophages have been explored in various biosensing applications focused to detect the microorganism due to their chemical and physical properties. They do not require labeling, which creates advantages of reduces cost, time, high sensitivity, widespread availability (food, soil, water, and environment) and specificity. Various biosensor designs using phages to detect the analytes have been reported so far. Figure 1.7 shows a SERS and colorimetric technique combined biosensor that detects *Salmonella Enteritidis* using F5–4 bacteriophage as a bioreceptor and [83].

1.4.6 MIPs

Diagnostic techniques ELISA, PCR, and cell culture require BRE, trained specialists, complex instruments, and sample preparation. They include mimicking various BRE that include NA, proteins, amino acids, cells, peptides, viruses, and

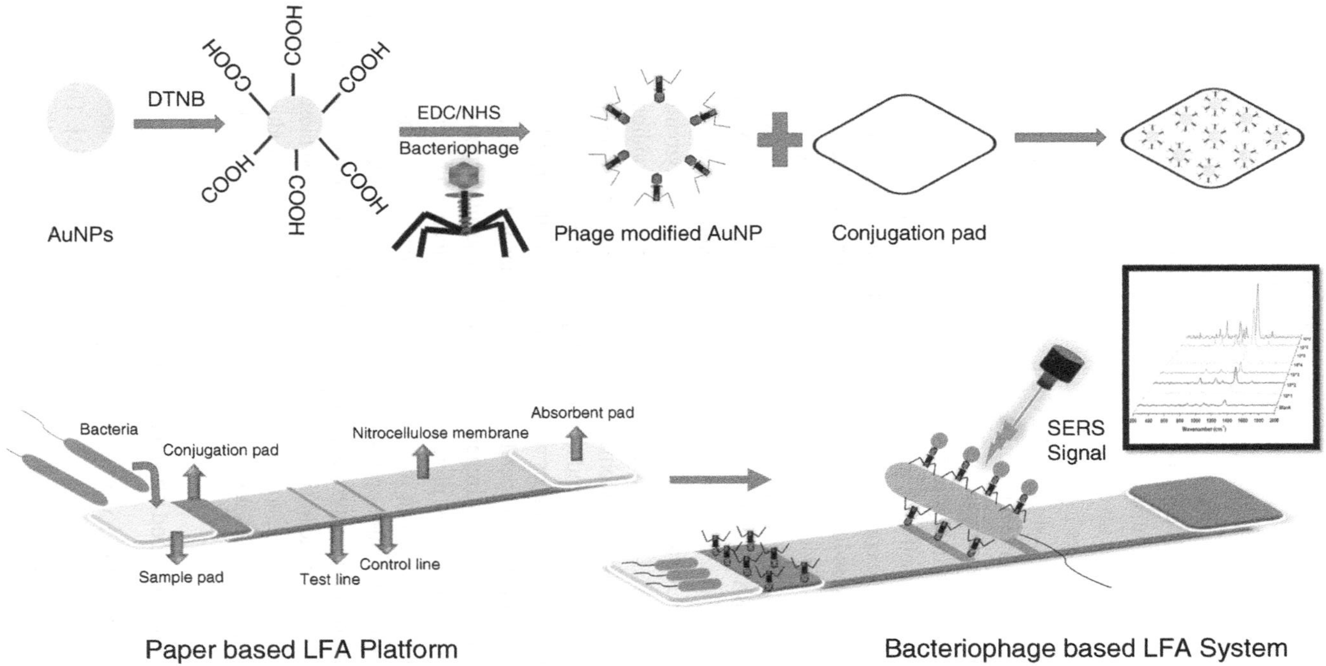

Figure 1.7 Graphic illustration of the F5-4 bacteriophage-based colorimetric lateral flow assay and SERS biosensor structure. *Source:* [83]/with permission of Elsevier.

bacteria that help to facilitate the easy isolation and investigation of complex samples. Molecular imprinting is a technique to develop the functionality of biomaterials into artificial materials, as naturally occurring materials are expensive and restricted in robustness with predefined specificity and selectivity [84]. MIP possesses better chemical stability, is temperature insensitive, requires less preparation time at a low cost, is easy to modify with chemicals, can be directly fabricated on the surface of the transducer, and has high physical and mechanical properties [85]. MIP synthesis involves reactive functional monomers that form specific complexes, cross-linkers for functional group immobilization on imprinted molecules, and initiators to shorten the cycle reaction in the usual way.

Functional monomer and target-based imprinting can be categorized in three ways that depend on their interaction: (i) covalent; (ii) semi-covalent; (iii) noncovalent imprinting, as shown in Figure 1.8 [86]. Figure 1.8a shows the stepwise synthesis of MIP, which includes self-assembly, polymerization, and template removal. Similarly, Figure 1.8b shows the commonly used ingredients that include initiators, functional monomers, and cross-linkers. Functional monomers are the polymers building block – for example, methacrylic acid (MAA), 4-vinyl pyridine (4-VP), acrylic acid (AA), 2-vinyl pyridine (2-VP) and cross-linkers involve trimethylolpropane-tri methacrylate (MBA), ethylene glycol dimethacrylate (EGDMA), divinylbenzene (DVB), and methylene acrylamide (TMPTM). An initiator is used to start the polymerization process, such as benzoyl peroxide (BPO), azobisisobutyronitrile (AIBN), and azodiisopentanyl (AIHN). Covalent imprinting uses a reverse bonding functional unit and template that distributes binding sites in a uniform mode [88]. Semi-covalent imprinting involves covalent and noncovalent polymerization approaches that can be achieved via covalent bonding as well as noncovalent methods [89]. During noncovalent bonding, interaction between functional monomer and sensing analyte is weak in nature that occur via ionic hydrogen bonding, and dipole interaction [90]. Out of these three imprinting techniques, noncovalent imprinting technique is most often used to synthesize the MIP, as shown in Figure 1.8b [91]. Numerous biosensor designs using MIP technology that include optical, ECL, and quartz crystal microbalance biosensors have been reported with improved performance for diverse analytes that include molecules from small to large in size [92]. Until recently, MIP-based biosensors have not been commercialized due to difficulties in large-scale MIP production, complete removal of templates, low selectivity, and less efficient synthesis methods [93].

1.4.7 Biosensors Based on Whole Cells

Biosensors that include whole cells employ different microbes that include viruses, bacteria, protozoa, fungi, and algae as bioreceptors [53]. These bioreceptors can self-replicate, are handled easily compared to plants and animal cells, are

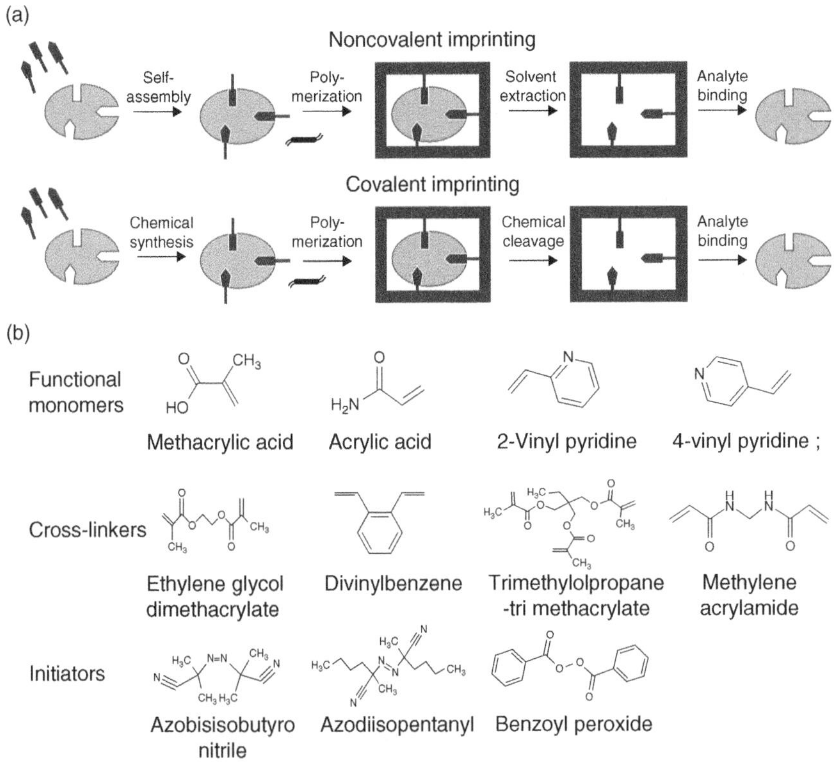

Figure 1.8 Graphic illustration of (a) various steps involved in covalent and noncovalent molecularly imprinted polymer technique. *Source:* [86]/MDPI/CC BY 4.0. (b) Some commonly used initiators, functional monomers, and cross-linkers during MIP fabrication. *Source:* [87]/Frontiers Media S.A/CC BY 4.0.

fast-proliferating, and do not require any extraction or purification methods to produce other bioreceptors such as antibodies [94]. Various biosensor designs based on whole cells have been reported that exhibit good sensitivity and specificity values to detect the different analytes [56, 95, 96]. Figure 1.9 shows the mechanism of a whole-cell-based biosensor that includes molecular bioreceptor immobilizing bacteria or live cells on the substrate to detect the specific target. The target binds itself to the surface of immobilized receptor that modulates the output signal or gene expression and can be measured using different transduction mechanism [96].

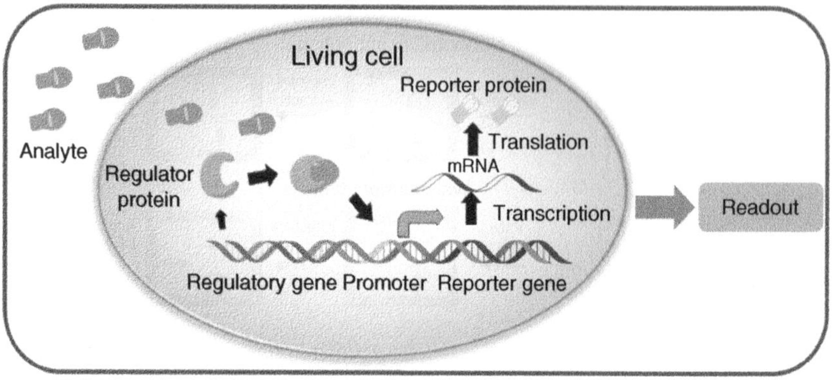

Figure 1.9 Biosensor design based on whole cell. *Source:* [96]/MDPI/CC BY 4.0.

1.5 Sensing Techniques

1.5.1 ECL Biosensors

An ECL (ECL) biosensor is made up of an interface for the analyte reaction, a receptor for binding the target molecule through BRE, and a device known as transducer that alters the interaction signal to a measurable electrical signal. This signal can be measured in the form of impedance, current, voltage, and conductance. ECL biosensors measure changes in electrical properties that result from a specific biochemical reaction. The principle of electrochemistry involves the connection between chemical reaction such as oxidation and reduction into electrical energy. The detection of biomarkers involves the use of an electrode modified with target that specifically binds to the disease biomarker. As the biomarker binds to the target molecule, this attachment changes in the measurable electrical signal. Electrochemical impedance spectroscopy (EIS) is an example that measures the output electrical signal as target cancer cells binds to bioreceptors, such as their size and surface charge. EIS can be used to monitor cancer cell growth and invasion and to detect cancer biomarkers in blood samples [97, 98].

In ECL biosensors, electrodes are utilized as transducers and reaction sites that sense the analyte by reducing or oxidizing it [99]. Reference electrode and working electrode are two main components during ECL sensor design. Silver (Ag) and silver chloride (AgCl) are used to fabricate the reference electrode, which forms a connection with the electrolyte solution and is kept at a distance to maintain the potential at a stable value. Reference electrode using graphite, gold (Au), platinum (Pt), and compounds made from silicon (Si) have been reported so far.

ECL sensors are classified into amperometric, potentiometric, conductometric, field effect transistor, and impedimetric. Amperometric sensors measure the signal in the form of a current generated from ECL reaction, potentiometric sensors measure voltage generated at electrode surface, and impedimetric sensors measure impedance [100].

Clark reported using ECL biosensors to measure glucose solutions [63]. In the case of potentiometric ions in solution, BRE is measured after being converted to potential. Impedimetric biosensor measure the impedance to detect the presence of various analytes [101–105]. ECL biosensors have a short lifespan (i.e. 1–3 years), and components must be replacement. Some ECL sensor designs involve using electrolyte solutions to enhance performance and lifespan; however, refilling the solution regularly is another drawback. Figure 1.10 shows a manganese oxide-fluorescent polymer dot–based ECL biosensor to detect Madin-Darby canine kidney (MDCK) and MD Anderson-metastatic breast (MDAMB) cancer cells cancer cells [106].

1.5.2 Optical Biosensors

Light is used in optical biosensors to detect the various analytes that possess advantages such as high sensitivity with low detection limits, fast speed, and shorter detection time. Optical biosensors detect changes in the optical properties of a sample resulting from a chemical reaction. Output is measured using optical transducers (i.e. colorimetric). Other examples of optical biosensors for cancer detection include fluorescence, Raman spectroscopy, and light scattering [39, 107, 108]. The classification of various optical sensor designs and their descriptions based on underlying operational principles and sensing applications are discussed in detail.

1.5.2.1 Plasmonic Biosensors

With the growing demand for portable, reliable, fast-responding, and highly sensitive detection mechanisms, plasmonic biosensors that consist of surface plasmon resonance (SPR) and localized surface plasmon resonance (LSPR) have become a favorable alternative technology to detect the various biochemicals. In recent years, considerable progress has been witnessed in the field of plasmonic biosensors and their commercialization in the different application areas. More precisely, the unique properties of the SPR phenomenon are focused on a variety of applications such as the guiding of light, nanoscale manipulation, overcoming the difficulty to provide good resolution below the diffraction limit, and single molecule detection [109].

Prism-based Kretschmann's configuration and fiberoptic structures are widely explored for various applications [110]. A surface plasmon (SP) phenomenon is

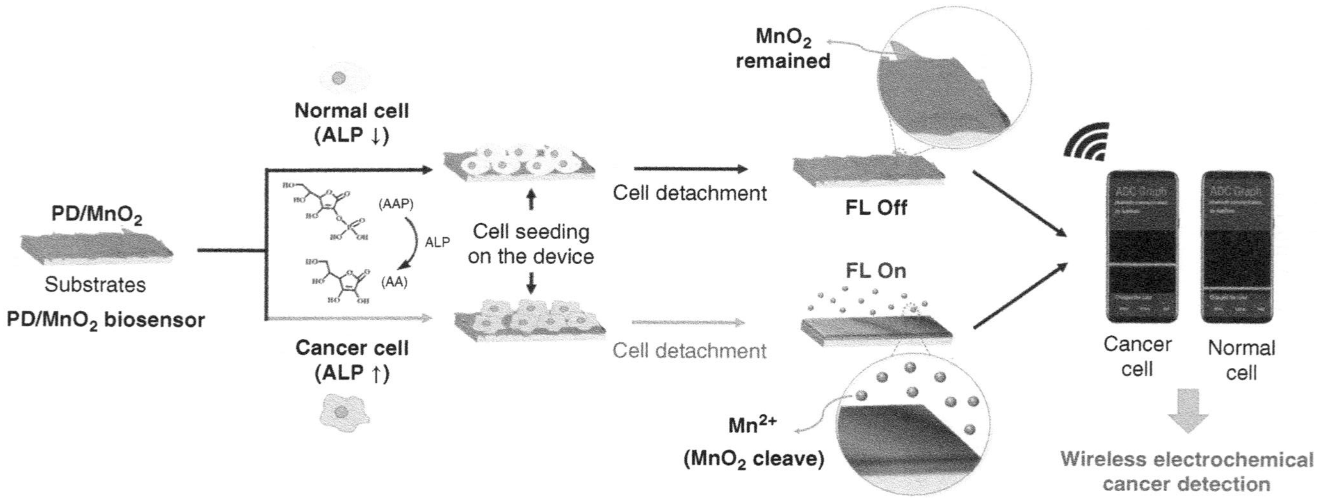

Figure 1.10 A fluorescent polymer dot-manganese oxide complex–based ECL sensor to detect the cancer cells. *Source:* [106]/with permission of Elsevier.

excited using a transverse magnetic wave whose electric field exists along the interface of two materials with opposite permittivity values fulfilled by metal and dielectric material. Figures 1.11a and b show penetration depth in metals (δ_m), dielectric (δ_s), and their numeric values in the case of most widely explored plasmonic metals Au and Ag [111]. As the wave vector and momentum of an oscillating charge are always greater than those of a massless photon, it is difficult to excite the surface plasmons' incident light directly, but the light can be excited by different techniques that increase their momentum.

Excitation methods include prism, Bragg, and fiber configuration. In these methods, the incident electromagnetic light is coupled through prisms for biosensing applications. For practical purposes, the Otto configuration was not found suitable, as it was not possible to maintain the few nm gaps between the metal layer and the prism material. Otto configuration was modified and reported by Kretschmann and Raether by depositing the plasmonic active metal layer on the base of prism [112]. This configuration has been explored for various applications and lays the foundation for rapid growth of prism-based SPR sensors. Figures 1.12a

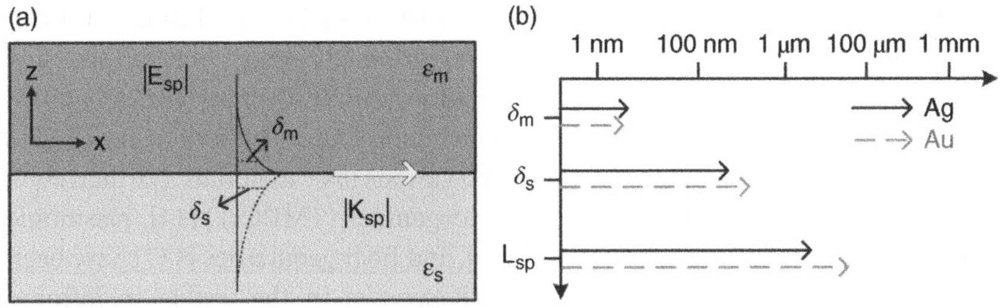

Figure 1.11 Schematic illustration of (a) surface plasmons existence at the interface of the metal and dielectric indication penetration depth in metals (δ_m), dielectric (δ_s) of the electromagnetic field and propagation length (L_{sp}) of surface plasmons; (b) numerical values of δ_m, δ_s, and L_{sp} for plasmonic active Ag and Au metals that are commonly used in biosensing applications.

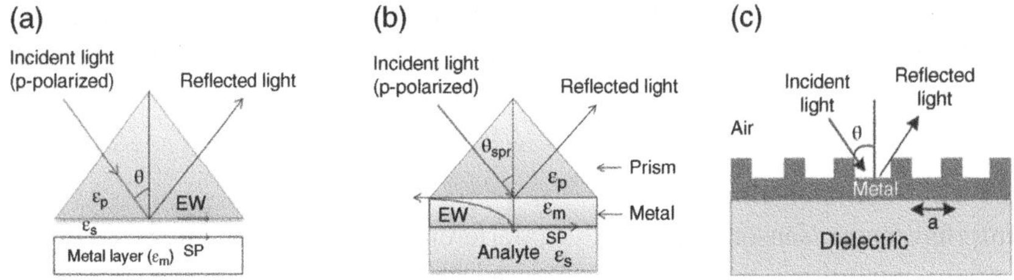

Figure 1.12 Schematic of light coupling in a plasmonic-based sensor using (a) Otto, (b) Kretschmann, and (c) Bragg grating configuration.

and b show the structure reported by Otto and Kretschmann for sensing purposes. SPR requires precise wave vector matching of incident light with surface plasmons at a specific angle known as resonance angle, denoted as θ_{SPR} [51]:

$$\frac{2\pi}{\lambda} n_{prism} \sin\theta_{SPR} = Real\left(\frac{2\pi}{\lambda}\sqrt{\frac{\varepsilon_m \varepsilon_s}{\varepsilon_m + \varepsilon_s}}\right) \tag{1.1}$$

Eq. (1.1) represents the evanescent wave-vector (k_{ev}), with dielectric permittivity (ε_s) and metal permittivity (ε_m). At resonance conditions, a decrease in intensity of reflected light is detected at resonance angle denoted as θ_{SPR}. This θ_{SPR} is responsive to any change in RI of sensing medium and shows angular shift ($\delta\theta_{SPR}$) for other analytes, which is the principle behind SPR sensing [112, 113]. Phase-matching condition with grating of holes or grooves having lattice constant a can be expressed as (Figure 1.12c).

$$\beta = \frac{2\pi}{\lambda} n_s \sin\theta \pm \nu \frac{2\pi}{a} \tag{1.2}$$

β, ν and n_s are the wave vector of surface plasmons (Eq. 1.2), diffraction order, and analyte RI. Fiberoptic-based sensors possess the advantages of small size, low cost, remote sensing, electromagnetic radiation immunity, long-term reliability, miniaturization, and online monitoring. Plasmonic sensors have been explored to detect the analytes such as gases, liquids, and various toxic materials. Furthermore, different strategies, transition metal dichalcogenides (TMDCs) [114], plasmonic nanocomposites [115], glass materials [116], and fiber geometries [117] have been used to improve the performance of SPR sensors in the visible to infrared region [118]. Discovery of other 2D materials and their unique properties has further triggered research in the field of SPR sensing [119]. Out of the four interrogation methods, wavelength and angular methods are most commonly used for the detection of various biochemical substances as they are simple to fabricate and provide superior resolution at a low cost [120]. Figure 1.13 shows the fiberoptic configuration used for various sensing applications.

Prism-based configurations utilize the phenomenon of total internal reflection (TIR) to excite SPs; therefore, a prism (due to its bulky size) can be replaced with a core of optical fiber for sensing purposes, as shown in Figure 1.13.

1.5.2.2 Interferometric Sensors

Interferometric sensors explore the interference phenomenon to measure the various quantities that include disease-related analytes, temperature, and humidity. Fabry-Perot (FPI), Mach-Zehnder (MZI), Sagnac, and Michelson interferometers are four types of interferometers used for many biochemical

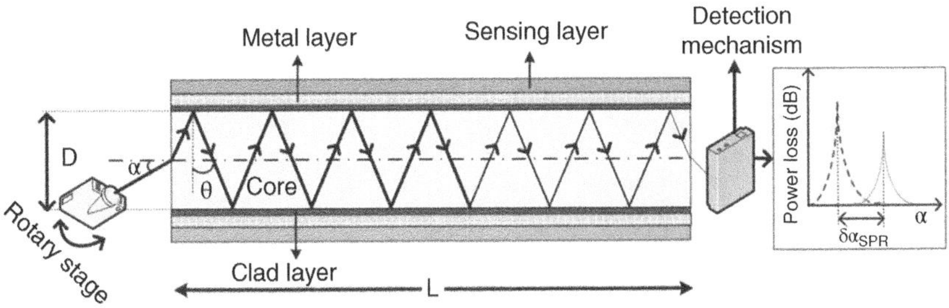

Figure 1.13 Schematic of fiberoptic configuration.

sensing applications. In interferometry, light is split into components that are further combined to produce maxima and minima series. The MZI interferometer is based on interference obtained by division of amplitude. Light can be split into its components using a beam splitter that covers the different path lengths and phases, which are further recombined with the help of another beam splitter [121]. Figure 1.14a shows the MZI interferometer structure that consist of laser light source, sensing arm with reference arm, input, output waveguide, and detector system.

In FPI, an etalon is used to separate the two surfaces that are parallel to each other by a certain distance. Incident and reflected light interfere multiple times at these parallel surfaces [125]. Figures 1.14b and c show the schematics of the FPI and Michelson interferometers. Michelson interferometers have the same principle of working as MZI, except for the reflector difference. In a Sagnac interferometer, a light beam travels with different polarizations along a loop fabricated using an optical fiber, as shown in Figure 1.14d [126]. The advantage of interferometric sensors lies in the fact that they can be applied via heavy optical components, optical fiber structures, and planar guides that involve mirrors as well as reflectors [127].

1.5.2.3 Colorimetric Sensors

Colorimetric sensors are widely used because changes are easily visible to the naked eye. They have easy use, low cost, high sensitivity, and high selectivity to detect the analytes. The sensors change color during interaction between analyte and ligand, having the advantage of parallel sensing [39]. Colorimetric sensors examine the chemical reaction of the analytes that yield high-sensitivity designs lying in the range of parts per billion to parts per trillion. Chemical properties detection is useful in toxic analytes because toxics are very reactive and can be detected easily with very low concentrations lying in the range of sub parts per million [128]. These days, colorimetric sensors are combined with different effects that include plasmonics, thin metallic layers, and 2D materials to improve biosensor performance. Figure 1.15 shows a AuNPs-based colorimetric Aptasensor to

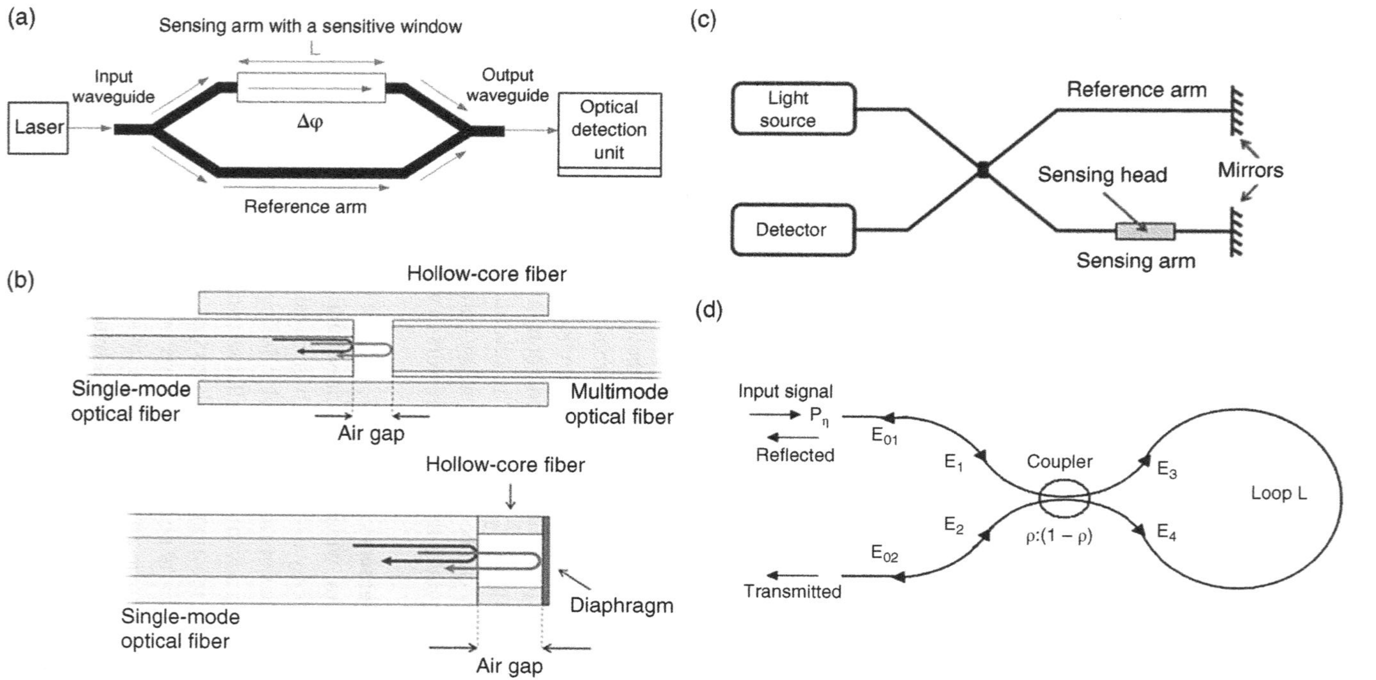

Figure 1.14 Schematic of (a) MZI-based biosensor design. *Source:* [122]/MDPI/CC BY 4.0. (b) FPI sensor. *Source:* [123]/Springer Nature/CC BY 4.0. (c) Michelson interferometric sensor. *Source:* [123]/Springer Nature/CC BY 4.0. and (d) Sagnac configuration. *Source:* [124]/with permission of Elsevier.

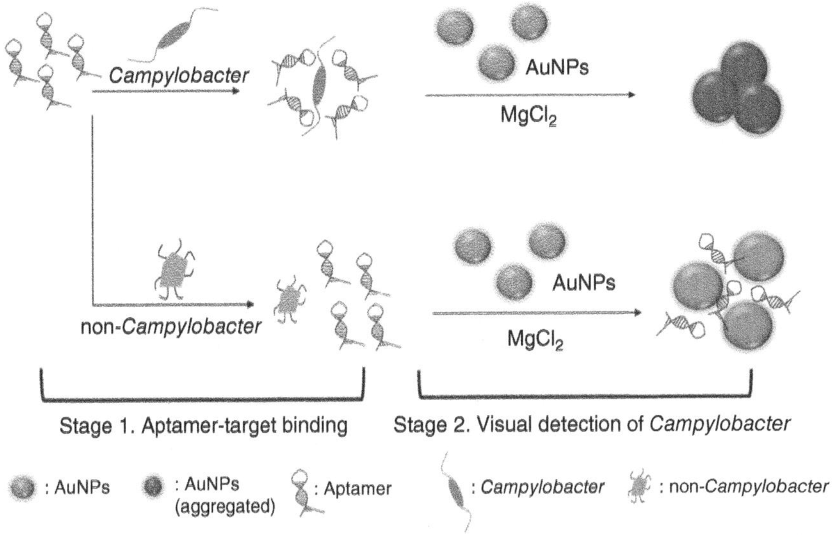

Figure 1.15 Schematic of AuNPs and aptamer-based colorimetric biosensor designs to detect campylobacteriosis that spread due to *Campylobacter jejuni* and *Campylobacter coli*. *Source:* [129]/with permission of Elsevier.

detect the foodborne disease campylobacteriosis that spread due to *Campylobacter jejuni* and *Campylobacter coli bacteria*. The biosensor structure includes gold nanoparticles functionalized with a specific aptamer that changes color and causes aggregation [129]. Colorimetric sensors have been widely explored to detect metal ions, toxics, biosamples, dyes, medicines, pesticides, and pollutants with high performance through the naked eye [130]. Two methods are commonly used to design colorimetric sensors: the first is direct binding (receptor-spacer-reporter), and the second is competitive binding–based sensors that include indicator displacement assays. In receptor-spacer-reporter–based sensor design, a spacer is used to bind the reporter and a receptor moiety. Binding of target with bioreceptor through the spacer changes output signal.

Indicator displacement assay sensor designs form a receptor-indicator assembly that generates competition among the target analyte and the indicator. As the indicator shows the displacement, a signal change is observed in the output signal [103].

1.5.2.4 SERS-Based Biosensors

The concept of inelastic scattering of incident light with a molecule that changes its frequency due to their interaction is used in SERS [131]. The output Raman signal is enhanced due to adsorption of molecules on the metal surface [131, 132].

This method enables the detection of a single molecule, ultra-sensitivity, high selectivity due to a narrow bandwidth of 0.1 nm, multiplexing detection in simple assay designs, a longer lifetime due to photo-bleaching resistance, and a lower detection limit. Various biosensing applications based on SERS have been reported so far [133–138]. SERS biosensors can be labeled or label-free. Labeled biosensors involve a target with an external Raman molecule, as shown in Figure 1.16 [140]. Label-free biosensor design involves direct interaction of the target with BRE; a shift in the Raman signal can be observed. Enhancing the Raman signal intensity depends on cross-section and the number of adsorbed molecules on the metal surface [138]. The electromagnetic and chemical enhancement mechanisms are two approaches responsible for Raman signal enhancement. During the interaction of the molecule with light in the electromagnetic mechanisms, a molecule is a point dipole that produces dipole moment, and charge distribution increases the field intensity near metal surface.

In case of chemical enhancement, a chemical interaction of metal and molecules generates the molecular polarizability. In addition, resonance due to incident light and the molecule's electron transition, resonance of the incident light molecule with the metal-molecule transition, and ground state of metal and molecule overlap with each other, leading to signal enhancement (the nonresonance effect).

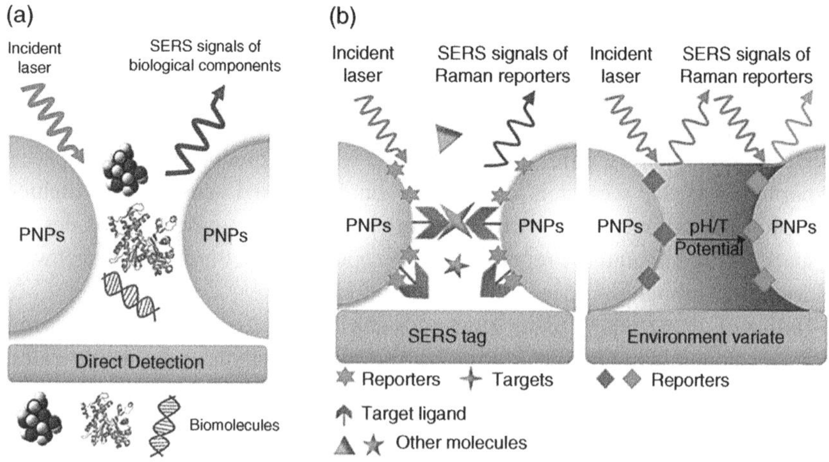

Figure 1.16 Schematic illustration of (a) label-free and (b) labeled SERS biosensors. *Source:* [139]/with permission of Elsevier.

The chemical effect contributes less as compared to the electromagnetic effect, and this effect is the least studied due to experimental quantification. The electromagnetic effect is independent of the analyte but depends directly on the metal roughness [139, 141].

1.5.2.5 Fluorescence-Based Biosensors

Fluorescence-based biosensors make use of light emitted by the fluorescent material as they absorb electromagnetic light depending on their state; they can be fluorescent in one state but not fluorescent in another state. For example, nicotinamide adenine dinucleotide + hydrogen (H) is fluorescent while NAD^+ does not emit light [142].

The absorbed photon has high energy as compared to released photon; therefore, a photon that excites dye has a lower wavelength as compared to an emitted photon. Dyes can be excited in the range of wavelengths (known as the "spectrum") as they are not excitable at a single wavelength. In the fluorescence technique, there is a light source to excite the light, a fluorophore that emits light after excitation, filters to filter wavelength, and a light detector to measure the intensity. Nucleic acids, flavin nucleotides, and green fluorescent proteins are some commonly used inherent fluorescent molecules for biosensing applications [144, 145]. Fluorescence biosensors are widely explored for various biochemical and other sensing applications. On the other hand, analytes or target molecules are nonfluorescent; therefore, these are labeled with fluorescent molecules to detect them easily using some reactive groups that include amino, hydroxyl, and carboxyl groups that form bonding with tag and target molecules [146, 147]. The requirement of a clear analyte solution to overcome interference and complex components makes it difficult to implement for commercial purposes [148]. Another drawback is that the binding site of the fluorescent tag suffers from photobleaching, and interaction of the tag with a specific target could lead to incorrect results. Fluorescence biosensors have less capability for multiplexing, a long detection time, and phototoxicity [39].

Figure 1.17 shows the fluorescently labeled biosensor used to detect the target molecule. Förster resonance energy transfer (FRET) is a distance-dependent interaction between two light-sensitive molecules (a donor and an acceptor fluorophore) that transfer energy in nonradiative way among each other. Fluorescence lifetime imaging is used to measure the fluorophores molecule decay time during fluorescence. Changes in fluorescence intensity measure the variation of light intensity emitted by the fluorophore molecule to investigate the molecular interactions. Fluorescence correlation spectroscopy measures the variation in intensity of a solution that comprises fluorescent molecules.

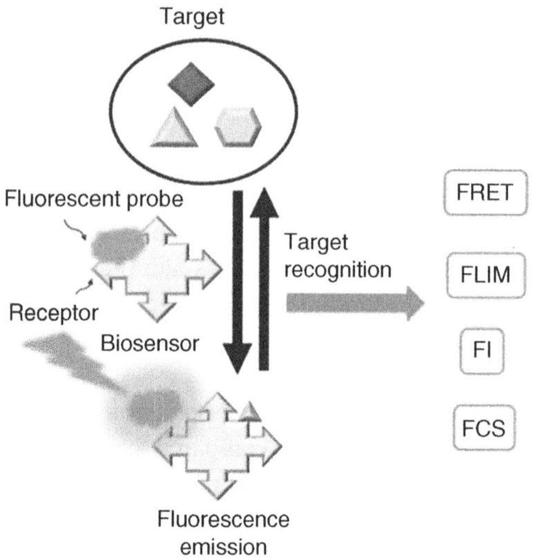

Figure 1.17 Schematic picture of a fluorescence-based sensing mechanism that involve molecular interaction methods Förster resonance energy transfer (FRET), fluorescence lifetime imaging (FLIM), changes in fluorescence intensity (FI), and fluorescence correlation spectroscopy (FCS). *Source:* [143]/MDPI/CC BY 4.0.

1.5.2.6 Photonic Crystal-Fiber–Based Biosensors

A photonic crystal consists of nanostructures arranged in periodic order that interact with incident light according to their wavelength and periodicity. PCF structures can be fabricated in all three possible dimensions using different techniques that change the refractive index in a periodic manner. PCFs are being implemented on different sensing platforms for various applications. PCF consists of small air holes that confine the light fabricated along the length of fiber. Two effects called photonic bandgap and index guiding effects are responsible for guiding the light in PCFs [149]. The effective RI of the core is higher than clad-effective RI in index guiding mechanism. In the core region, air holes are arranged in a periodic manner such that it makes the core effective RI more than air hole surrounding them. The size of clad air hole is kept large as compared to core region surrounding air holes. There is contrast RI difference between core and clad that guides the light via total internal reflection phenomenon inside the core [150]. The operating principle of PCF and traditional optical fiber is almost the same except for a higher effective RI contrast between core and cladding, which leads to much stronger confinement for different applications. In a photonic bandgap PCF, the light is confined by a photonic bandgap generated using the microstructured cladding [66]. Different materials, which include silica, polymers, chalcogenides, and glasses, are used to fabricate the PCFs. Figure 1.18 shows that various types of PCF structures are explored to detect the different analytes that include DNA, RNA, viruses, bacteria, and various diseases [151–154].

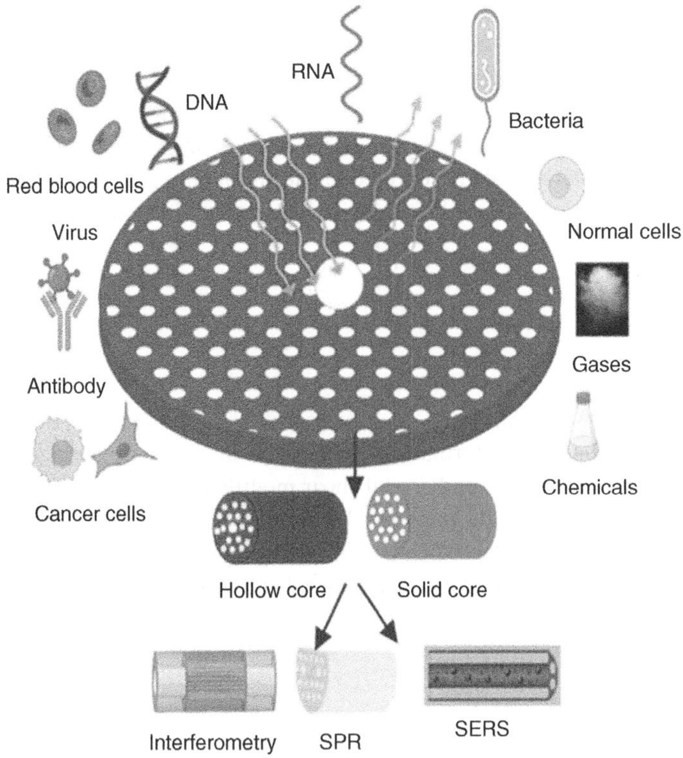

Figure 1.18 Schematic demonstration of different types of PCFs for numerous analytes detection. *Source:* [28] with permission of Elsevier.

1.5.3 Mass Biosensors

Mass-based biosensors can measure the changes in the mass of the crystal as it vibrates on applying an electric field. It can be piezoelectric and magnetoelastic according to the crystal type. For example, quartz crystal microbalance biosensors measure changes in resonance frequency that result from the binding of a cancer biomarker to an immobilized receptor. Other examples of mass-based biosensors for cancer detection include surface acoustic wave (SAW) biosensors and micro-cantilever biosensors [155, 156]. Piezoelectric biosensors include quartz crystal microbalances that consist of thin quartz layers sandwiched between a pair of electrodes and surface acoustic-based devices. On the application of electric voltage mechanical vibrations are generated due to excitation of the structure. The crystal resonant frequency and the deposited layer near the surface are connected to each other and expressed in eq. (1.3). The frequency of vibration decreases as the deposit attaches to the crystal surface. The frequency of vibration becomes proportional to the mass of the deposit material as its thickness becomes very thin and rigid. Therefore, the mass of the deposit can be determined using the Sauerbrey relation. In surface-acoustic wave-based sensor design, guided sound-waves travel parallel to the elastic material surface with decaying displacement amplitude inside the material and are confined to within roughly one wavelength of the surface. Surface-acoustic wave-based devices activate at ultrasonic frequencies in the substrate.

$$\Delta f = -\frac{2 f_0^2}{A\sqrt{\rho_{q\mu_q}}}\Delta m \tag{1.3}$$

In eq. (1.3), the symbols f_o, Δf, Δm, A, $\rho_q\mu_q$ represents the fundamentals mode resonant frequency, change in normalized frequency, mass, piezoelectrically active crystal area, quartz density, and crystal shear modulus [157]. In piezoelectric biosensors, piezoelectric crystal is modified with bioreceptors, as mechanical stress is applied that generate electric charge and binding of analyte on crystal surface produce change in mass that can be measured at transducer in the form of

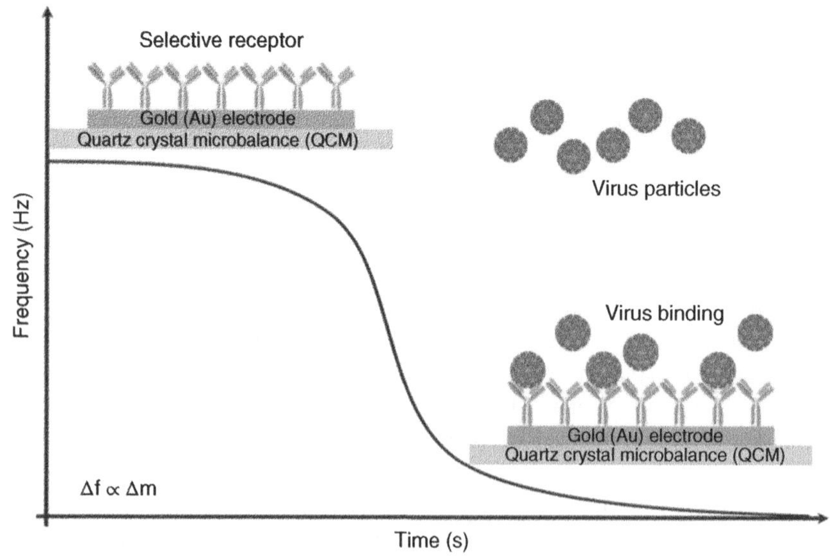

Figure 1.19 Schematic of frequency vs. time plot and structure of Au and quartz crystal-based biosensor to detect the virus. As virus binds to bioreceptor surface, it changes the mass, which changes the frequency that can be selected with diverse techniques. *Source:* [158]/MDPI/CC BY 4.0.

electrical signal [61]. In magnetoelastic biosensors, a magnetic field is used to excite the sensor by generating the magnetic flux through amorphous ferromagnetic ribbons or wires. As no direct connection is required, the sensing coil can be placed at a distance, so magnetoelastic biosensors can be used for wireless monitoring. Figure 1.19 shows the structure of a quartz crystal and Au-based biosensor and a change in frequency can be observed after binding of virus with bioreceptor in frequency vs. time plot [159, 160].

References

1 Javaid, M., Haleem, A., Rab, S. et al. (2021). Sensors for daily life: a review. *Sens. Int.* 2: 100121. https://doi.org/10.1016/j.sintl.2021.100121.

2 Evtugyn, G. (n.d.). *Biosensors: Essentials, Lecture Notes in Chemistry 84.* Berlin Heidelberg: Springer-Verlag *2014. - 265 c.*

3 Sharma, A.K., Jha, R., and Gupta, B.D. (2007). Fiber-optic sensors based on surface plasmon resonance: a comprehensive review. *IEEE Sensors J.* 7 (8): 1118–1129. https://doi.org/10.3323/jcorr1974.30.5_265.

4 Calcerrada, M., García-Ruiz, C., and González-Herráez, M. (2015). Chemical and biochemical sensing applications of microstructured optical fiber-based systems. *Laser Photonics Rev.* 9 (6): 604–627. https://doi.org/10.1002/lpor.201500045.

5 Langer, J., Jimenez de Aberasturi, D., Aizpurua, J. et al. (2020). Present and future of surface-enhanced Raman scattering. *ACS Nano* 14 (1): 28–117. https://doi.org/10.1021/acsnano.9b04224.

6 Chen, Z. and Lu, C. (2005). Humidity sensors: a review of materials and mechanisms. *Sens. Lett.* 3 (Section 2): 274–295. https://doi.org/10.1166/sl.2005.045.

7 Rajibul Islam, M., Mahmood Ali, M., Lai, M.H. et al. (2014). Chronology of Fabry-Perot interferometer fiber-optic sensors and their applications: a review. *Sensors* 14 (4): 7451–7488. https://doi.org/10.3390/s140407451.

8 Brongersma, M.L. and Kik, P.G. (2007). *Surface Plasmon Nanophotonics.* Netherlands: Springer.

9 Clark, L.C. and Lyons, C. (1962). Electrode systems for continuous monitoring in cardiovascular surgery. *Ann. N. Y. Acad. Sci.* 102 (1): 29–45. https://doi.org/10.1111/j.1749-6632.1962.tb13623.x.

10 Updike, S.J. and Hicks, G.P. (1967). The enzyme electrode. *Nature* 214: 986–988. https://doi.org/10.1038/214986a0.

11 Guilbault, G.G. and Montalvo, J.G. (1969). Urea-specific enzyme electrode. *J. Am. Chem. Soc.* 19: 2164–2165.

12 Bergveld, P. (1972). Development, operation, and application of the ion-sensitive field-effect transistor as a tool for electrophysiology. *IEEE Trans. Biomed. Eng.* 5: 342–351. https://doi.org/10.1109/TBME.1972.324137.

13 Janata, J. (1975). Immunoelectrode. *J. Am. Chem. Soc.* 97 (10): 2914–2916.

14 Caras, S. and Janata, J. (1980). Field effect transistor sensitive to penicillin. *Anal. Chem.* 52 (12): 1935–1937. https://doi.org/10.1021/ac50062a035.

15 Kubáň, V. (1993). Continuous precipitation techniques in flow injection analysis - a review. *Fresen. J. Anal. Chem.* 346 (10–11): 873–881. https://doi.org/10.1007/BF00322743.

16 Soleymani, J. (2015). Advanced materials for optical sensing and biosensing of neurotransmitters. *TrAC, Trends Anal. Chem.* 72: 27–44. https://doi.org/10.1016/j.trac.2015.03.017.

17 Mobed, A., Hasanzadeh, M., Ahmadalipour, A., and Fakhari, A. (2020). Recent advances in the biosensing of neurotransmitters: material and method overviews towards the biomedical analysis of psychiatric disorders. *Anal. Methods* 12 (4): 557–575. https://doi.org/10.1039/c9ay02390a.

18 Hasanzadeh, M., Shadjou, N., and Guardia, M.d.l. (2017). Current advancement in electrochemical analysis of neurotransmitters in biological fluids. *TrAC, Trends Anal. Chem.* 86: 107–121. https://doi.org/10.1016/j.trac.2016.11.001.

19 Sangubotla, R. and Kim, J. (2018). Recent trends in analytical approaches for detecting neurotransmitters in Alzheimer's disease. *TrAC, Trends Anal. Chem.* 105: 240–250. https://doi.org/10.1016/j.trac.2018.05.014.

20 Moon, J.M., Thapliyal, N., Hussain, K.K. et al. (2018). Conducting polymer-based electrochemical biosensors for neurotransmitters: a review. *Biosens. Bioelectron.* 102 (December 2017): 540–552. https://doi.org/10.1016/j.bios.2017.11.069.

21 Chauhan, N., Soni, S., Agrawal, P. et al. (2020). Recent advancement in nanosensors for neurotransmitters detection: Present and future perspective. *Process Biochem.* 91 (September 2019): 241–259. https://doi.org/10.1016/j.procbio.2019.12.016.

22 Arumugasamy, S.K., Chellasamy, G., Gopi, S. et al. (2020). Current advances in the detection of neurotransmitters by nanomaterials: an update. *TrAC, Trends Anal. Chem.* 123: 115766. https://doi.org/10.1016/j.trac.2019.115766.

23 Eddin, F.B.K. and Fen, Y.W. (2020). The principle of nanomaterials based surface plasmon resonance biosensors and its potential for dopamine detection. *Molecules* 25 (12): 1–20. https://doi.org/10.3390/molecules25122769.

24 Siddeeg, S.M. (2020). Electrochemical detection of neurotransmitter dopamine: a review. *Int. J. Electrochem. Sci.* 15 (1): 599–612. https://doi.org/10.20964/2020.01.61.

25 Yadav, D. and Kumar, P. (2022). Restoration and targeting of aberrant neurotransmitters in Parkinson's disease therapeutics. *Neurochem. Int.* 156: 105327. https://doi.org/10.1016/j.neuint.2022.105327.

26 Wood, R.W. (1902). On a remarkable case of uneven distribution of light in a diffraction grating spectrum. *Proc. Phys. Soc. Lond.* 18 (1): 269–275. Retrieved from http://stacks.iop.org.ezproxy.usherbrooke.ca/1478-7814/18/i=1/a=325.

27 Rayleigh, L. (1907). On the dynamical theory of gratings. *Proc. R. Soc. A: Math. Phys. Eng. Sci.* 79: 399–416. https://doi.org/10.1098/rspa.1907.0051.

28 Zenneck, J. (1907). Uber d i e Tortpflanxung ebener elektromngnetdscher Wellen. *Annalen der Physik* 328 (10): 846–866.

29 Otto, A. (1968). Excitation of nonradiative surface plasma waves in silver by the method of frustrated total reflection. *Zeitschrift ffir Physik* 216: 398–410.

30 Liedberg, B., Nylander, C., and Lundstrom, I. (1983). Surface plasmon resonance for gas detection and biosensing. *Sensors Actuators* 4: 299–304. https://doi.org/10.1016/0250-6874(83)85036-7.

31 Jorgenson, R.C. and Yee, S.S. (1993). A fiber-optic chemical sensor based on surface plasmon resonance. *Sensors Actuators B Chem.* 12 (3): 213–220. https://doi.org/10.1016/0925-4005(93)80021-3.

32 Wang, J. (2008). Electrochemical glucose biosensors. *Chem. Rev.* 108: 814–825. https://doi.org/10.1016/B978-012373738-0.50005-2.

33 Mittal, S., Kaur, H., Gautam, N., and Mantha, A.K. (2017). Biosensors for breast cancer diagnosis: a review of bioreceptors, biotransducers and signal amplification strategies. *Biosens. Bioelectron.* 88: 217–231.

34 Pashchenko, O., Shelby, T., Banerjee, T., and Santra, S. (2018). A comparison of optical, electrochemical, magnetic, and colorimetric point-of-care biosensors for infectious disease diagnosis. *ACS Infect. Dis.* 4 (8): 1162–1178. https://doi.org/10.1021/acsinfecdis.8b00023.A.

35 Kumar, V. and Guleria, P. (2020). Application of DNA-Nanosensor for environmental monitoring: recent advances and perspectives. *Curr. Pollut. Rep.* https://doi.org/10.1007/s40726-020-00165-1.

36 Lobnik, A., Turel, M., and Urek, Š.K. (2012). Optical chemical sensors: design and applications. In: *Advances in Chemical Sensors* (ed. W. Wang), 4–28.

37 Nagel, B., Dellweg, H., and Gierasch, L.M. (1992). Glossary for chemists of terms used in biotechnology. *Pure Appl. Chem.* 64 (1): 143–168.

38 Kaur, B., Kumar, S., and Kumar, B. (2022). Advances in photonic crystal fiber: sensing and supercontinuum generation applications. *Opt. Fiber Technol.* 72: 102982.

39 Kaur, B., Kumar, S., and Kaushik, B.K. (2022). Recent advancements in optical biosensors for cancer detection. *Biosens. Bioelectron.* 197: 113805.

40 Sharma, A.K., Pandey, A.K., and Kaur, B. (2018). A review of advancements (2007–2017) in plasmonics-based optical fiber sensors. *Opt. Fiber Technol.* 43: 20–34. https://doi.org/10.1016/j.yofte.2018.03.008.

41 Fu, Y. and Ma, Q. (2020). Recent developments in electrochemiluminescence nanosensors for cancer diagnosis applications. *Nanoscale* 12 (26): 13879–13898. https://doi.org/10.1039/d0nr02844d.

42 Xing, G., Zhang, W., Li, N. et al. (2022). Recent progress on microfluidic biosensors for rapid detection of pathogenic bacteria. *Chin. Chem. Lett.* 33 (4): 1743–1751. https://doi.org/10.1016/j.cclet.2021.08.073.

43 Shang, Y., Xiang, X., Ye, Q. et al. (2022). Advances in nanomaterial-based microfluidic platforms for on-site detection of foodborne bacteria. *TrAC, Trends Anal. Chem.* 147: 116509. https://doi.org/10.1016/j.trac.2021.116509.

44 Yoo, S.M. and Lee, S.Y. (2016). Optical biosensors for the detection of pathogenic microorganisms. *Trends Biotechnol.* 34 (1): 7–25. https://doi.org/10.1016/j.tibtech.2015.09.012.

45 Grandview Research (2023). Biosensors market size, share & trends analysis report by technology (electrochemical, thermal, piezoelectric), by application, by end-user, and segment forecasts 2024–2030. https://www.grandviewresearch.com/industry-analysis/biosensors-market

46 Ranjan, P., Yadav, S., Sadique, M.A., and Khan, R. (2021). Nanomaterials for the electrochemical biosensors. *Biosensors* 2021 11: 414. 1–34.

47 Purohit, B., Vernekar, P.R., Shetti, N.P., and Chandra, P. (2020). Biosensor nanoengineering: design, operation, and implementation for biomolecular analysis. *Sens. Int.* 1 (July): 100040. https://doi.org/10.1016/j.sintl.2020.100040.

48 Mahato, K., Srivastava, A., and Chandra, P. (2017). Paper based diagnostics for personalized health care: emerging technologies and commercial aspects. *Biosens. Bioelectron.* 96: 246–259. https://doi.org/10.1016/j.bios.2017.05.001.

49 Zourob, M., Elwary, S., and Turner, A. (2018). *Principles of Bacterial Detection.* Springer.

50 Kumar, P., Vallabhan, C.P.G., Nampoori, V.P.N. et al. (2002). A fibre optic evanescent wave sensor used for the detection of trace nitrites in water. *J. Opt. A Pure Appl. Opt.* 4 (3): 247–250. https://doi.org/10.1088/1464-4258/4/3/305.

51 Maier, S.A. (2007). *Plasmonics : Fundamentals and Applications*, 1ste. New York, NY: Springer.

52 Haus, J. (2010). *Optical Sensors: Basics and Applications.* Wiley-VCH https://doi.org/10.1002/9783527629435.

53 Naresh, V. and Lee, N. (2021). A review on biosensors and recent development of nanostructured materials-enabled biosensors. *Sensors* 21 (4): 1–35. https://doi.org/10.3390/s21041109.

54 Chang, D., Zakaria, S., Esmaeili Samani, S. et al. (2021). Functional nucleic acids for pathogenic bacteria detection. *Acc. Chem. Res.* 54 (18): 3540–3549. https://doi.org/10.1021/acs.accounts.1c00355.

55 Ning, Y., Hu, J., and Lu, F. (2020). Aptamers used for biosensors and targeted therapy. *Biomed. Pharmacother.* 132: 110902. https://doi.org/10.1016/j.biopha.2020.110902.

56 Ahmed, A., Rushworth, J.V., Hirst, N.A., and Millner, P.A. (2014). Biosensors for whole-cell bacterial detection. *Clin. Microbiol. Rev.* 27 (3): 631–646. https://doi.org/10.1128/CMR.00120-13.

57 Ertürk, G. and Mattiasson, B. (2017). Molecular imprinting techniques used for the preparation of biosensors. *Sensors* 17 (2): 1–17. https://doi.org/10.3390/s17020288.

58 Azab, M.Y., Nasr, A.M., Obayya, S.S.A., and Hameed, M.F.O. (2021). DNA hybridization detection based on plasmonic photonic crystal fiber. *Appl. Comput. Electromagn. Soc. J.* 36 (3): 229–234. https://doi.org/10.47037/2020.ACES.J.360301.

59 Odeh, F., Nsairat, H., Alshaer, W. et al. (2019). Aptamers chemistry: chemical modifications and conjugation strategies. *Molecules* 25 (3): 1–51.

60 Di, Y., Wang, P., Li, C. et al. (2020). Design, bioanalytical, and biomedical applications of aptamer-based hydrogels. *Front. Med.* 7: 1–15. https://doi.org/10.3389/fmed.2020.00456.

61 Inamuddin, R.K., Mohammad, A., and Asiri, A.M. (2019). *Advanced Biosensors for Health Care Applications*. Amsterdam, Netherlands: Elsevier.

62 Miao, X., Zhu, Z., Jia, H. et al. (2020). Colorimetric detection of cancer biomarker based on enzyme enrichment and pH sensing. *Sensors Actuators B Chem.* 320: 128435.

63 Nguyen, H.H., Lee, S.H., Lee, U.J. et al. (2019). Immobilized enzymes in biosensor applications. *Materials* 12 (1): 1–34. https://doi.org/10.3390/ma12010121.

64 Sun, W., Yuan, S., Huang, H. et al. (2017). A label-free biosensor based on localized surface plasmon resonance for diagnosis of tuberculosis. *J. Microbiol. Methods* 142: 41–45. https://doi.org/10.1016/j.mimet.2017.09.007.

65 Carneiro, M.C.C.G., Sousa-Castillo, A., Correa-Duarte, M.A., and Sales, M.G.F. (2019). Dual biorecognition by combining molecularly-imprinted polymer and antibody in SERS detection. Application to carcinoembryonic antigen. *Biosens. Bioelectron.* 146: 111761.

66 Danlard, I. and Akowuah, E.K. (2020). Assaying with PCF-based SPR refractive index biosensors: from recent configurations to outstanding detection limits. *Opt. Fiber Technol.* 54 (October 2019): 102083. https://doi.org/10.1016/j.yofte.2019.102083.

67 Chen, J. and Nugen, S.R. (2019). Detection of protease and engineered phage-infected bacteria using peptide-graphene oxide nanosensors. *Anal. Bioanal. Chem.* 411: 2487–2492. https://doi.org/10.1007/s00216-019-01766-6.

68 Farooq, U., Yang, Q., Ullah, M.W., and Wang, S. (2018). Bacterial biosensing: recent advances in phage-based bioassays and biosensors. *Biosens. Bioelectron.* 118 (July): 204–216. https://doi.org/10.1016/j.bios.2018.07.058.

69 Mack, J.D., Yehualaeshet, T., Park, M.K. et al. (2017). Phage-based biosensor and optimization of surface blocking agents to detect salmonella typhimurium on Romaine lettuce. *J. Food Saf.* 37 (2): https://doi.org/10.1111/jfs.12299.

70 Peng, H. and Chen, I.A. (2019). Rapid colorimetric detection of bacterial species through the capture of gold nanoparticles by chimeric phages. *ACS Nano* 13 (2): 1244–1252. https://doi.org/10.1021/acsnano.8b06395.

71 Samota, S., Rani, R., Chakraverty, S., and Kaushik, A. (2022). Biosensors for simplistic detection of pathogenic bacteria: a review with special focus on field-effect transistors. *Mater. Sci. Semicond. Process.* 141 (August 2021): 106404. https://doi.org/10.1016/j.mssp.2021.106404.

72 Ali, Q., Zheng, H., Rao, M.J. et al. (2022). Advances, limitations, and prospects of biosensing technology for detecting phytopathogenic bacteria. *Chemosphere* 296: 133773. https://doi.org/10.1016/j.chemosphere.2022.133773.

73 Ikuta, K.S., Swetschinski, L., Aguilar, G. et al. (2022). Global mortality associated with 33 bacterial pathogens in 2019: a systematic analysis for the Global Burden of Disease Study 2019. *Lancet* 400 (10369): 2221–2248. https://doi.org/10.1016/S0140-6736(22)02185-7.

74 Silhavy, T.J., Kahne, D., and Walker, S. (2010). The bacterial cell envelope. *Cold Spring Harb. Perspect. Biol.* 2: 1–16. Retrieved from https://www.ncbi.nlm.nih.gov/pmc/articles/PMC2857177/pdf/cshperspect-PRK-a000414.pdf.

75 Cani, P.D. (2018). Human gut microbiome: hopes, threats and promises. *Gut* 67 (9): 1716–1725. https://doi.org/10.1136/gutjnl-2018-316723.

76 Kabiraz, M.P., Majumdar, P.R., Mahmud, M.M.C. et al. (2023). Conventional and advanced detection techniques of foodborne pathogens: a comprehensive review. *Heliyon* 9 (4): e15482. https://doi.org/10.1016/j.heliyon.2023.e15482.

77 Qin, J., Wang, W., Gao, L., and Yao, S.Q. (2022). Emerging biosensing and transducing techniques for potential applications in point-of-care diagnostics. *Chem. Sci.* 13 (10): 2857–2876. https://doi.org/10.1039/d1sc06269g.

78 Kadadou, D., Tizani, L., Wadi, V.S. et al. (2022). Recent advances in the biosensors application for the detection of bacteria and viruses in wastewater. *J. Environ. Chem. Eng.* 10 (1): https://doi.org/10.1016/j.jece.2021.107070.

79 Cesewski, E. and Johnson, B.N. (2020). Electrochemical biosensors for pathogen detection. *Biosens. Bioelectron.* 159 (April): 112214. https://doi.org/10.1016/j.bios.2020.112214.

80 Park, J.H., Cho, Y.W., and Kim, T.H. (2022). Recent advances in surface plasmon resonance sensors for sensitive optical detection of pathogens. *Biosensors* 12 (3): https://doi.org/10.3390/bios12030180.

81 Cui, F., Ye, Y., Ping, J., and Sun, X. (2020). Carbon dots: current advances in pathogenic bacteria monitoring and prospect applications. *Biosens. Bioelectron.* 156 (February): https://doi.org/10.1016/j.bios.2020.112085.

82 Bhardwaj, S.K., Singh, H., Khatri, M. et al. (2022). Advances in MXenes-based optical biosensors: A review. *Biosens Bioelectron* 202: 113995. https://pubmed.ncbi.nlm.nih.gov/35065477/.

83 Ilhan, H., Tayyarcan, E.K., Caglayan, M.G. et al. (2021). Replacement of antibodies with bacteriophages in lateral flow assay of salmonella enteritidis. *Biosens. Bioelectron.* 189: 113383. https://doi.org/10.1016/j.bios.2021.113383.

84 Sarafraz-Yazdi, A. and Razavi, N. (2015). Application of molecularly-imprinted polymers in solid-phase microextraction techniques. *TrAC, Trends Anal. Chem.* 73: 81–90. https://doi.org/10.1016/j.trac.2015.05.004.

85 El-Schich, Z., Zhang, Y., Feith, M. et al. (2020). Molecularly imprinted polymers in biological applications. *BioTechniques* 69 (6): 407–420. https://doi.org/10.2144/btn-2020-0091.

86 Lusina, A. and Cegłowski, M. (2022). Molecularly imprinted polymers as state-of-the-art drug carriers in hydrogel transdermal drug delivery applications. *Polymers* 14 (3): 640. https://doi.org/10.3390/polym14030640.

87 Gao, M., Gao, Y., Chen, G. et al. (2020). Recent advances and future trends in the detection of contaminants by molecularly imprinted polymers in food samples. *Front. Chem.* 8: 1–20. https://doi.org/10.3389/fchem.2020.616326.

88 Chen, Y., Zhou, S., Li, L. et al. (2017). Nanomaterials-based sensitive electrochemiluminescence biosensing. *Nano Today* 12: 98–115. https://doi.org/10.1016/j.nantod.2016.12.013.

89 Ansari, S. (2017). Combination of molecularly imprinted polymers and carbon nanomaterials as a versatile biosensing tool in sample analysis: recent applications and challenges. *TrAC, Trends Anal. Chem.* 93: 134–151. https://doi.org/10.1016/j.trac.2017.05.015.

90 Ashley, J., Shahbazi, M.A., Kant, K. et al. (2017). Molecularly imprinted polymers for sample preparation and biosensing in food analysis: Progress and perspectives. *Biosens. Bioelectron.* 91 (November 2016): 606–615. https://doi.org/10.1016/j.bios.2017.01.018.

91 Song, X., Xu, S., Chen, L. et al. (2014). Recent advances in molecularly imprinted polymers in food analysis. *J. Appl. Polym. Sci.* 131 (16): 1–18. https://doi.org/10.1002/app.40766.

92 Sharma, S., Shrivastav, A.M., and Gupta, B.D. (2020). Lossy mode resonance based Fiber optic creatinine sensor fabricated using molecular imprinting over nanocomposite of MoS_2/SnO_2. *IEEE Sensors J.* 20 (8): 4251–4259. https://doi.org/10.1109/JSEN.2020.2964262.

93 Zhang, J., Wang, Y., and Lu, X. (2021). Molecular imprinting technology for sensing foodborne pathogenic bacteria. *Anal. Bioanal. Chem.* 413 (18): 4581–4598. https://doi.org/10.1007/s00216-020-03138-x.

94 Hansen, M.L., He, Z., Wibowo, M., and Jelsbak, L. (2021). A whole-cell biosensor for detection of 2,4- Diacetylphloroglucinol (DAPG)-producing bacteria from grassland soil. *Appl. Environ. Microbiol.* 87 (3): 1–12. https://doi.org/10.1128/AEM.01400-20.

95 Cao, Y., Zhang, B., Zhu, Z. et al. (2021). Microfluidic based whole-cell biosensors for simultaneously on-site monitoring of multiple environmental contaminants. *Front. Bioeng. Biotechnol.* 9 (March): 1–6. https://doi.org/10.3389/fbioe.2021.622108.

96 Gui, Q., Lawson, T., Shan, S. et al. (2017). The application of whole cell-based biosensors for use in environmental analysis and in medical diagnostics. *Sensors* 17 (7): 1–17. https://doi.org/10.3390/s17071623.

97 Sanli, S., Moulahoum, H., Ugurlu, O. et al. (2020). Screen printed electrode-based biosensor functionalized with magnetic cobalt/single-chain antibody fragments for cocaine biosensing in different matrices. *Talanta* 217 (April): 121111. https://doi.org/10.1016/j.talanta.2020.121111.

98 Hartati, Y.W., Irkham, I., Zulqaidah, S. et al. (2022). Recent advances in hydroxyapatite-based electrochemical biosensors: applications and future perspectives. *Sens. Biosensing. Res.* 38 (August): 100542. https://doi.org/10.1016/j.sbsr.2022.100542.

99 Chen, Z., Ma, L., Bu, S. et al. (2021). CRISPR/Cas12a and immuno-RCA based electrochemical biosensor for detecting pathogenic bacteria. *J. Electroanal. Chem.* 901 (October): https://doi.org/10.1016/j.jelechem.2021.115755.

100 Grieshaber, D., MacKenzie, R., Vörös, J., and Reimhult, E. (2008). Electrochemical biosensors - sensor principles and architectures. *Sensors* 8 (3): 1400–1458. https://doi.org/10.3390/s8031400.

101 Guilbault, G.G., Kramer, D.N., and Cannon, P.L. (1962). Electrochemical determination of organophosphorous compounds. *Anal. Chem.* 34 (11): 1437–1439. https://doi.org/10.1021/ac60191a027.

102 Muñoz-San Martín, C., Gamella, M., Pedrero, M. et al. (2020). Magnetic beads-based electrochemical immunosensing of HIF-1α, a biomarker of tumoral hypoxia. *Sensors Actuators B Chem.* 307: 127623. https://doi.org/10.1016/j.snb.2019.127623.

103 Castle, L.M., Schuh, D.A., Reynolds, E.E., and Furst, A.L. (2021). Electrochemical sensors to detect bacterial foodborne pathogens. *ACS Sensors* 6 (5): 1717–1730. https://doi.org/10.1021/acssensors.1c00481.

104 Shafiei, F., Saberi, R.S., and Mehrgardi, M.A. (2021). A label-free electrochemical aptasensor for breast cancer cell detection based on a reduced graphene oxide-chitosan-gold nanoparticle composite. *Bioelectrochemistry* 140: 107807. https://doi.org/10.1016/j.bioelechem.2021.107807.

105 Khanmohammadi, A., Aghaie, A., Vahedi, E. et al. (2020). Electrochemical biosensors for the detection of lung cancer biomarkers: a review. *Talanta* 206: 120251. https://doi.org/10.1016/j.talanta.2019.120251.

106 Won, H.J., Robby, A.I., Jhon, H.S. et al. (2020). Wireless label-free electrochemical detection of cancer cells by MnO_2decorated polymer dots. *Sensors Actuators B Chem.* 320: 128391. https://doi.org/10.1016/j.snb.2020.128391.

107 Kaur, B., Kumar, S., and Kaushik, B.K. (2022). MXenes-based fiber-optic SPR sensor for colorectal cancer diagnosis. *IEEE Sensors J.* 22 (7): 6661–6668.

108 Kaur, B., Kumar, S., and Kaushik, B.K. (2022). Antimonene, CNT and MoS_2 based SPR-Fiber-optic probe for tuberculosis detection. *IEEE Sensors J.* 22 (15): 14903–14910.

109 Francis, T.S.Y. and Shizhuo, Y. (2002). *Fiber Optic Sensors*. New York, NY: Marcel Dekker AG https://doi.org/10.1109/ULTSYM.1980.197490.

110 Samuel, V.R. and Rao, K.J. (2022). A review on label free biosensors. *Biosens. Bioelectron.: X* 11: 100216. https://doi.org/10.1016/j.biosx.2022.100216.

111 Gupta, B.D., Srivastava, S.K., and Verma, R. (2015). *Fiber Optic Sensors Based on Plasmonics*. Singapore: World Scientific publishing.

112 Kretschmann, E. and Raether, H. (1968). Radiative decay of nonradiative surface plasmons excited by light. *Zeitschrift für Naturforschung A* 23 (12): 2135–2136. https://doi.org/10.1515/zna-1968-1247.

113 Wolfbeis, O.S. (1991). *Fiber Optic Chemical Sensors and Biosensors*, vol. 1. USA: CRC press.

114 Le Person, J., Colas, F., Compère, C. et al. (2008). Surface plasmon resonance in chalcogenide glass-based optical system. *Sensors Actuators B Chem.* 130 (2): 771–776. https://doi.org/10.1016/j.snb.2007.10.067.

115 Santos, I.P., Kinnear, C., Jorge, P.J. et al. (2018). Plasmonic polymer nanocomposites. *Nat. Rev. Mater.* 3 (10): 375–391. https://doi.org/10.1038/s41578-018-0050-7.

116 Tao, G., Heidepriem, E.H., Stolyarov, A.M., and Danto, S. (2015). *Infrared fibers. Adv. Opt. Photonics* 7: 379–458. https://doi.org/10.1364/AOP.

117 Gupta, B.D. and Verma, R.K. (2009). Surface plasmon resonance-based fiber optic sensors: principle, probe designs, and some applications. *J Sens* 2009: 1–12. https://doi.org/10.1155/2009/979761.

118 Aliofkhazraei, M., Ali, N., William, I.M. et al. (2016). *Graphene Science Handbook*. New York: CRC Press https://doi.org/10.1201/b19642-35.

119 Naik, G.V., Shalaev, V.M., and Boltasseva, A. (2013). Alternative plasmonic materials: beyond gold and silver. *Adv. Mater.* 25 (24): 3264–3294. https://doi.org/10.1002/adma.201205076.

120 Srivastava, S.K. and Gupta, B.D. (2013). Fiber optic plasmonic sensors: past, present and future. *The Open Opt. J.* 7 (1): 58–83. https://doi.org/10.2174/1874328501307010058.

121 Miliou, A. (2021). In-fiber interferometric-based sensors: overview and recent advances. *Photonics* 8 (7): 265. https://doi.org/10.3390/photonics8070265.

122 Yuan, D., Dong, Y., Liu, Y., and Li, T. (2015). Mach-Zehnder interferometer biochemical sensor based on silicon-on-insulator rib waveguide with large cross section. *Sensors* 15 (9): 21500–21517. https://doi.org/10.3390/s150921500.

123 Teixeira, J.G.V., Leite, I.T., Silva, S., and Frazão, O. (2014). Advanced fiber-optic acoustic sensors. *Photonic Sens.* 4 (3): 198–208. https://doi.org/10.1007/s13320-014-0148-5.

124 Ferreira, A.C., Costa, M.B.C., Coêlho, A.G. et al. (2012). Analysis of the nonlinear optical switching in a Sagnac interferometer with non-instantaneous Kerr effect. *Opt. Commun.* 285 (6): 1408–1417. https://doi.org/10.1016/j.optcom.2011.10.026.

125 Lee, B.H., Kim, Y.H., Park, K.S. et al. (2012). Interferometric fiber optic sensors. *Sensors* 12 (3): 2467–2486. https://doi.org/10.3390/s120302467.

126 Li, H.C., Leng, Y.K., Liao, Y.C. et al. (2022). Tapered microfiber MZI biosensor for highly sensitive detection of *staphylococcus aureus*. *IEEE Sensors J.* 22 (6): 5531–5539. https://doi.org/10.1109/JSEN.2022.3149004.

127 Liu, Q., Shin, Y., Kee, J.S. et al. (2015). Mach-Zehnder interferometer (MZI) point-of-care system for rapid multiplexed detection of microRNAs in human urine specimens. *Biosens. Bioelectron.* 71: 365–372. https://doi.org/10.1016/j.bios.2015.04.052.

128 Li, Z., Askim, J.R., and Suslick, K.S. (2019). The optoelectronic nose: colorimetric and fluorometric sensor arrays. *Chem. Rev.* 119 (1): 231–292. https://doi.org/10.1021/acs.chemrev.8b00226.

129 Kim, Y.J., Kim, H.S., Chon, J.W. et al. (2018). New colorimetric aptasensor for rapid on-site detection of campylobacter jejuni and campylobacter coli in chicken carcass samples. *Anal. Chim. Acta* 1029: 78–85. https://doi.org/10.1016/j.aca.2018.04.059.

130 Liu, B., Zhuang, J., and Wei, G. (2020). Recent advances in the design of colorimetric sensors for environmental monitoring. *Environ. Sci. Nano* 7 (8): 2195–2213. https://doi.org/10.1039/d0en00449a.

131 Tahir, M.A., Dina, N.E., Cheng, H. et al. (2021). Surface-enhanced Raman spectroscopy for bioanalysis and diagnosis. *Nanoscale* 13 (27): 11593–11634. https://doi.org/10.1039/d1nr00708d.

132 Blanco-Formoso, M. and Alvarez-Puebla, R.A. (2020). Cancer diagnosis through Sers and other related techniques. *Int. J. Mol. Sci.* 21 (6): https://doi.org/10.3390/ijms21062253.

133 Veloso, A.B., Longo, J.P.F., Muehlmann, L.A. et al. (2017). SERS investigation of cancer cells treated with PDT: quantification of cell survival and follow-up. *Sci. Rep.* 7 (1): 1–12. https://doi.org/10.1038/s41598-017-07469-1.

134 Guerrini, L., Pazos-Perez, N., Garcia-Rico, E., and Alvarez-Puebla, R. (2017). Cancer characterization and diagnosis with SERS-encoded particles. *Cancer Nanotechnol.* 8 (1): https://doi.org/10.1186/s12645-017-0031-3.

135 Zhai, W., You, T., Ouyang, X., and Wang, M. (2021). Recent progress in mycotoxins detection based on surface-enhanced Raman spectroscopy. *Compr. Rev. Food Sci. Food Saf.* 20 (2): 1887–1909. https://doi.org/10.1111/1541-4337.12686.

136 Eravuchira, P.J., Banchelli, M., D'Andrea, C. et al. (2020). Hollow core photonic crystal fiber-assisted Raman spectroscopy as a tool for the detection of Alzheimer's disease biomarkers. *J. Biomed. Opt.* 25 (07): 1. https://doi.org/10.1117/1.jbo.25.7.077001.

137 Dinish, U.S., Beffara, F., Humbert, G. et al. (2019). Surface-enhanced Raman scattering-active photonic crystal fiber probe: towards next generation liquid biopsy sensor with ultra high sensitivity. *J. Biophotonics* 12 (11): https://doi.org/10.1002/jbio.201900027.

138 Szaniawska, A. and Kudelski, A. (2021). Applications of surface-enhanced Raman scattering in biochemical and medical analysis. *Front. Chem.* 9: 1–7. https://doi.org/10.3389/fchem.2021.664134.

139 Li, P., Long, F., Chen, W. et al. (2020). Fundamentals and applications of surface-enhanced Raman spectroscopy–based biosensors. *Curr. Opin. Biomed. Eng.* 13: 51–59. https://doi.org/10.1016/j.cobme.2019.08.008.

140 Sha, M.Y., Xu, H., Penn, S.G., and Cromer, R. (2007). SERS nanoparticles: a new optical detection modality for cancer diagnosis. *Nanomedicine* 2 (5): 725–734. https://doi.org/10.2217/17435889.2.5.725.

141 Kahrizi, M. and Sohi, P.A. (2020). *Surface-Enhanced Raman Scattering: Introduction and Applications*. London, UK: IntechOpen Retrieved from https://www.intechopen.com/books/advanced-biometric-technologies/liveness-detection-in-biometrics.

142 Sharma, A., Khan, R., Catanante, G. et al. (2018). Designed strategies for fluorescence-based biosensors for the detection of mycotoxins. *Toxins* 10 (5): 1–19. https://doi.org/10.3390/toxins10050197.

143 Chen, Y.T., Lee, Y.C., Lai, Y.H. et al. (2020). Review of integrated optical biosensors for point-of-care applications. *Biosensors* 10 (12): 1–22. https://doi.org/10.3390/BIOS10120209.

144 Elahi, N., Kamali, M., Baghersad, M.H., and Amini, B. (2019). A fluorescence Nano-biosensors immobilization on iron (MNPs) and gold (AuNPs) nanoparticles for detection of shigella spp. *Mater. Sci. Eng. C* 105: 110113. https://doi.org/10.1016/j.msec.2019.110113.

145 Odom, T.W. and Schatz, G.C. (2011). *Introduction to Plasmonics*, vol. 111. New York, NW: Pan stanford CRC Press https://doi.org/10.1021/cr2001349.

146 Zhao, X., Dai, X., Zhao, S. et al. (2021). Aptamer-based fluorescent sensors for the detection of cancer biomarkers. *Spectrochim. Acta A Mol. Biomol. Spectrosc.* 247: 119038. https://doi.org/10.1016/j.saa.2020.119038.

147 Bruinink, A. (2020). Biosensor-bearing wound dressings for continuous monitoring of hard-to-heal wounds: now and next. *Biosens. Bioelectron. Open Access* 100017. https://doi.org/10.29011/bboa-117.100017.

148 Tian, X., Murfin, L.C., Wu, L. et al. (2021). Fluorescent small organic probes for biosensing. *Chem. Sci.* 12 (10): 3406–3426. https://doi.org/10.1039/d0sc06928k.

149 Inan, H., Poyraz, M., Inci, F. et al. (2017). Photonic crystals: emerging biosensors and their promise for point-of-care applications. *Chem. Soc. Rev.* 46 (2): 366–388. https://doi.org/10.1039/c6cs00206d.

150 Russell, P. (2003). Photonic crystal fibers. *Science* 299: 358–362.

151 Villatoro, J. and Zubia, J. (2016). [INVITED] new perspectives in photonic crystal fibre sensors. *Opt. Laser Technol.* 78: 67–75. https://doi.org/10.1016/j.optlastec.2015.07.025.

152 Paul, B.K., Ahmed, K., El, H.J. et al. (2020). The design and analysis of a dual-diamond-ring PCF-based sensor. *J. Comput. Electron.* 19: 1288–1294.

153 Mittal, S., Sharma, T., and Tiwari, M. (2021). Surface plasmon resonance based photonic crystal fiber biosensors: a review. *Mater. Today: Proc.* 43: 3071–3074. https://doi.org/10.1016/j.matpr.2021.01.405.

154 Parvin, T., Ahmed, K., Alatwi, A.M., and Rashed, A.N.Z. (2021). Differential optical absorption spectroscopy-based refractive index sensor for cancer cell detection. *Opt. Rev.* 28 (1): 134–143. https://doi.org/10.1007/s10043-021-00644-w.

155 Khatami, S.H., Karami, S., Siahkouhi, H.R. et al. (2022). Aptamer-based biosensors for Pseudomonas aeruginosa detection. *Mol. Cell. Probes* 66 (June): 101865. https://doi.org/10.1016/j.mcp.2022.101865.

156 Ghosh, G. (2020). Early detection of cancer: focus on antibody coated metal and magnetic nanoparticle-based biosensors. *Sens. Int.* 1 (June): 100050. https://doi.org/10.1016/j.sintl.2020.100050.

157 Mandal, D. and Banerjee, S. (2022). Surface acoustic wave (SAW) sensors: physics, materials, and applications. *Sensors* 22: 820.

158 Afzal, A., Mujahid, A., Schirhagl, R. et al. (2017). Gravimetric viral diagnostics: QCM based biosensors for early detection of viruses. *Chemosensors* 5 (1): 1–25. https://doi.org/10.3390/chemosensors5010007.

159 Iarossi, M., Schiattarella, C., Rea, I. et al. (2018). Colorimetric immunosensor by aggregation of photochemically functionalized gold nanoparticles. *ACS Omega* 3 (4): 3805–3812. https://doi.org/10.1021/acsomega.8b00265.

160 Bhattacharya, D., Rathore, P. K., & Majumdar, S. (2018). Non-invasive piezoelectric sensor for detection of lung cancer. *Proceedings of the 3rd International Conference on Communication and Electronics Systems, ICCES 2018*, 418–421. https://doi.org/10.1109/CESYS.2018.8723897

2

Immobilization Techniques for Bioreceptors

2.1 Introduction

Immobilization technique is restricting the movement of bio-recognition elements (BREs) that include enzyme, cells, and aptamers on the suitable support or substrate. Several techniques have been reported to immobilize different bioreceptors that include antibodies, aptamers, nucleic acid (NA), bacteriophage, enzymes, and molecularly imprinted polymer (MIP). Immobilized techniques have been explored for various applications [1, 2]. Nelson and Griffin, in 1916, observed the catalytic active property of invertase enzyme immobilized on charcoal, which led to the development of immobilization techniques. These techniques are broadly classified into three phases [3].

The early phase or pre-1950s included adsorption, filtration, and irreversible covalent. Immobilization of various biomolecules, including enzymes, on different supports of charcoal, metals, clay, cellulose, and glass, was reported as shown in Figure 2.1. These methods suffer from low efficiency, nonspecificity, and leaching of the immobilized molecules [4].

In the second phase, between the 1950s and the 1980s, covalent attachment, entrapment, and cross-linking techniques developed. With the advent of these technologies, stability, multi-immobilization, orientation control, and activity of immobilized biomolecules have led to the development of various biosensing and other applications [5, 6]. The industrial use of enzyme immobilization was reported by Sato, which includes the covalent immobilization of Aspergillus oryzae l-aminoacylase onto halogenoacetylcelluloses [7].

Biosensors: Nanomaterials, Approaches, and Performance-Enhancement Strategies,
First Edition. Baljinder Kaur, Santosh Kumar, and Brajesh Kumar Kaushik.

Published 2025 by John Wiley & Sons, Inc.
Companion website: www.wiley.com/go/kaur

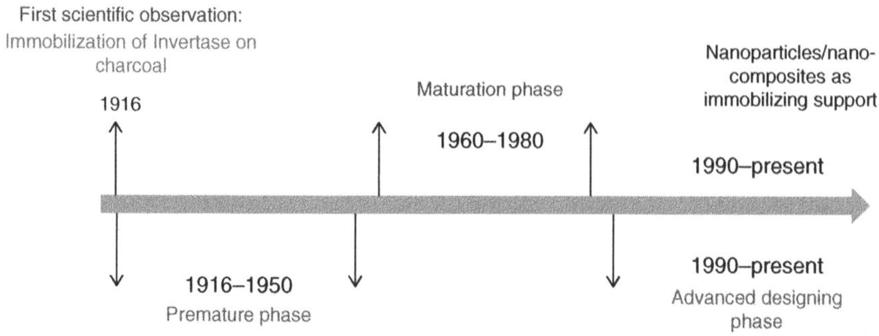

Figure 2.1 The schematic of year-wise progress of immobilization techniques. *Source:* [3]/with permission Springer Nature.

The third phase, from 1990 to the present, includes more advanced immobilization techniques, such as layer-by-layer assembly, self-assembled monolayers, and surface plasmon resonance. These techniques have allowed for the precise control of biomolecule immobilization and the development of novel applications such as biomolecular recognition and nanobiotechnology [8].

Adsorption or electrostatic interaction, covalent binding, entrapment, and cross-linking are the most common immobilization techniques for bioreceptors [9]. It is important to choose a suitable immobilization technique that depends on the molecule and supports nature. In reversible immobilization, the process can be reversed under certain conditions, while irreversible immobilizations are irreversible in nature [10]. Immobilization methods can be reversible or irreversible, depending on the attachment [11]. Among all techniques, adsorption is reversible and covalent coupling, entrapment, and crosslinking are irreversible in nature [12]. Reversible immobilization does not require chemical modification; activated biomolecules during use can be replaced in reversible immobilization; and the rapid accomplishment of the immobilization process using adsorption is advantageous as compared to irreversible techniques [13]. The schematic of different techniques of bioreceptor immobilization is shown in Figure 2.2.

This chapter is divided into five sections to discuss available immobilization techniques. Following this introduction, Section 2.2 discusses the need for immobilization technologies and their cons and pros. Section 2.3 explores the details of various immobilization methods and recent developments in these technologies and sensor design. Details of support materials and their selection criteria among immobilized techniques are discussed in Section 2.4. Section 2.5 discusses the possibilities of immobilization technology in the biosensing field.

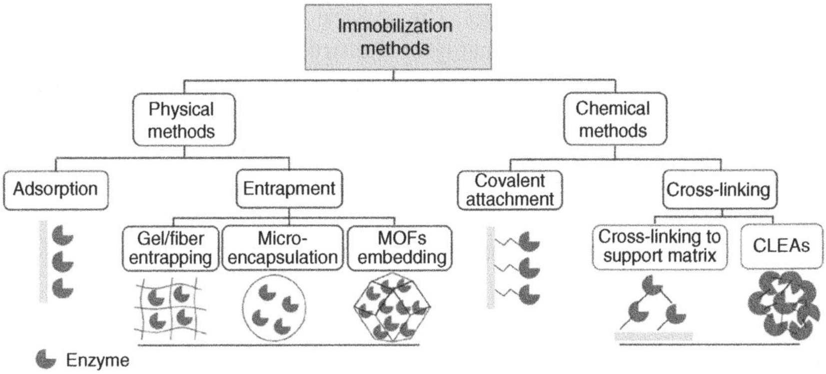

Figure 2.2 Classification of different techniques for bioreceptor immobilization. *Source:* [10]/with permission of Elsevier.

2.2 Requirements of Immobilization

Immobilization techniques allow effective attachment of BREs on the surface of sensor, stability, and long-term functionality. They have various applications in research, biomedical fields, and agriculture industries. These techniques can restrict the movement of molecules and control their orientation [14–16]. Immobilization of biomolecules on a solid support is relatively more stable as compared to free-floating counterparts, protected from degradation and other factors that can break them down [10, 17]. Immobilization also plays a significant role in activity and selectivity enhancement of biomolecules as it can reduces the diffusion rate and local concentration increment [16]. This can be particularly important for enzymes and other catalysts, which need to be highly concentrated to be effective [18]. The other advantage of using immobilization technology is easy isolation of components among the mixture and availability of vast variety of different methods that include filtration and chromatography. This makes them valuable tools for separation and purification processes in biotechnology and other fields [19–21].

The possibility of reusing immobilized biomolecules or bioreceptor decreases the cost of immobilization and makes it environment friendly compared to free-floating counterparts, which are typically used once and then discarded [13, 22, 23]. Due to this, continuous use of BRE is possible. The other advantages of immobilization include reduced cost as purification steps are not required, less needed labor, less reaction time with small contamination; improved process control, a high enzyme substrate ratio, reduced aggregate and foaming, and the ability to stop reactions at different stages. The physical methods are simple, low cost, and preferred to maintain originality of the structure of the sample. Physical methods suffer from low loading capacity and limited efficiency [17]. Covalent immobilization is preferred in cases that require high loading capacity and better stability [19]. The use of complicated steps in the case of covalently bonded immobilization limits its use. There are some drawbacks associated with each immobilization technique, including loss of biological activity of an immobilized biomolecule, cost as it requires complex equipment, and instability [18].

2.3 Immobilization Methods

2.3.1 Adsorption Immobilization or Electrostatic Interaction Method

In the adsorption method, a molecule on the substrate surface can be attached by various interaction such as hydrogen and Van der Waals bond. Figure 2.3 shows the schematic of enzyme immobilization through adsorption process on the support surface. Adsorption can be physical, affinity, and ion adsorption. Physical adsorption is the most widely explored immobilization technique for various application. Adsorption is the easiest, oldest, and simplest technique to immobilize various bioreceptor molecules that include enzymes, antibodies, and DNA probes. In this case, bioreceptors are adsorbed directly onto a transducer's solid surface or polymer matrix (conducting electrode such as Au or nanostructured materials) through different weak binding [24].

The bonding between the immobilized molecule and solid support is not permanent, reversible and weak in nature due to the presence of adsorption target. The binding forces are vulnerable to any changes in pH, temperature, and ionic strength that lead to poor stability of immobilized molecule [25]. This method suffers from the leaching problem that detaches it from the bonding surface. This problem can be resolved by coating corresponding functional groups [26]. It does not require additional coupling or linker agents. Adsorption-based immobilization techniques cause less disruption to enzymes and require fewer reagents and clean-up steps. However, it suffers from several drawbacks, such as weak interaction, environmental susceptibility, and a limited lifetime [3].

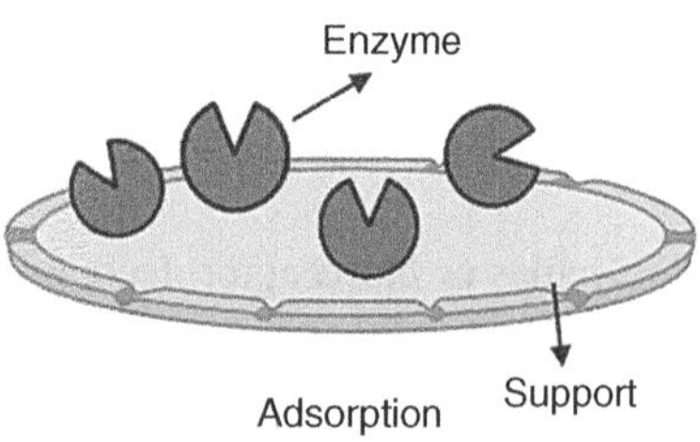

Figure 2.3 The schematic illustration of adsorption immobilization includes the adsorption of enzymes on the support surface.

2.3.2 Entrapment

Entrapment is an irreversible technique to immobilize a molecule of that include caging of a bioreceptor using a polymer network or fiber networks via covalent or noncovalent interactions. The polymer network controls the leakage of molecule via its pore size. A monomer solution is used to suspend the immobilizable bioreceptors and is further polymerized using a gel before entrapment, as shown in Figure 2.4a. Polymers can be attached to surface using thermal methods and photochemical methods with the help of dip-coating procedures. Immobilized molecules in entrapment methods maintain chemical activity of the molecule or entity and minimize the chance of matrix leaching [26].

The process of entrapment immobilization can be accomplished in a variety of ways, depending on the material used for immobilization. The solution of polymer – for instance, alginate or any other polymer – is mixed with biological material, and then calcium ion-rich solution is added to crosslink it and form a matrix that entraps the biomaterial. The pores of the membranes are smaller than the biomaterial and thus entrap it inside physically. This has been widely explored for various applications that include enzyme immobilization in industry, enzyme isolation from the mixture, and cell immobilization for tissue engineering applications [25].

2.3.3 Membrane Encapsulation

The encapsulation immobilization method involves immobilizing of bioreceptors using a semipermeable material, that restricts the motion of bioreceptors inside the membrane and can move inside the capsule as shown in Figure 2.4b. Hydrogels are used to cross-link polymer networks that entrap the bioreceptors inside the

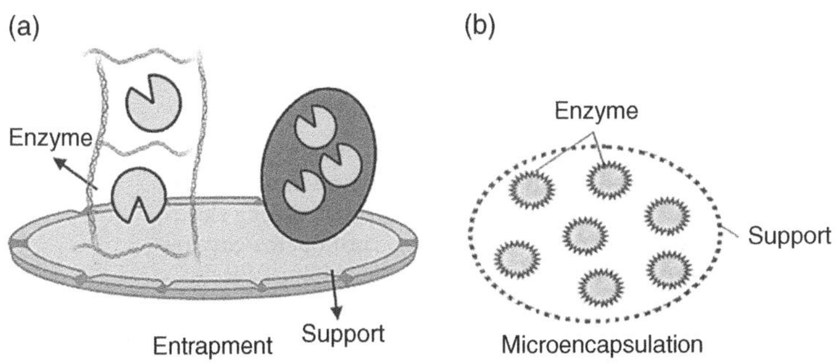

Figure 2.4 Schematic illustration of (a) entrapment and (b) covalent immobilization-based immobilization techniques for bioreceptors.

porous structure. Hydrogels are synthesized using natural polymers (alginate, collagen, chitosan), synthetic polymers, and liposomes. Liposomes are spherical-shaped vesicles made up of a lipid bilayer formed from different compositions of lipids, and their size and shape can be controlled to optimize the encapsulation efficiency and stability of the biomolecules [27]. Encapsulation immobilization can prevent denaturation and provide a protective microenvironment for the bioreceptors to hold native conformations. Additionally, it can provide a way to spatially organize multiple biomolecules, enabling synergistic or complementary interactions between them. Encapsulation immobilization can also have drawbacks, such as limited diffusion of substrates and products, which can lead to mass transfer limitations and reduced reaction rates. Additionally, the encapsulation material can affect the performance of the biomolecules, such as by altering the pH or temperature optima, or by inducing steric hindrance or diffusion barriers. Therefore, careful process of optimizing the encapsulation ensures the better immobilization of the biomolecules.

Table 2.1 summarizes the various advantages and disadvantages of the immobilization techniques during immobilize the different bioreceptors. Reversible

Table 2.1 Advantages and drawbacks associated with immobilization techniques.

Schemes	Advantages	Drawbacks	Ref.
Adsorption	Simple, direct steps, as it does not require linkers, reversible, easy recovery of biomolecules	Release of an adsorbed substance, nonspecific adsorption, weak bonding, low reproducibility	[3, 27]
Covalent immobilization	Independent of diffusion, small response time, strong interaction, stable toward heat, irreversible	Matrix cannot be reconstructed, can pair with toxic products, shows significant loss in molecule activity, has nonrenewable support materials, involves use of linker molecules, is irreversible	[2, 28]
Entrapment	Chemically stable, multi-immobilization is possible in the same polymer, maintain density of cells and allow operation continuously	Leakage and stability issue, requires extra monomer concentration during electro polymerization, toxicity, low molecule loading capacity	[20, 29]
Affinity	Orientation can be controlled, high specificity, reversible	Affects pH values, needs specific group such as biotin in enzyme immobilization	[26, 30, 31]

immobilization techniques are used in the applications that requires reusable and recoverable entities while or irreversible techniques are preferred that require stability, long life, requires permanent attachment [9].

2.3.4 Covalent Immobilization

Bioreceptors are attached via chemical methods that also support the matrix through stable covalent bonding [32]. The stable covalent bonds yield a stable and durable immobilized bioreceptor as compared to other immobilization techniques. Support matrix surface can also be functionalized with reactive groups, as bioreceptors are added that interact with the surface groups via covalent bonding to form stable attachment. High stability, increased resistance toward environmental conditions of change in pH, temperature, excellent durability, and reusability are advantages associated with covalent immobilization to use over a wide range of applications [7].

Immobilization of the horseradish peroxidase (HRP) enzyme via covalent bonding is shown in Figure 2.5a in case of chemiluminescent sensor design [27]. However, covalent immobilization can be more complex and time-consuming than other immobilization techniques and may not be suitable for all biological materials. Covalent immobilization is commonly used in biotechnology and biomedical research for applications such as enzyme immobilization, biosensors, and immunoassays. There are several advantages of covalent immobilization: it provides stability to support matrix and can increase their resistance to harsh environmental conditions, making them useful for industrial processes. Qu et al. explored applied cobalt-nitrilotriacetic acid chemistry to immobilize hexahistidine-tagged proteins as bioreceptors on the surface plasmon resonance (SPR)-based fiber bio-sensor, as shown in Figure 2.5b [33]. In biosensors and immunoassays, covalent immobilization can be used to attach biomolecules such as antibodies or DNA probes to a support matrix that can detect the analytes with high sensitivity and specific detection of target molecules.

Copolymerization or cross-linking is a type of covalent immobilization and irreversible method that immobilizing biomolecules, such as enzymes, antibodies, or DNA, onto a solid support through covalent bonding [10]. A cross-linking agent is used to connect the biomolecules and the support to form a stable network of cross-linked molecules. Cross-linking immobilization is stable and can be used in harsh environmental conditions, control the orientation and density of the immobilized bioreceptors, provide high specificity, and be robust in nature [24]. Figure 2.6 shows an ECL biosensor that utilize cross-linking immobilization with lactate dehydrogenase and pyruvate oxidase to detect the L-lactate [21]. There are several drawbacks associated with cross-linking immobilization that include non-specific binding and structure alteration risk and activity of the immobilized

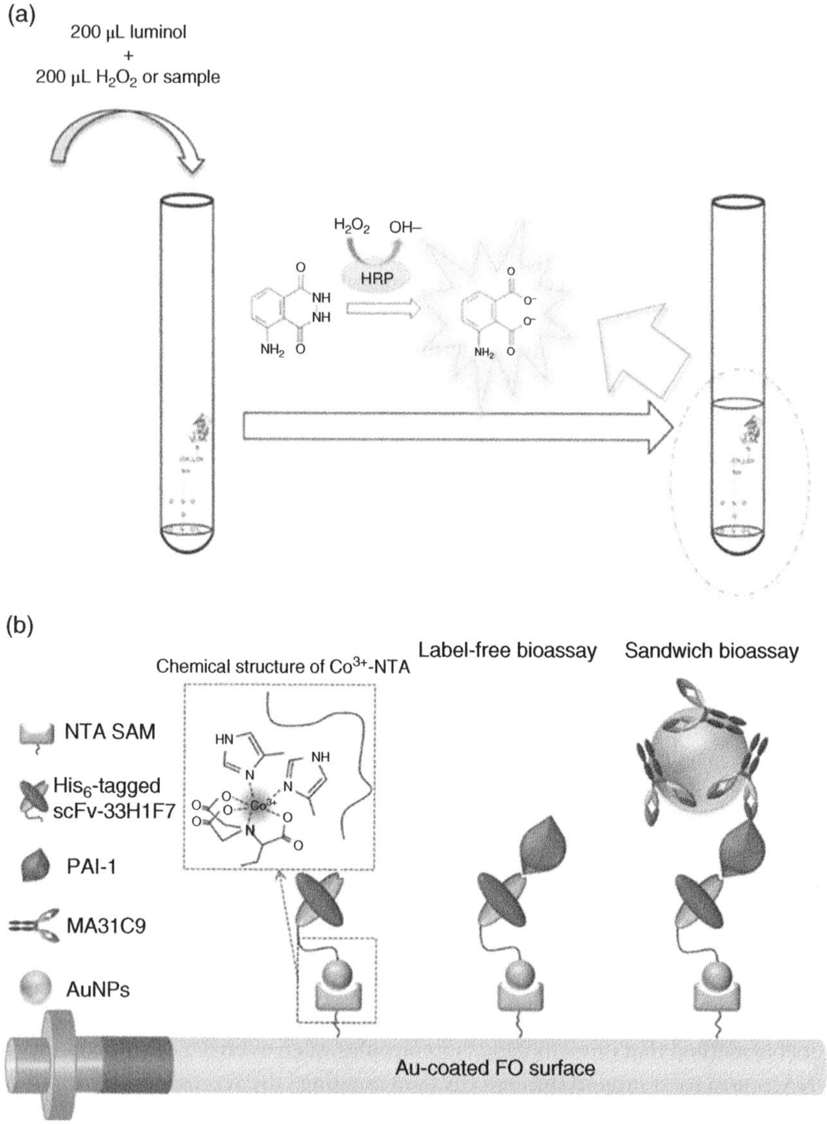

Figure 2.5 Schematic illustration of (a) HRP enzyme through covalent immobilization in the chemiluminescent sensor design. *Source:* [27]/with permission of American Chemical Society. (b) Hexahistidine-tagged proteins in the case of SPR sensor. *Source:* [33]/with permission of American Chemical Society.

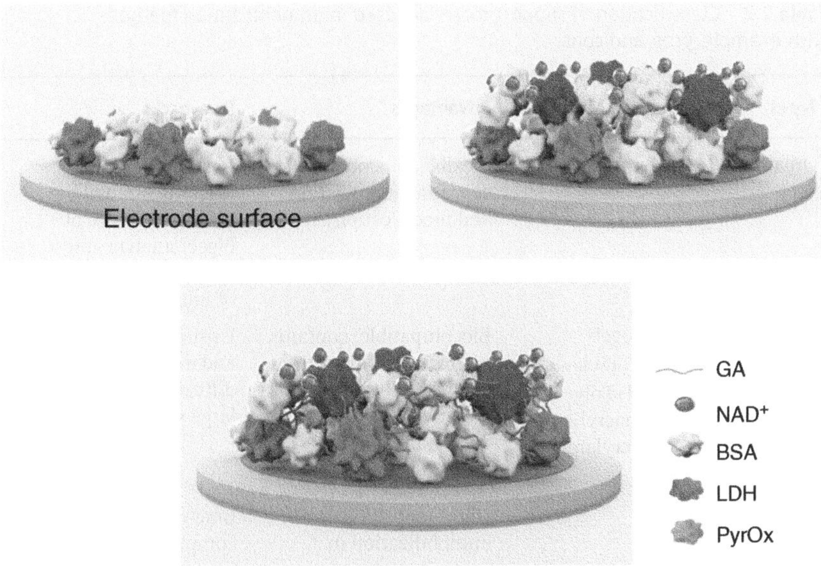

Figure 2.6 Lactate dehydrogenase /pyruvate oxidase using cross-linking immobilization-based ECL biosensors to detect the L-lactate. *Source:* [21]/with permission of Elsevier.

bioreceptors. Therefore, careful optimization of the cross-linking conditions is necessary to ensure the best possible performance of the immobilized biomolecules (Table 2.1).

2.4 Materials Used in Different Immobilization Techniques and Supports

A variety of materials have used immobilization techniques as a support material, including glass, polymers, hydrogels, SAM, metals, nanoparticles, and membranes. The selection of support material depends on the particular are of application, properties, and nature of the detectable analyte. Various cells, biomolecules, or analytes are immobilized on the surface of supports materials [17]. These materials are classified as organic, inorganic, and biomaterials. Their pros, cons, and examples are summarized in the Table 2.2.

Organic, inorganic, and biomaterials have been widely explored in various applications; among them, inorganic materials are flexible, scalable, inert, and stable, making them ideal candidates for use in harsh environments and high temperatures. As compared to inorganic materials, organic materials are complex

Table 2.2 Classification of support materials used in immobilization methods with example, pros, and cons.

Types	Support Materials	Advantages	Drawbacks
Organic	Polymers	Flexible, biocompatible, easy functionalization and modification	Restricted stability, leaching, limited by diffusion in case of bigger analyte and nonspecific adsorption of interfering substance
	Hydrogels Poly (ethylene glycol) Poly (methacrylic acid) Polyacrylamide Alginate	Biocompatible, contains high water content to enable easily maintaining biomolecular activity, mass transport due to porous structure	Unstable due to swelling and dehydration and diffusion issue with large size analytes
	SAM	Highly specific immobilization in a controlled manner, stability, monolayers uniformity, handy surface chemistry	time-consuming and complex preparation, inadequate load capability of sample
	Synthetic peptides	Highly specific binding of target and affinity	complex synthesis and purification steps
Inorganic	Silica-based materials (glass, zeolite, silica gels)	Stable with inert surface, large surface area; allow multiple groups functionalization	Limited diffusion and leaching issue
	AuNPs	Large surface that amplifies signal; stable and easy functionalization, supported by strong plasmonic effects	Costly and easy aggregation
	Magnetic NPs	Easy separation and manipulation using magnetic fields that allow target localization, huge surface area with good binding capacity	Suffer from interference effect arise due to magnetic fields
	Carbon-based materials	Good electrical and mechanical properties; enhances performance, chemically stable	Cytotoxic and non-biocompatible, high cost

Table 2.2 (Continued)

Types	Support Materials	Advantages	Drawbacks
Biomaterials	Cellulose	Good porosity; inert surface and biocompatible	Stability issue in harsh environment
	Chitosan	Biodegradable, nontoxic, stable, can immobilize a large number of biomolecules, biocompatible, antibacterial, and antimicrobial properties	Expensive, difficult to purify, and limited by variable reproducibility
	Collagen, gelatin	Natural, better adhesion properties, tissue biocompatible, appropriate for bio-samples of native structure	Limited stability; degrades with passage of time
	Proteins	High affinity, negligible nonspecific binding, compatible; can detect the small changes in the analyte concentration due to high sensitivity	Expensive and limited to antibody immobilization; instability at high temperatures or harsh chemicals

and costly. While organic materials are easy to work with, they are limited by instability and are not resistant in harsh chemical environment as compared to inorganic materials. Biomaterials are biocompatible, biodegradable hybrid materials that allow their use in applications associated with living tissues. As compared to organic and inorganic materials, these have more specificity and sensitivity [29–31]. Glass, an optically transparent and inert material, is widely explored in various applications that include microscopy, industry, and sensors [10, 30, 31, 34]. Polymers possess tunable physical and chemical properties that make them versatile for use in immobilization [27]. Polymers can be shaped into various geometries – for example, hydrogels [28]. Metals and their nanoparticles, such as copper (Cu), aluminum (Al), gold (Au), and silver (Ag), have been explored as supports in case of plasmonic, colorimetric, and SERS biosensors [35–39]. They provide a conductive surface for electrical or optical measurements and can be modified with various functional groups to achieve the specific binding interactions [13].

Nanoparticles (NPs) such as gold and silica nanoparticles can serve as both immobilization supports and immobilization materials attributed to small size that provide large surface area [64–68]. NPs include nanowires, nanotubes, and nano-capsules [25]. Membranes that involve cellulose acetate and polycarbonate membranes, have been reported in encapsulation techniques to act as a semipermeable barrier to control the diffusion of molecules during exchange of nutrients and waste in a process [14–68]. Hydrogels are commonly used in biomedical applications as they can trap molecules or cells within their structure due to water-swollen networks of cross-linked polymers. Hydrogels are synthesized to achieve specific properties that include stiffness, porosity, and degradation rates that make them better candidates for various applications [25]. Overall, material selection for immobilization depends on the specific application and the properties required for the immobilized material [69]. Table 2.3 details various reported biosensors based on support materials immobilized using different techniques.

Zhang et al. reported an ECL biosensor to detect the human epidermal growth factor (HER2) protein, a biomarker for breast cancer. This biosensor is based on a peptide hydrogel that is immobilized on a poly(3,4-ethylenedioxythiophene) film. This functionalized group makes the peptide hydrophilic, preventing aggregation and forming a thick layer on the poly(3,4-ethylenedioxythiophene) (PEDOT) film. The peptide hydrogel also contains a high density of negative charges, which helps to repel other negatively charged biomolecules. The peptide hydrogel is designed to be antifouling, meaning that it resists the nonspecific binding of proteins and other molecules. This sensor reaches the range of detection of 0.1 ng/ml–1.0 μg/ml and limit of detection (LOD) of 45 pg/ml [70].

A hydrogel-based suspension array that uses HRP-mediated Ag precipitation within antibody-immobilized hydrogel microparticles was reported and shown in Figure 2.7. The hydrogel microparticles are prepared by polymerizing a PEGDA monomer using a cross-linking agent. The resulting microparticles have a tunable porosity that allows them to be loaded with a high concentration of antibodies. The antibodies are then immobilized on microparticles surface by covalent connection [70]. Table 2.4 summarizes various reported ECL, optical, and mass-based biosensors, analytes, immobilized molecules, and immobilization methods.

2.5 Future Prospects and Possibilities in Immobilization Technology

The field of immobilization techniques is constantly evolving, and improving these technologies to enhance biosensor performance and other applications is the focus of researchers. One way to improve this technology is to develop new methods with improved stability and higher biomolecules load capacity, surface

Table 2.3 Various reported biosensors based on different support materials immobilized using different techniques.

Sensor Structure	Transduction Method	Analyte	LOD	Ref.
Carbon QDs-glucose oxidase/cellulose acetate complex-based sensor	Fluorescence	Glucose	25.79 nM	[40]
Cellulose-hydroxyapatite carbon electrode composite-based sensor	ECL	Plumbum ions	0.11 μg/L	[41]
Tricyanofuran-hydrazone and urease enzyme in nano-whiskers biosensor	Colorimetric	Urea	50–1100 ppm	[42]
Cellulose nano-whiskers and AgNPs-based sensor	Colorimetric	H_2O_2	0.014 and 112 μM	[43]
Polysorbate crosslinked cellulose-Ag–Cu nanohybrid sensor from bitter leaf stem	Colorimetric	Urea	0.8102 ppm	[44]
Carboxy-methyl cellulose and AgNPs-based sensor	Colorimetric	Hg^{2+}	5 nM	[45]
Micro-fibrillated cellulose aerogel sensor	Colorimetric	Sweat	n.r.[a]	[46]
Kenaf cellulose and dimethylglyoxime-based sensor	Colorimetric	Ni^{2+}	40 lg/l	[47]
Microporous cellulose xerogel-based sensor	Colorimetric	Ammonia gas	9.0×10^{-2} ppb	[48]
Congo red on triacetyl cellulose films via epichlorohydrin using covalent immobilization	Colorimetric	pH	n.r.[a]	[49]
Cotton cellulose nanocrystals and protease peptide-based sensor	Colorimetric	Human neutrophil elastase	50 mU	[50]
Dialdehyde cellulose-based sensor	Colorimetric	Ag^+	10^{-6} mol/l	[51]
2,5-dithiourea deposited on biomass cellulose	Colorimetric	Ag^+ Cu^{2+}	10^{-3} mol/l 10^{-4} mol/l	[52]
Cellulose-based colorimetric sensor	Colorimetric	Cu^{2+}	10^{-7} mol/l	[53]

(Continued)

Table 2.3 (Continued)

Sensor Structure	Transduction Method	Analyte	LOD	Ref.
Cellulose and 1-(2-pyridylazo)-2-naphthol-based sensor	Colorimetric	Zn^{2+}, Cu^{2+}	100 ppb	[54]
Cellulose fiber-Au NP composites	SERS and Colorimetric	Malachite green and water	10 ppb	[55]
Poly(acrylamide)-based self-driven DNA hydrogel	Optical	microRNA	n.r.[a]	[56]
Poly (ethylene glycol)	Optical	Collagenase	2 nM	[57]
Poly (vinyl alcohol) and 3D-nanoporous ZnO-based sensor	ECL	Glucose	0.2 mM	[58]
Poly (methacrylic acid) and MIP-based quartz crystal microbalance (QCM) biosensor	QCM	L-tryptophan	0.73 ng/ml	[59]
Hydrogel-based QCM biosensor	QCM	Swelling and sorption measurements	n.r.[a]	[60]
Chitosan matrix and naphthalimide fluorophore-based sensor	Fluorescence	p-nitrophenol and 2, 4, 6-trinitrophenol	0.28 μM	[61]
Chitosan and sodium alginate-based sensor	ECL	Glucose and insulin	22 mM	[62]
Dextran-based spiral microelectrode sensor	ECL	Alzheimer's disease	0.15 pg/ml	[63]

[a] Not reported.

modification strategies, and SAM with better control over surface chemistry. Developing new and advanced materials set of materials, such as metal–organic frameworks, 2D materials, hydrogels, and nanoparticles can improve the efficiency of biosensors in future. Integration with other technologies such as microfluidics channels could provide more control on sample detection. Advancements in bioactive surface engineering that include tailored surface chemistries, surface patterning techniques, and easily scalable technology can be used in industrial applications. The use of 3D printing to fabricate the sensor geometries with customizable microenvironments can improve the sensor performance. The new application areas such as food science, agriculture, and energy production can be

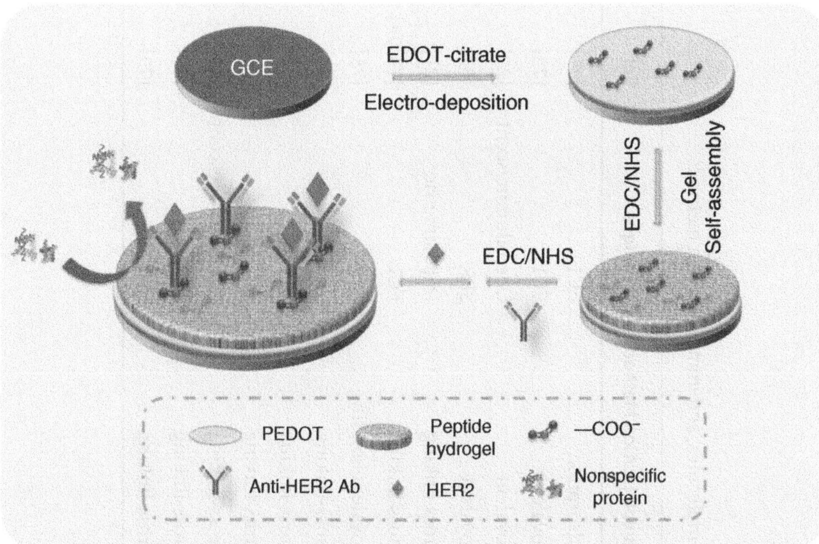

Figure 2.7 Schematic depiction of the hydrogel-based ECL sensor for HER2 detection. *Source:* [70]/with permission of American Chemical Society.

explored using these techniques. The combination of bioinformatics, multi-analyte sensing, machine learning, and data integration can aid in optimizing immobilization protocols.

Figure 2.8 shows the numbers of scientifically published articles and their trends at different sensing platforms in the years 2010–2018, as reported by Nguyen et al. using different bioreceptors. It shows that enzyme-based biosensor designs are widely explored, and it is at first place in the plot. Antibody-based biosensors are second-most widely explored field. Phage-based biosensors are the least explored area for different applications. Whole-cell, aptamer, and nucleic acids are the next dominant areas after phage biosensors.

2.6 Summary

In this chapter, the fundamentals of immobilization techniques and their types on different sensing platforms, including ECL, optical, piezoelectric, and affinity-based sensors, are discussed in detail. Each bioreceptor has different properties such as instability, high costs, and difficult recovery of active molecules from reaction mixture. Immobilization techniques overcome the various difficulties associated with biosensing applications, such as specificity and low intensity of the

Table 2.4 Reported ECL, optical, and mass-based biosensors, analytes, immobilized molecules, and immobilization methods.

Substrates	Immobilized Enzymes	Immobilization Methods	Technique	Ref.
H_2O_2	Catalyst	Adsorption	ECL	[71]
Glucose	Glucose oxidase	Covalent	ECL	[72]
H_2O_2	HRP	Covalent	Chemiluminescent	[27]
Plasminogen activator inhibitor1	Hexahistidine tagged proteins	Covalent	SPR	[33]
L-lactate selective	Lactate dehydrogenase /pyruvate oxidase	Cross-linking	Impedimetric	[21]
Porous polytetrafluoroethylene	Urease	Cross-linking	ECL	[73, 74]
Glucose	Glucose oxidase	Covalent bonding	SPR	[75]
Lactose	Glucose oxidase, β-galactosidase	Cross-linking	Colorimetric	[76]
Polydopamine-modified substrate	H_2O_2	Cross-linking	ECL	[77]
Organophosphates	Acetylcholinesterase	Cross-linking	ECL	[26]
Acetylcholine	Acetylcholinesterase	Cross-linking	Chemiluminescent	[19]
Butyrylcholine	Butyrylcho-linesterase	Cross-linking	SPR	[78]
Glucose	Glucose oxidase	Cross-linking	ECL	[79]

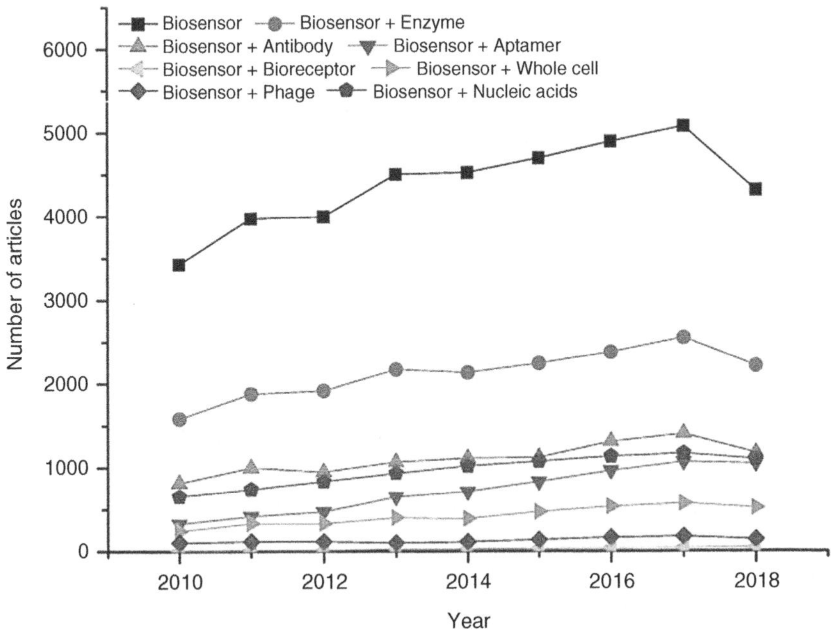

Figure 2.8 Numbers of articles published on different platforms based on bioreceptor-assisted biosensors between the years 2010 and 2018. It clearly indicates that throughout these years, enzyme-based biosensors have dominated this field with a large number of publications. *Source:* [14]/MDPI/CC BY 4.0.

output signal, and they improve the overall performance of the sensor. The advantages and disadvantages of each immobilization technique have been discussed in detail. The choice of immobilizing technique in each type of bioreceptor molecules play important role in the biosensor's fabrication. The development of nanostructures that include nanofibers, two-dimensional nanomaterials, carbon nanotubes, and metal nanoparticles leads to better and more efficient support. With their high porosity, optical and electrical properties, and high surface area, nanostructures could more often be considered as carriers. Covalent immobilization is a commonly used method to immobilize bioreceptors to provide stable and repeatable signal for several uses.

References

1 Kaur, B., Kumar, S., and Kaushik, B.K. (2023). *Biomedical Sensors: Advanced Materials, Approaches and Enhancement*, 1e, 1–13. IEEE Press Series on Sensors.

2 Ligler, F.S. and Taitt, C.R. (2018). *Optical Biosensors Today and Tomorrow, Second*. Elsevier B.V https://doi.org/10.1016/B978-044453125-4.50003-6.

3 Tripathi, A. (2021). *Jose Savio Melo, Gels Horizons: From Science to Smart Materials*. Singapore: Springer https://www.mdpi.com/2310-2861/7/3/110/htm.

4 Li, J., Liu, X., Sun, H. et al. (2021). A new type of optical fiber glucose biosensor with enzyme immobilized by electrospinning. *IEEE Sensors J.* 21: 16078–16085. https://doi.org/10.1109/JSEN.2021.3075553.

5 Bounegru, A.V. and Apetrei, C. (2023). Tyrosinase immobilization strategies for the development of electrochemical biosensors—a review. *Nanomaterials* 13: 760. https://doi.org/10.3390/nano13040760.

6 Yang, L.F., Ling, M., Kacherovsky, N., and Pun, S.H. (2023). Aptamers 101: aptamer discovery and in vitro applications in biosensors and separations. *Chem. Sci.* 14: 4961–4978. https://doi.org/10.1039/d3sc00439b.

7 Sato, T., Mori, T., Tosa, T., and Chibata, I. (1971). Studies on immobilized enzymes. IX. Preparation and properties of aminoacylase covalently attached to halogenoacetylcelluloses. *Arch. Biochem. Biophys.* 147: 788–796. https://doi.org/10.1016/0003-9861(71)90440-1.

8 De Girolamo, A., McKeague, M., Pascale, M. et al. (2018). Immobilization of aptamers on substrates. In: *Aptamers for Analytical Applications*, 85–126. Wiley-VCH Verlag GmbH & Co. KGaA https://doi.org/10.1002/9783527806799.ch3.

9 Maghraby, Y.R., El-Shabasy, R.M., Ibrahim, A.H., and Azzazy, H.M.E.S. (2023). Enzyme immobilization technologies and industrial applications. *ACS Omega* 8: 5184–5196. https://doi.org/10.1021/acsomega.2c07560.

10 Liu, D.M., Chen, J., and Shi, Y.P. (2018). Advances on methods and easy separated support materials for enzymes immobilization. *TrAC – Trends Anal. Chem.* 102: 332–342. https://doi.org/10.1016/j.trac.2018.03.011.

11 Guisan, J.M. (2013). Immobilization of enzymes and cells IN series editor. *Immobil. Enzym. Cells.* 1051: 1–375. https://doi.org/10.1007/978-1-62703-550-7.

12 Shanbhag, M.M., Manasa, G., Mascarenhas, R.J. et al. (2023). *Fundamentals of Bio-Electrochemical Sensing*. Elsevier B.V https://doi.org/10.1016/j.ceja.2023.100516.

13 Feng, Y., Xu, Y., Liu, S. et al. (2022). Recent advances in enzyme immobilization based on novel porous framework materials and its applications in biosensing. *Coord. Chem. Rev.* 459: https://doi.org/10.1016/j.ccr.2022.214414.

14 Nguyen, H.H., Lee, S.H., Lee, U.J. et al. (2019). Immobilized enzymes in biosensor applications. *Materials (Basel)* 12: https://doi.org/10.3390/ma12010121.

15 Aslan, Y., Atabay, M., Chowdhury, H.K. et al. (2023). Aptamer-based point-of-care devices: emerging technologies and integration of computational methods. *Biosensors* 13: 569. https://doi.org/10.3390/bios13050569.

16 Krishnamoorthi, S., Banerjee, A., and Roychoudhury, A. (2015). Immobilized enzyme technology: potentiality and prospects review. *Enzymol. Metab.* 1: 1–11.

17 Datta, S., Christena, L.R., and Rajaram, Y.R.S. (2013). Enzyme immobilization: an overview on techniques and support materials. *3 Biotech.* 3: 1–9. https://doi.org/10.1007/s13205-012-0071-7.

18 Bié, J., Sepodes, B., Fernandes, P.C.B., and Ribeiro, M.H.L. (2022). Enzyme immobilization and co-immobilization: main framework, advances and some applications. *Processes* https://doi.org/10.3390/pr10030494.

19 Chakraborty, S., Rusli, H., Nath, A. et al. (2016). Immobilized biocatalytic process development and potential application in membrane separation: a review. *Crit. Rev. Biotechnol.* 36: 43–48. https://doi.org/10.3109/07388551.2014.923373.

20 Moya-Ramírez, I., Kotidis, P., Marbiah, M. et al. (2022). Polymer encapsulation of bacterial biosensors enables coculture with mammalian cells. *ACS Synth. Biol.* 11: 1303–1312. https://doi.org/10.1021/acssynbio.1c00577.

21 Chan, D., Barsan, M.M., Korpan, Y., and Brett, C.M.A. (2017). L-lactate selective impedimetric bienzymatic biosensor based on lactate dehydrogenase and pyruvate oxidase. *Electrochim. Acta* 231: 209–215. https://doi.org/10.1016/j.electacta.2017.02.050.

22 Morales, M.A. and Halpern, J.M. (2018). Guide to selecting a biorecognition element for biosensors. *Bioconjug. Chem.* 29: 3231–3239. https://doi.org/10.1021/acs.bioconjchem.8b00592.

23 Balcar, H. and Roth, W.J. (2013). *Hybrid Catalysts for Olefin Metathesis and Related Polymerizations*. Elsevier B.V https://doi.org/10.1016/B978-0-444-53876-5.00001-5.

24 Lee, C.H., Jin, E.S., Lee, J.H., and Hwang, E.T. (2020). Immobilization and stabilization of enzyme in biomineralized calcium carbonate microspheres. *Front. Bioeng. Biotechnol.* 8: 1–8. https://doi.org/10.3389/fbioe.2020.553591.

25 Imam, H.T., Marr, P.C., and Marr, A.C. (2021). Enzyme entrapment, biocatalyst immobilization without covalent attachment. *Green Chem.* 23: 4980–5005. https://doi.org/10.1039/d1gc01852c.

26 Dong, Y. (2018). *Aptamers for Analytical Applications*. Wiley-VCH Verlag GmbH & Co. KGaA https://doi.org/10.1002/9783527806799.

27 Bocanegra-Rodríguez, S., Jornet-Martínez, N., Molins-Legua, C., and Campíns-Falcó, P. (2020). New reusable solid biosensor with covalent immobilization of the horseradish peroxidase enzyme: in situ liberation studies of hydrogen peroxide by portable chemiluminescent determination. *ACS Omega* 5: 2419–2427. https://doi.org/10.1021/acsomega.9b03958.

28 Hassan, M.E., Yang, Q., Xiao, Z. et al. (2019). Impact of immobilization technology in industrial and pharmaceutical applications. *3 Biotech* 9: 1–16. https://doi.org/10.1007/s13205-019-1969-0.

29 Asal, M., Özen, Ö., Şahinler, M. et al. (2019). An overview of biomolecules, immobilization methods and support materials of biosensors. *Sens. Rev.* 39: 377–386. https://doi.org/10.1108/SR-04-2018-0084.

30 Makaraviciute, A. and Ramanaviciene, A. (2013). Site-directed antibody immobilization techniques for immunosensors. *Biosens. Bioelectron.* 50: 460–471. https://doi.org/10.1016/j.bios.2013.06.060.

31 Abdel-Hameed, S.A.M., Ahmed, S.A., Mostafa, F.A. et al. (2022). Preparation and characterization of sugilite glass from basalt for α-amylase immobilization, statistical optimization of the immobilization process and description of free and immobilized enzyme. *Heliyon* 8: e09960. https://doi.org/10.1016/j.heliyon.2022.e09960.

32 Malhotra, B.D. and Ali, A. (2018). *Nanomaterials for Biosensors Fundamentals and Applications*, 1e. Amsterdam, Netherlands: Elsevier.

33 Qu, J.H., Horta, S., Delport, F. et al. (2020). Expanding a portfolio of (FO-) SPR surface chemistries with the co(III)-NTA oriented immobilization of His6-tagged bioreceptors for applications in complex matrices. *ACS Sensors* 5: 960–969. https://doi.org/10.1021/acssensors.9b02227.

34 Sharmin, F., Rakshit, S.K., and Jayasuriya, H.P.W. (2007). Enzyme immobilization on glass surface for the development of phosphate detection biosensors. *Agric. Eng. Int.* IX: 1–15.

35 Chaudhary, V.S., Kumar, D., and Kumar, S. (2022). Au-TiO_2 coated photonic crystal Fiber based SPR refractometric sensor for detection of cancerous cells. *IEEE Trans. Nanobioscience* 6–13. https://doi.org/10.1109/TNB.2022.3219104.

36 Bordbar, M.M., Samadinia, H., Sheini, A. et al. (2022). A colorimetric electronic tongue based on bi-functionalized AuNPs for fingerprint detection of cancer markers. *Sensors Actuators B Chem.* 368: 132170. https://doi.org/10.1016/j.snb.2022.132170.

37 Muhammad, M. and Huang, Q. (2021). A review of aptamer-based SERS biosensors: design strategies and applications. *Talanta* 227: 122188. https://doi.org/10.1016/j.talanta.2021.122188.

38 Cui, F., Zhou, Z., and Zhou, H.S. (2020). Review-measurement and analysis of cancer biomarkers based on electrochemical biosensors. *J. Electrochem. Soc.* 167: 037525.

39 Singh, S., Podder, P.S., Russo, M. et al. (2022). Tailored point-of-care biosensors for liquid biopsy in the field of oncology. *Lab Chip* 71: 44–61. https://doi.org/10.1039/d2lc00666a.

40 Yu, S., Ding, L., Lin, H. et al. (2019). A novel optical fiber glucose biosensor based on carbon quantum dots-glucose oxidase/cellulose acetate complex sensitive film. *Biosens. Bioelectron.* 146: 111760. https://doi.org/10.1016/j.bios.2019.111760.

41 Ajab, H., Ali Khan, A.A., Nazir, M.S. et al. (2019). Cellulose-hydroxyapatite carbon electrode composite for trace plumbum ions detection in aqueous and palm oil mill effluent: interference, optimization and validation studies. *Environ. Res.* 176: 108563. https://doi.org/10.1016/j.envres.2019.108563.

42 Khattab, T.A., Fouda, M.M.G., Rehan, M. et al. (2020). Novel halochromic cellulose nanowhiskers from rice straw: visual detection of urea. *Carbohydr. Polym.* 231: 115740. https://doi.org/10.1016/j.carbpol.2019.115740.

43 Teodoro, K.B.R., Migliorini, F.L., Christinelli, W.A., and Correa, D.S. (2019). Detection of hydrogen peroxide (H_2O_2) using a colorimetric sensor based on cellulose nanowhiskers and silver nanoparticles. *Carbohydr. Polym.* 212: 235–241. https://doi.org/10.1016/j.carbpol.2019.02.053.

44 Nwosu, F.O., Saliu, O.D., Oyinlola, K.A., and Ojo, E.O. (2020). Colorimetric based polysorbate crosslinked cellulose-Ag–Cu nanohybrid sensor for urea sensing applications. *J. Polym. Environ.* 28: 1475–1483. https://doi.org/10.1007/s10924-020-01703-0.

45 Sakly, N., Marzouk, W., Ben Ouada, H., and Majdoub, H. (2017). Enhancing performances of colorimetric response of carboxymethylcellulose-stabilized silver nanoparticles: a fully eco-friendly assay for Hg2+ detection. *Sensors Actuators B Chem.* 253: 918–927. https://doi.org/10.1016/j.snb.2017.07.035.

46 Khattab, T.A., Dacrory, S., Abou-Yousef, H., and Kamel, S. (2019). Smart microfibrillated cellulose as swab sponge-like aerogel for real-time colorimetric naked-eye sweat monitoring. *Talanta* 205: 120166. https://doi.org/10.1016/j.talanta.2019.120166.

47 Ruecha, N., Soatthiyanon, N., Aumnate, C. et al. (2020). Kenaf cellulose-based 3D printed device: a novel colorimetric sensor for Ni(II). *Cellulose* 27: 5211–5222. https://doi.org/10.1007/s10570-020-03141-6.

48 Khattab, T.A., Dacrory, S., Abou-Yousef, H., and Kamel, S. (2019). Development of microporous cellulose-based smart xerogel reversible sensor via freeze drying for naked-eye detection of ammonia gas. *Carbohydr. Polym.* 210: 196–203. https://doi.org/10.1016/j.carbpol.2019.01.067.

49 Salmani, M., Rounaghi, G.H., and Chamsaz, M. (2018). An optical sensor for determination of low pH values based on covalent immobilization of Congo red on triacetyl cellulose films via epichlorohydrin. *Sensors Actuators B Chem.* 254: 177–181. https://doi.org/10.1016/j.snb.2017.07.027.

50 Ling, Z., Xu, F., Edwards, J.V. et al. (2019). Nanocellulose as a colorimetric biosensor for effective and facile detection of human neutrophil elastase. *Carbohydr. Polym.* 216: 360–368. https://doi.org/10.1016/j.carbpol.2019.04.027.

51 Wang, L., Zhang, C., He, H. et al. (2020). Cellulose-based colorimetric sensor with N, S sites for Ag+ detection. *Int. J. Biol. Macromol.* 163: 593–602. https://doi.org/10.1016/j.ijbiomac.2020.07.018.

52 Guo, W., He, H., Zhu, H. et al. (2019). Preparation and properties of a biomass cellulose-based colorimetric sensor for Ag+ and Cu2+. *Ind. Crop. Prod.* 137: 410–418. https://doi.org/10.1016/j.indcrop.2019.05.044.

53 Zhou, S., He, H., Guo, W. et al. (2019). Structural design of a high sensitivity biomass cellulose-based colorimetric sensor and its in situ visual recognition mechanism for Cu2+. *Carbohydr. Polym.* 219: 95–104. https://doi.org/10.1016/j.carbpol.2019.04.094.

54 Zhang, M., Zhang, L., Tian, H., and Lu, A. (2020). Universal preparation of cellulose-based colorimetric sensor for heavy metal ion detection. *Carbohydr. Polym.* 236: 116037. https://doi.org/10.1016/j.carbpol.2020.116037.

55 Yu, Q., Kong, X., Ma, Y. et al. (2018). Multi-functional regenerated cellulose fibers decorated with plasmonic Au nanoparticles for colorimetry and SERS assays. *Cellulose* 25: 6041–6053. https://doi.org/10.1007/s10570-018-1987-9.

56 Wang, H., Wang, H., Li, Y. et al. (2020). Capillarity self-driven DNA hydrogel sensor for visual quantification of microRNA. *Sensors Actuators B Chem.* 313: 128036. https://doi.org/10.1016/j.snb.2020.128036.

57 Watkinson, M., Becer, C.R., Gautrot, J.E., and Krause, S. (2019). Peptide cross-linked poly (ethylene glycol) hydrogel films as biosensor coatings for the detection of collagenase. *Sensors* 19: 1677.

58 Khazaei, S., Mozaffari, S.A., and Ebrahimi, F. (2021). Polyvinyl alcohol as a crucial omissible polymer to fabricate an impedimetric glucose biosensor based on hierarchical 3D-NPZnO/chitosan. *Carbohydr. Polym.* 266: 118105. https://doi.org/10.1016/j.carbpol.2021.118105.

59 Prabakaran, K., Jandas, P.J., Luo, J. et al. (2021). Molecularly imprinted poly(methacrylic acid) based QCM biosensor for selective determination of L-tryptophan. *Colloids Surfaces A Physicochem. Eng. Asp.* 611: 125859. https://doi.org/10.1016/j.colsurfa.2020.125859.

60 Hernandez-martinez, A.R. (2021). Poly(2-Hydroxyethyl methacrylate-co-N,N-dimethylacrylamide)-coated quartz crystal microbalance sensor: membrane characterization and proof of concept. *Gels* 7: 151.

61 Xiong, S., Marin, L., Duan, L., and Cheng, X. (2019). Fluorescent chitosan hydrogel for highly and selectively sensing of p-nitrophenol and 2, 4, 6-trinitrophenol. *Carbohydr. Polym.* 225: 115253. https://doi.org/10.1016/j.carbpol.2019.115253.

62 Zhou, J., Ma, Z., Hong, X. et al. (2019). Top-down strategy of implantable biosensor using adaptable, porous hollow fibrous membrane. *ACS Sensors* 4: 931–937. https://doi.org/10.1021/acssensors.9b00035.

63 Kim, H.J., Choi, W., San Lee, J. et al. (2022). Clinical application of serological Alzheimer's disease diagnosis using a highly sensitive biosensor with hydrogel-enhanced dielectrophoretic force. *Biosens. Bioelectron.* 195: 113668. https://doi.org/10.1016/j.bios.2021.113668.

64 Goud, K.Y., Sandhu, S.S., Teymourian, H. et al. (2021). Textile-based wearable solid-contact flexible fluoride sensor: toward biodetection of G-type nerve agents. *Biosens. Bioelectron.* 182: 113172. https://doi.org/10.1016/j.bios.2021.113172.

65 Abellán-Llobregat, A., Jeerapan, I., Bandodkar, A. et al. (2017). A stretchable and screen-printed electrochemical sensor for glucose determination in human perspiration. *Biosens. Bioelectron.* 91: 885–891. https://doi.org/10.1016/j.bios.2017.01.058.

66 Deng, M., Song, G., Zhong, K. et al. (2022). Wearable fluorescent contact lenses for monitoring glucose via a smartphone. *Sensors Actuators B Chem.* 352: 131067. https://doi.org/10.1016/j.snb.2021.131067.

67 Kumar, V., Raghuwanshi, S.K., and Kumar, S. (2022). Recent advances in carbon nanomaterials based SPR sensor for biomolecules and gas detection-a review. *IEEE Sensors J.* 22: 15661–15672. https://doi.org/10.1109/JSEN.2022.3191042.

68 Huang, X., Feng, B., Liu, M. et al. (2022). Preclinical detection of lysophosphatidic acid: a new window for ovarian cancer diagnostics. *Talanta* 247: 123561. https://doi.org/10.1016/j.talanta.2022.123561.

69 Cass, A.E.G., Davis, G., Francis, G.D. et al. (1984). Ferrocene-mediated enzyme electrode for Amperometric determination of glucose. *Anal. Chem.* 56: 667–671. https://doi.org/10.1021/ac00268a018.

70 Wang, W., Han, R., Chen, M., and Luo, X. (2021). Antifouling peptide hydrogel based electrochemical biosensors for highly sensitive detection of cancer biomarker HER2 in human serum. *Anal. Chem.* 93: 7355–7361. https://doi.org/10.1021/acs.analchem.1c01350.

71 Shamsipur, M., Asgari, M., Maragheh, M.G., and Moosavi-Movahedi, A.A. (2012). A novel impedimetric nanobiosensor for low level determination of hydrogen peroxide based on biocatalysis of catalase. *Bioelectrochemistry* 83: 31–37. https://doi.org/10.1016/j.bioelechem.2011.08.003.

72 Shervedani, R.K., Mehrjardi, A.H., and Zamiri, N. (2006). A novel method for glucose determination based on electrochemical impedance spectroscopy using glucose oxidase self-assembled biosensor. *Bioelectrochemistry* 69: 201–208. https://doi.org/10.1016/j.bioelechem.2006.01.003.

73 Naresh, V. and Lee, N. (2021). A review on biosensors and recent development of nanostructured materials-enabled biosensors. *Sensors* 21: 1–35. https://doi.org/10.3390/s21041109.

74 Kim, J., Sung, G.Y., and Park, M. (2020). Efficient portable urea biosensor based on urease immobilized membrane for monitoring of physiological fluids. *Biomedicines* 8: 1–11. https://doi.org/10.3390/biomedicines8120596.

75 Purohit, B., Vernekar, P.R., Shetti, N.P., and Chandra, P. (2020). Biosensor nanoengineering: design, operation, and implementation for biomolecular analysis. *Sensors Int.* 1: 100040. https://doi.org/10.1016/j.sintl.2020.100040.

76 Gui, Q., Lawson, T., Shan, S. et al. (2017). The application of whole cell-based biosensors for use in environmental analysis and in medical diagnostics. *Sensors* 17: 1–17. https://doi.org/10.3390/s17071623.

77 Salazar, P., Martin, M., and Gonzalez, J.L. (2016). Polydopamine-modified surfaces in biosensor applications. *Polym. Sci. Res. Adv. Pract. Appl. Educ. Asp.* 1: 385–396. https://www.researchgate.net/publication/305044131_Polydopamine-modified_surfaces_in_biosensor_applications.

78 Wittwer, C.T. and Makrigiorgos, G.M. (2018). *Nucleic acid techniques*. Elsevier Inc. https://doi.org/10.1016/B978-0-12-816061-9.00004-7.

79 Shukla, M., Pramila, I.A., and Palani, V.S. (2017). Effect of immobilization technique on performance ZnO nanorods based enzymatic electrochemical glucose biosensor. *J. Phys. Conf. Ser.* 924: https://doi.org/10.1088/1742-6596/924/1/012013.

3

Nucleic Acid–Based Biosensors

3.1 Introduction

Nucleic acids are complex molecules that contain information about human genetics and carry information among the cells. They can be a type of DNA and RNA that depend on a single or double base of chains [1]. More specifically, DNA is made from nucleotide monomeric units, and it has a double-stranded structure that forms a double helix. DNA is made up of single- (cytosine: C, thymine: T) and double-ring purine (adenine: A, guanine: G) bases as shown in Figure 3.1. It provides the necessary instructions for the formation and preservation of an organism by encoding specific sequences of these bases [2].

By contrast, gene expression, protein synthesis, and other biological processes are completed by using RNA. The nitrogenous bases in RNA are C, A, G, and uracil (U), having single-stranded structure usually and with the ability to fold into complex structures. RNA can be of different types depending on their function in the cell messenger RNA: mRNA, ribosomal RNA: rRNA, transfer RNA: t-RNA, small nuclear RNA, and nucleolar RNA [3]. The property of self-replication is present in DNA but not RNA; i.e. RNA does not replicate on its own. It is synthesized from DNA as required. RNA can easily break as compared to DNA, and its secondary structures are not stable generally [4].

Nucleic acids have been explored on various platforms, such as optical, ECL, and piezoelectric detection, to detect the various targets using specific nucleic acid sequences [5]. For biosensors, a nucleic acid probe is immobilized on substrate or metal surface [6]. This immobilized probe is complementary to the target sequence [7]. In the presence of a target sequence, it will bind to the probe and cause measurable changes at the output end. These biosensors, which utilize the

Biosensors: Nanomaterials, Approaches, and Performance-Enhancement Strategies,
First Edition. Baljinder Kaur, Santosh Kumar, and Brajesh Kumar Kaushik.

Published 2025 by John Wiley & Sons, Inc.
Companion website: www.wiley.com/go/kaur

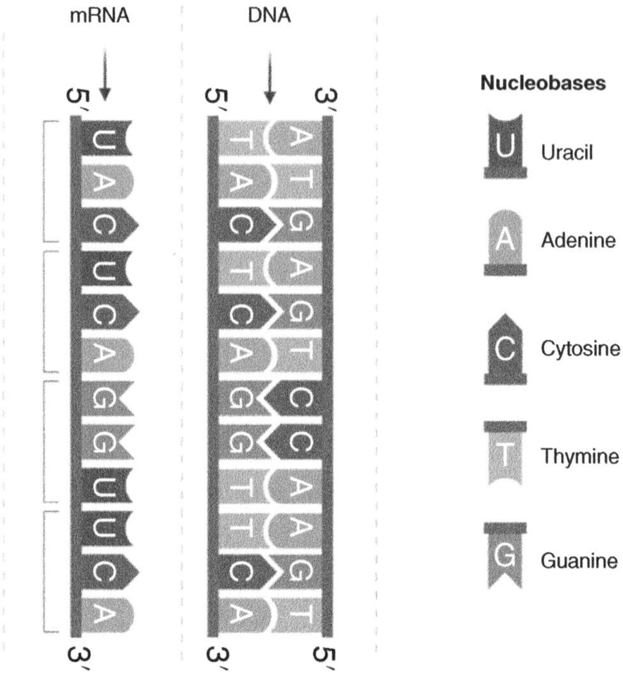

Figure 3.1 Schematic of structure of human genome DNA and RNA molecules with base pairs.

specific binding properties of DNA to detect complementary DNA sequences or specific genetic mutations, are being explored for various applications [8–11]. They include microbes such as bacteria, viruses, parasites, pollutants, tuberculosis, sepsis, cancer, and cystic fibrosis [12–21].

3.2 ECL Biosensor Designs

A reverse-phase polymerization method was used to synthesize the nanocomposite of polyaniline and graphene deposited on carbon electrode surface-based ECL sensor to detect the human immunodeficiency virus responsible for AIDS. Viruses can be detected in the concentration of 10^{-16}–1.0×10^{-10} M with lowest concentration of 10^{-16} M [22]. An AuNPs CRISPR-based nucleic acids-biosensor method requires amplification before detection and adding a CRISPR reaction separately by opening the reaction vessel that can cause contamination. Alone, CRISPR technology can detect the target with limit of detection (LOD) in the fM range only. Therefore, various methods have been suggested to prevent contamination and to achieve low LOD and high sensitivity values that include mixing of case enzyme and reagents for amplification to carry detection and nucleic acid amplification simultaneously [23]. The reagent is added from the bottom and CRISPR components on the tube wall to complete the reaction without opening the tube lid [24].

Another solution was to use a tube-in-tube structure and a one-pot CRISPR reaction solution. A one-pot CRISPR/Cas13a-based biosensor to detect the COVID-19 virus involved the inner and outer tube, with the inner tube containing two holes for amplification with a previously stored fluorescent agent. After amplification of nucleic acids, the mixture was sent to the outer tube through a hole and centrifuge technique. A blue LED was used to analyze the fluorescent signal that enables detection of COVID-19 virus with LOD and linear range of 3 copy/μL, 10^7–10^2 copy/mL [25]. Another ultra-sensitive and high-resolution biosensor using Ta_2C-MXene for SARS-CoV-2 detection was demonstrated. Ta_2C-MXene is a two-dimensional material composed of transition metal carbides and nitrides. This biosensor applies gold-coated-fiber Bragg grating and Ta_2C-MXene layer that measures the change in the SPR spectrum to detect the target. It can be detected in the lowest concentrations of 0.2 pg/ml of the SARS-CoV-2 target. A carbon dots-based ECL biosensor with catalytic hairpin assembly was developed to detect coronavirus. Catalytic hairpin assembly involves partially complementary DNA strands that can self-assemble into a hairpin structure. A nitrogen-doped carbon QDs, catalytic hairpin assembly for nucleic acid amplification on glassy carbon electrode modified with a SAM of thiolated DNA to detect the SARS-CoV-2 virus was designed. Figure 3.2a shows the schematic of a carbon QD-based ECL sensor. SARS-CoV-2 in the range of 50 fM to 200 pM with 20 fM LOD can be detected with QD-based biosensor in 40 minutes [26]. An Au-g-C_3N_4, CRISPR/Cas12a DNA tetrahedron on glassy carbon electrode surface based ECL biosensor was developed for detection of SARS-CoV-2 RNA polymerase gene. The biosensor utilizes a regenerative DNA tetrahedron structure, which is a self-assembled three-dimensional DNA nanostructure, as shown in Figure 3.2b. The DNA tetrahedron is a supporting structure for the attachment of various elements. The binding of RNA polymerase gene of SARS-CoV-2 with DNA tetrahedron initiates the CRISPR/Cas12a trans-activity to produce reactive oxygen species and output signal. SARS-CoV-2 can be sensed in the range of 1–100 pM and detection limit of 43.70 aM in half an hour [27]. An AuNP-based ECL biosensor was developed to detect the *Legionella pneumophila*. Cysteamine was deposited on a gold electrode surface, providing high surface area to the target DNA. *Legionella pneumophila* was detected in linear range of 1 μM–1 Zepto (Z) M and a low LOD of 1 ZM [28].

A paper-based biosensor that uses a modified cell phone camera to detect *Mycobacterium tuberculosis* (MTB) DNA in sputum samples is being developed.

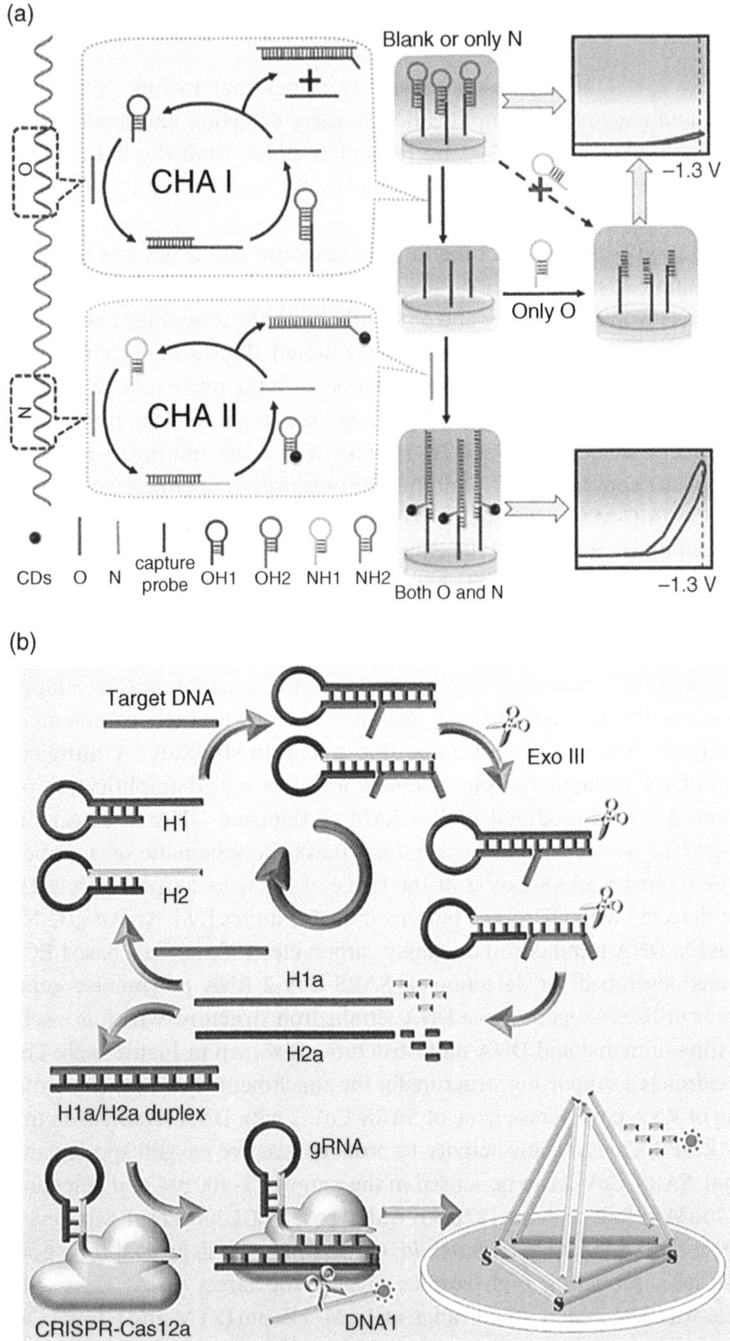

Figure 3.2 Schematic of (a) a dual-target responsive ECL sensor for COVID-19 detection. *Source:* [26]/with permission of Elsevier. (b) Au-g-C_3N_4, CRISPR/Cas12a DNA tetrahedron on glassy carbon electrode surface based ECL biosensor to detect the SARS-CoV-2. *Source:* [27]/with permission of Elsevier.

The biosensor is simple to use and provides results in less than an hour [29]. Wang et al. developed a sensitive and selective biosensor for the detection of MTB. The biosensor uses a graphene oxide-based field-effect transistor and can detect MTB DNA at a concentration as low as 10 fg/μl [30]. Table 3.1 presents the recently reported nucleic-acid based ECL biosensors to detect different targets.

3.3 Nucleic Acid-Based Colorimetric Biosensors

The performance of thiolate-modified AuNPs with hexadecyltrimethyl ammonium bromide and cysteamine capped-based biosensor to detect the hepatitis C virus RNA was compared and studied in detail. It can directly detect the virus without amplification. The study investigates the LOD and linear range of virus and found to be 4.57 U/μl and 10^6 U/ml. The sensor exhibits 93.3% sensitivity with a LOD of [43].

An oligonucleotide modified AuNPs-based colorimetric sensing platform through triplex formation with negligible background to detect the let-7a miRNA using three DNA hairpin probes (H1, H2, and H3) has been developed. The platform consists of a glass slide modified with a DNA probe, a hybridization slide, and a detection reagent. When the target molecule is not present, H1 and H2 hairpins form a complex with AuNPs-oligonucleotide probe, which reduces background noise and provides stability. In the presence of an miRNA target, it binds with the probe and can be detected with 10 pM LOD and concentration range of 20 pM–0.50 nM.

Another target known as platelet-derived growth factor BB was also detected in linear span of 20 pM–1.0 nM and detection limit of 20 pM [44]. An AuNPs-based logic gate was designed to detect miRNA. The chemical reduction method is used to produce AuNPs complementary to the miRNA targets that are attached to DNA probes with the help of DNA linkers. As the miRNA targets are available, they bind to the DNA probes and trigger a strand displacement reaction that leads to AuNPs aggregation. These aggregated NPs in the presence of the target cause a change in their localized surface plasmon resonance (LSPR) absorption that is detected by spectroscopy. miRNA can be detected with a detection limit of 10^{-12} M and a linear range of 0.01 to 0.2×10^{-9} M [45].

Figure 3.3a shows a hairpin DNA-AuNPs conjugate, polyethylene glycol-based colorimetric sensor that consists of a capture probe synthesized using the enzymatic method to detect aptamer-specific ligand. The hairpin DNA-AuNP conjugates are dispersed in the solution. miRNA-203 is used as a target, and aptamer-specific ligands are used as target molecules. As the target binds with capturing probe, it activates initiator sequence that initiates a hybridization

Table 3.1 Recently reported nucleic acid–based ECL biosensors.

Sensor structure	Analyte	Nucleic acid	LOD	Linear range	Refs.
Paper-based ECL sensor	miRNA-492 adenocarcinoma	PNA	6 nM	0.1–100 nM	[31]
CRISPR/Cas13a and AuNF-based ECL sensor	SARS-CoV-2	ssDNA	4.4×10^{-2} fg/ml	10^{-1}–10^{5} fg/ml	[32]
DNAzyme-based ECL sensor	Various	DNA	n.r.	100 pM–10 nM	[33]
Metal-organic frameworks-based ECL sensor	Mycoplasma ovine pneumonia	ssDNA	1 pM	10^{-10} to 10^{-6} M	[34]
Electric field-enhanced ECL CRISPR	Human papillomavirus-16	ssDNA	10 pM	100 pM–10 nM	[35]
Three-way junction DNA-based MicroRNAs detection	MicroRNAs	ssDNA	77 aM	100 Am–100 pM	[36]
DNA junction scaffold for multiple targets detection	Various	DNA	10 fM	100 nM–1 μM	[37]
CRISPR/Cas14a and PtPd@PCN-224 nano-enzymes-based ECL sensor	*Burkholderia pseudomallei*	ssDNA	12.8 aM	0.125 Mm–4 μM	[38]
Universal DNA-hairpin, Au needle and methylene blue–based ECL biosensor	SARS-CoV-2 RNA	ssDNA	5.0 ag/μl S and 6.8 ag/μl	641–1.34×10^{11} copies/ ml	[39]
Peptide nucleic acids, hairpin assembly and Au electrode–based ECL sensor	miRNA21 miRNA155 (cancer biomarker)	ssDNA	2.49 fM miRNA21 11.63 fM miRNA155	10 fM–5 nM (miRNA21) 50 fM–50 nM (miRNA155)	[40]
Duplex-specific nuclease-based ECL sensor	SARS-CoV-2 RdRp RNA	ssDNA	21.69 aM	30–400 aM	[41]
Microscale 35 fM ECL DNA	Hand, foot, and mouth disease-related gene	ssDNA	35 fM	100 fM–1 nM	[42]

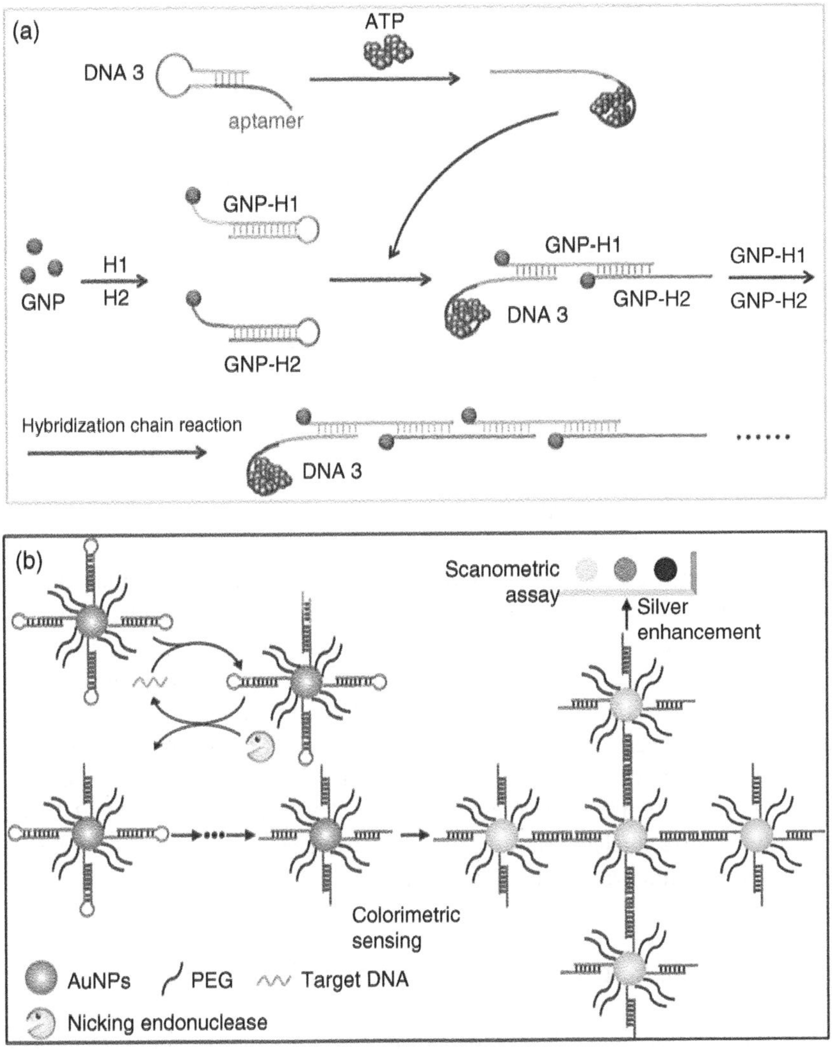

Figure 3.3 Schematic of (a) hairpin DNA-AuNPs conjugates colorimetric sensors for aptamer-specific ligand. *Source:* [46]/with permission of Elsevier. (b) AuNPs-DNA snow-ball assembly based colorimetric sensor to detect the thrombin and DNA. *Source:* [47]/with permission of Elsevier.

chain reaction, leading to aggregation of the AuNPs. A color change was observed in the output spectra due to aggregation of the AuNPs. Linear range, sensitivity, and LOD of target DNA was 10^{-11}–10^{-10} M, 1.0×10^{-8} M, and 1.0×10^{-11} M [46]. An AuNPs functionalized with DNA forming snow-ball assembly-based biosensor driven by Nt.BbvCI enzyme to detect the thrombin and DNA sample was reported as shown in Figure 3.3b. It includes the incubation of the hairpin DNA- AuNPs-target DNA with BbvCI enzyme to cleave the target DNA that detaches the hairpin DNA from nanoparticles. The released hairpin DNA molecules bind themselves to another palindromic DNA sequences to form snowball structure assembly (Figure 3.3b). Sensors can detect target DNA and thrombin with a LOD and concentration in the ranges of 9.2, 8.3, and 10–70 nM, 10–100 nM. This method is single temperature method, amplifying the signal, and can be used at various biosensing platforms [47].

A multiplex paper-based colorimetric DNA sensor that consists of pyrrolidinyl peptide nucleic acid (PNA) and AgNPs was developed for the simultaneous detection of Middle East respiratory syndrome coronavirus, *Mycobacterium tuberculosis*, and human papillomavirus. This technique involves a peptide nucleic acid–based probe instead of DNA or RNA, and is capable of hybridization with high efficiency, easy of synthesis, and stability. A peptide nucleic acid probe consists of a single positive charge that causes aggregation of AgNPs in the nonavailability of target DNA. As goal DNA is available, the probe and AgNPs form a duplex that changes color due to metal nanoparticles dispersion. The LOD and linearity of coronavirus, *Mycobacterium tuberculosis*, and human papillomavirus are 1.53, 1.27, 1.03 nM, and 20–1000, 50–2500, 20–2500 nM [48]. Table 3.2 lists recently reported nucleic-acid based colorimetric biosensors to detect the target such as ions, Influenza A virus, and COVID-19.

3.4 Nucleic Acid–Based Fluorescent Biosensor

A RNA-based fluorescent biosensor for detection of small bacterial RNAs was reported. These biosensors are based on the principle of riboswitches, which are natural RNA structures that regulate gene expression in response to small molecules. The activity of bacteria was analyzed using fluorescence resonance energy transfer as a mechanism to report the presence and activity of sRNAs in real time. This biosensor provides good response in the concentration range of 0.5–10 μM [54]. A multitag-regulated cascade reaction-based amplification that involves multiple elements to control and monitor the reaction occurring in series for detecting miR let-7a was reported as shown in Figure 3.4b. Streptavidin was used to functionalize the transducer and accommodate numerous elements or

Table 3.2 Recently reported nucleic-acid based colorimetric biosensors.

Sensor structure	Analyte	LOD	Linear range	Refs.
AuNPs with hybridization chain reaction–based colorimetric	miRNA	10^{-12} M	0.01–0.2× 10^{-9} M	[45]
AuNPs with hybridization chain reaction–based colorimetric	Pb^{2+}	59.39 pM	0–1 pM	[49]
Peptide nucleic acid biosensor	Influenza A virus	2.3 ng	2–20 pM pmol	[50]
AuNPs with CRISPR/Cas12a-based colorimetric biosensor	Prostate-specific antigen (PSA)	0.1 ng/ml	0–400.0 nM	[51]
RNA polymerization actuating NA membrane–based biosensor	COVID-19	100	1–10^8 aM	[52]
CRISPR-Cas12a and hydrogel-2D-MOF fluorescence/colorimetric biosensor	Estradiol PSA	0.015 ng/ml Estradiol 0.14 ng/ml PSA	2–20 ng/ml Estradiol 20–200 ng/ml PSA	[53]

tags, also ensuring uniform distance from the signal. The study investigated the detection limit of miR at levels as low as 0.8 fM and a concentration region of 1 fM–71 pM [56]. A fluorescent biosensor assisted with polymerase chain reaction on an optical fiber platform immobilized with Cy5-tagged deoxycytidine triphosphates as a tag to target DNA to detect the microcystin synthetase A that produces *M. aeruginosa* (Figure 3.4a). The probe was designed in silico that provide 10 pM LOD, for the linear range of 10 pM to 00 nM [55]. Various nucleic acid–based fluorescence biosensors are summarized in Table 3.3.

3.5 Nucleic Acid–Based Plasmonic Biosensor

A prism-based SPR biosensor used Au film, double-layer DNA tetrahedrons, hairpin, fluorescent dye to detect the human immune deficiency virus. A 48 fM LOD and linear range of 1 pM–150 nM was achieved to detect the virus [64]. Hossain and Rana present a DNA hybridization detection method using an SPR prism-based biosensor on graphene and Au substrates. They used a resonance frequency readout technique to detect hybridization events. The sensor's performance was evaluated through experiments and compared to simulations, demonstrating its potential for sensitive DNA detection. The graphene layer acts as a sensing surface for DNA hybridization, and the graphene layer number is varied from 1 to 10 to tune the sensor's performance. The hybridization process

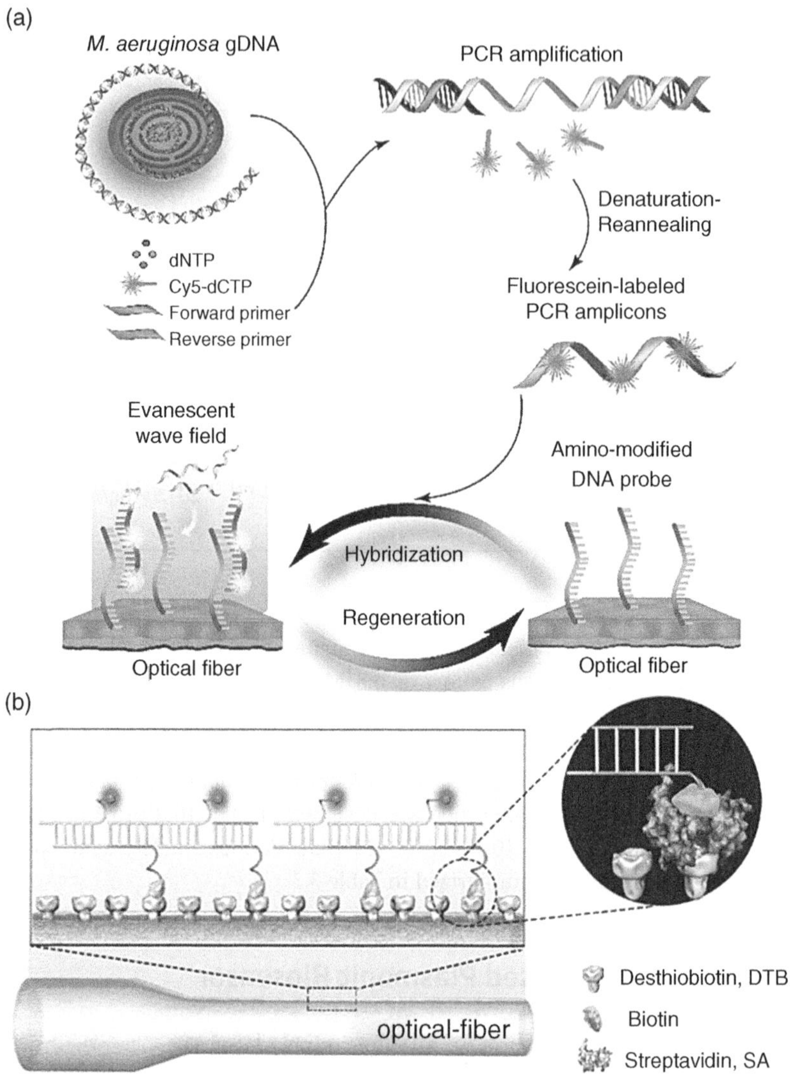

Figure 3.4 Schematic of (a) fluorescent biosensor assisted with polymerase chain reaction for detection of the microcystin synthetase A gene. *Source:* [55]/with permission of American Chemical Society. (b) multitag-regulated cascade-based optical-fiber biosensor. *Source:* [56]/with permission of American Chemical Society.

Table 3.3 Recently reported nucleic acid-based fluorescence biosensors.

Sensor structure	Analyte	LOD	Linear range	Refs.
DNA hydrogel-coated 2D-metal organic framework	Estradiol PSA	0.015 ng/ml 0.14 ng/ml	2–20 ng/ml 20–200 ng/ml	[53]
CRISPR/Cas12a-based portable biosensor	CaMV35S promoter and Lectin gene	n.r.	n.r.	[57]
Target nucleic acid sequence-triggered transcription	COVID-19	0.96 copy/μl	1 fM–5 nM	[58]
One-pot CRISPR/Cas13a-based fluorescent biosensor	SARS-Cov-2	3 copy/μl	3×10^7–10^2 copy/ml	[25]
Aptamer-based Cas14a1 biosensor for	*S. aureus*	400 CFU/ml	150–300 μL	[59]
CRISPR/Cas12a-based fluorescence biosensors	Hypochlorous acid and myeloperoxidase	0.33 μM	1–5 μM	[60]
CRISPR/Cas12a-mediated and amplification-free biosensor	*Salmonella typhimurium*	1.8×10^3 CFU/ml	10^2–10^5 CFU/ml	[61]
CRISPR/Cas12a-powered evanescent wave fluorescence nano-biosensing platform	*S. aureus*	592 CFU/ml	50–500 nM	[62]
Multifunctional DNA nano-dumbbell lock biosensor with hybridization chain reaction	miR-141, miR-375, miR-21, ATP, cortisol, insulin	145 fM-miR-141 10 nM-miR-375 and miR-21 11 pM-ATP 240 pM-cortisol 240 pM-Insulin	500 fM–10 nM miR-141 100 pM–10 μM ATP, 1 nM to 10 μM cortisol 1 nM to 10 μM Insulin	[63]

changes resonance angle due to a change in refractive index that can be measured to detect the analyte.

It has been observed that adding a graphene layer enhances sensitivity [65]. A modeling study was conducted with a highly sensitive fiber sensor structure designed using Ag metal and hybrid structure of MoS_2-graphene for DNA hybridization detection and single-nucleotide polymorphisms. The structure of the Ag-MoS_2-graphene hybrid based SPR sensor is shown in Figure 3.5a. The sensor's performance was optimized by varying the number of graphene and MoS_2 layers. The biosensor exhibits sensitivity, detection accuracy, and quality factor of 105.71°/RIU, 1.626/RIU, and 23.23/RIU for the concentrations of target 1000–1100 nM [66]. A black phosphorus (BP), Ag, graphene, and silicon-based prism SPR sensor was demonstrated to detect the single strand.

Vasimalla et al. focused on enhancing the performance of prism-based SPR biosensors for DNA hybridization detection [70]. The study explores the use of black phosphorus, silver, and silicon materials to improve the sensitivity and reliability of SPR-based DNA biosensors. The BP layer provides a high refractive index contrast, which enhances the SPR signal. The Ag layer provides high conductivity, which increases the sensitivity of the sensor. The Si layer provides high biocompatibility, which makes the sensor suitable for biological applications. The sensor consists of a thin layer of BP deposited on a Si substrate. Other structures have been studied in detail, including Ag/BP/Gr, Ag/Si/BP/Gr, Ag/Gr, and Ag. The number of graphene and BP layers is varied from 1 to 10 and compared. The BP layer is then covered with a layer of Ag DNA hybridization. The number of graphene and black phosphorus layers were varied from 0 to 15 and its impact on the performance of sensor was analyzed. The sensitivity, detection accuracy, quality factor, and figure of merit of the sensor with Ag-silicon-black phosphorus-graphene structure were found to be 53.08°/RIU, 69, 1061.6/RIU, 554.58 and with Ag/BP/Gr are 91.54°/RIU, 3.6, 54.81/RIU, 54.78 [70].

Yi developed an evanescent wave Förster resonance energy transfer (FRET) biosensor using a fiber structure to detect lead (Pb^{2+}) by taking a human serum sample. The sensing element consists of a DNAzyme probe immobilized on the fiber surface and Cyanine 3 as a fluorescent dye to label substrate and GR-5 DNAzyme sequence as a quencher label. LOD can be detected 9.34 nM with an RSD of 14.8% for the detection range of 0–120 nM [71]. An AuNPs-based optical fiber SPR biosensor made up of hollow-core fiber sandwiched between multimode fibers to determine the DNA hybridization detection was reported. The multimode fiber acts as a channel to guide the light and hollow-core fiber enhances the SPR signal. To fabricate the structure, hollow-core fiber was spliced between two multimode fibers with an inner and outer diameter of 20 and 125 μm. The detection limit for the concentration span of target was found to be 1 pM, 4.04 nm/log (μM) and 1 pM–10 nM [72]. Triple-helix molecular switches and G-quadruplex nanowires-based biosensors were developed to detect the hepatitis A virus and microRNA-31, as shown in Figure 3.5b. The triple-helix molecular switch is a DNA molecule that bind to specific nucleic acid, can form a stable triple-helix structure in the presence of target. The G-quadruplex nanowires are created using DNA sequences having the property of self-assembling into nanowires. The interaction of target nucleic acid and triple-helix molecular switch triggers the release

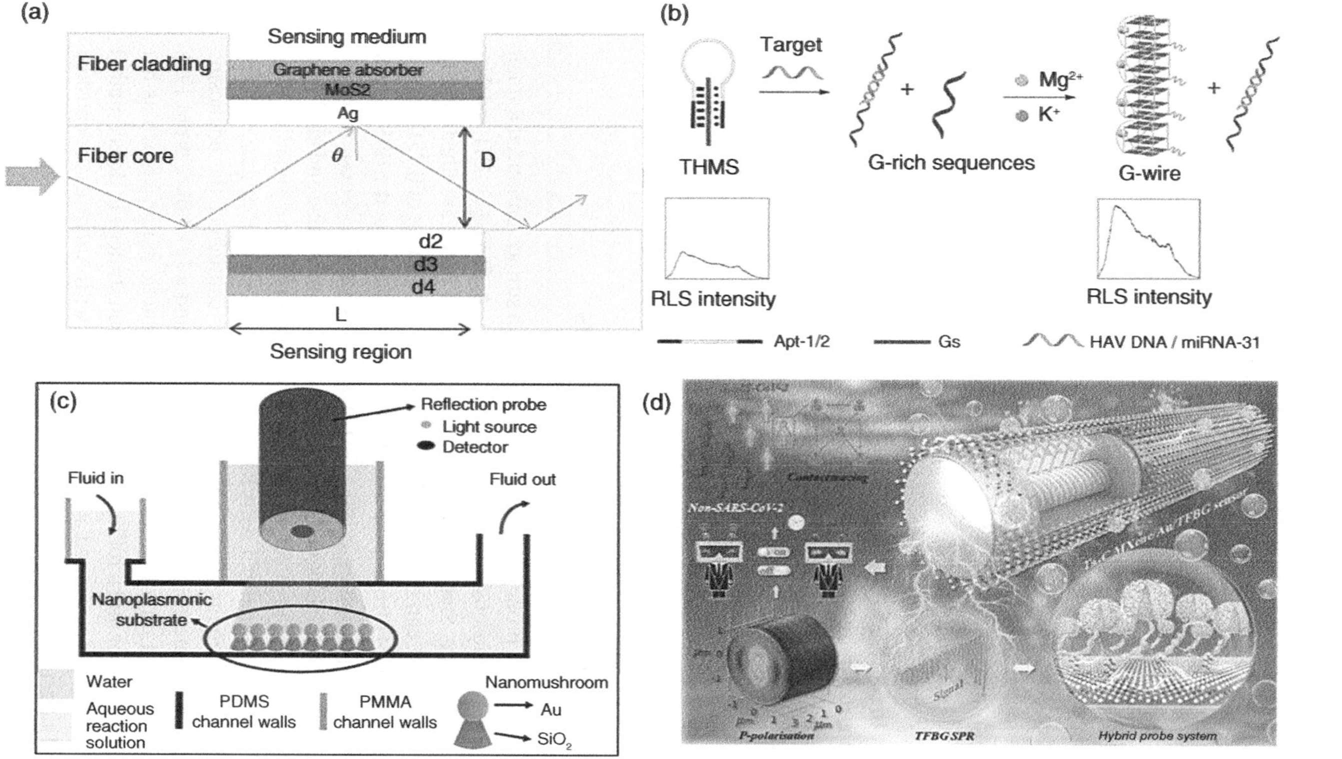

Figure 3.5 Schematic of (a) Ag-MoS_2-graphene hybrid SPR biosensor. *Source:* [66]/with permission of Elsevier. (b) Triple-helix molecular switches and G-quadruplex nanowires-based biosensor was developed to detect the Hepatitis A Virus and microRNA-31. *Source:* [67]/with permission of Elsevier. (c) Polydimethylsiloxane (PDMS) and Polymethyl Methacrylate (PMMA) substrate-based nano-plasmonic microfluidic chip–based LSPR-based sensor. *Source:* [68]/with permission of Elsevier. and (d) Identification of SARS-CoV-2 Omicron using Ta_2C-MXene layer and Au-based fiber Bragg grating sensor. *Source:* [69]/with permission of Elsevier.

of G-quadruplex nanowires from the switch that causes a change in the output signal of the biosensor. Hepatitis A virus and microRNA-31 were detected with LOD 7.1 pM and a linear range of 50 pM–300 nM [67].

Figure 3.5c shows a polydimethylsiloxane microfluidic and AuNPs-based LSPR sensor with 1-Hexadecanethiol spacer to detect the DNA polymerase activity. The platform consists of a microfluidic channel to control fluid flow, Au functionalized with ssDNA complementary to the target DNA and a polymerase enzyme to catalyze the polymerization of nucleotides. LOD and sensitivity of polymerase are 54 6 nm/RIU and 0.0625 U/ml [68]. An active helical Au nanorod enhances sensitivity, and three hairpins (H1, H2, and H3) detect the target hepatitis B virus. Helical Au nanorods to enhance the sensitivity were functionalized with specific DNA probes complementary to the hepatitis B virus, as shown in Figure 3.5d. The virus target can be detected in the concentration range and LOD of 0.05–10 pM, 30.15 fM [73]. A Ta_2C-MXene layer and Au-based fiber Bragg grating sensor are used to detect the SARS-CoV-2 RNA. Ta_2C-MXene was explored due to biocompatibility, supporter in immobilization and better conductivity, and sufficient surface area. The Ta_2C-MXene layer is then modified with DNA probes specific to the target pathogen and allowed to load a greater number of target molecules. SARS-CoV-2 RNA was detected in the concentration range of 0.2–100 pg/ml [69]. Recently reported nucleic acid–based plasmonic biosensors are summarized in Table 3.4.

3.6 SERS-Based Nucleic Acid Biosensors

A core-shell NPs based probe was developed to construct surface-enhanced Raman spectroscopy (SERS) biosensor for detecting miRNA-21. $Ag/TiO_2@3'-NH_2$-ssDNA was used as a substrate. Steps involved in developing the probe are illustrated in Figure 3.6a. miRNA-21 can be detected with lowest concentration of 0.75 fM and a linear range of 1.0 fM–1.0 nM [94]. An AuNPs aggregation-based SERS sensor detects adenosine triphosphate using a 3-D DNA nanomachine. These nanomachines consist of carefully designed DNA strands that can recognize and bind with ATP, a critical molecule involved in cellular energy transfer and signaling. The DNA strands are functionalized with Raman-active molecules that generate distinctive SERS signals upon excitation. This biosensor can detect the adenosine triphosphate linear concentration range of $1–10^5$ pM and a LOD of 0.29 pM [95]. The biosensor is based on a high-intensity electromagnetic region known as hot spot–based SERS sensor and a rolling circle amplification strategy to detect methyl transferase activity. SiO_2 was used as a SERS substrate, with AuNP array deposited on its top and target DNA sequence. DNA probes are labeled with Raman reporters. The analyte methyl transferase activity was detected with sensitivity,

Table 3.4 Recently reported nucleic-acid-based plasmonic biosensors.

Sensor structure	Analyte/disease	LOD/linear range	Refs.
Graphene and sapphire-based graphene field-effect transistor	DNA hybridization	100 fM/100 fM–1 nM	[74]
Homogeneous Au electrode with bovine serum albumin modified ECL biosensor	*Cryptococcus neoformans*	800 fM/5 pM–1 nM	[75]
Reduced GO decorated Sm_2O_3 NPs on carbon electrode for DNA-hybridization ECL biosensor	Amyotrophic lateral sclerosis	10^{-14} mol/l/ 10^{-13}–10^{-8} mol/l	[76]
3D DNA walker and hybridization chain reaction-based fluorescence sensor	microRNA let-7a	7.9 fM/10 fM–1 nM	[77]
Graphene oxide quantum dots as fluorescent molecule and GO quencher for DNA hybridization	NOS terminator gene sequences	0.008 nM/ 0.05–50 nM	[78]
SF10 glass-Au-WS_2 and graphene-coated SPR biosensor	DNA hybridization	25.19/RIU/1000–1100 nM	[79]
Au nanorods and hair pin assembly-based DNA colorimetric biosensor	DNA hybridization	1.47 nM/0–60 nM	[80]
Ethyl green–based ECL DNA-biosensor	Cadmium ions	0.3 pM/ 1.0 pM–1.0 μM	[81]
Label-free pencil graphite electrode-based ECL biosensor	Influenza A and B	35 and 21 nM	[82]
Cysteamine and AuNPs-based ECL biosensor	*Legionella pneumophila*	1 Zeptomolar (Z)/1 μM–1 ZM	[28]
6-mercapto-1-hexanol and Au electrode-based ECL biosensor	miRNA-25	0.3334 fM/ 1 fM–10 pM	[83]
3D cloth- multiwalled CNT-electrochemiluminescence biosensor	K-ras gene	0.13 fM/0.001–2500 pM	[84]
Mercaptopropionic acid and Au-based thermodynamically designed target-specific DNA probe ECL	*E. coli*	10–400 nM	[85]
Luminol functionalized AuNPs-based Electrochemiluminescence sensor	p53 gene	0.02 fM/0.0001–1000 pM	[86]

(*Continued*)

Table 3.4 (Continued)

Sensor structure	Analyte/disease	LOD/linear range	Refs.
AuNPs and hairpin assembly-based LSPR biosensor	miR-17	1 pM/0–1000 nM	[87]
Mercaptohexanol, screen-printed Au nanostructured electrode and methylene blue disposable ECL DNA biosensor	*Bacillus thuringiensis*	10^{-12} M/10^{-6} M–10^{-12} M	[88]
Multi-walled CNT-polypyrrole and hydroxyapatite NPs-based ECL DNA biosensor	*Mycobacterium tuberculosis*	0.141 nM/0.25–200 nM	[89]
Dithiothreitol, AuNPs-based dual strip ECL biosensors	Hepatitis B virus	0.05 nM/ 5 pM–0.1 nM	[90]
Manganese/nickel layered double hydroxide ECL biosensor	Uracil-DNA glycosylase	10^{-4} U/ml/ 0.001–1 U/ml	[91]
MXene-platinum-carbon nanocomposite-based ECL biosensor	COVID-19	0.4 aM/ 1 aM–100 nM	[92]
AuNPs/reduced GO/g-C_3N_4 nanocomposite ECL biosensor	DNA methylation	0.74 fM/10^{-7} M–10^{-15} M	[93]

concentration range, and LOD as 2.37×10^{-4}, 0.005 to 50, 2.37×10^{-4}, and 2.51×10^{-4} U/ml in phosphate-buffered saline buffer and human serum solution [96]. A gold nano-flowers substrate that generates provides hot spots, streptavidin, cyanine-5, hairpin assembly with biotin-based SERS biosensor using hybridization chain reaction amplification can be used to detect the genetically modified organism's DNA in maize sample. Increase in the intensity of electromagnetic field was confirmed using finite-difference time-domain based results. The target DNA concentration range of 0.01–10 000 fM and 6.31 aM LOD was detected [97]. ^{18}O stable isotope labeling-based SERS biosensors revealed changes in physiological information of cells to detect *E. coli* bacteria [98]. SERS sensors consist of Ag nano, amplification of signal with nicking endonuclease and Raman reporter of 4-mercaptobenzoic acid, as shown in Figure 3.6b. A LOD of 3.1 fM with concentrations from 10 fM to 0.1 nM and an RSD of 4.6–7.6% was detected [99].

3.7 Interferometric NA Biosensors

A fiber-based Mach-Zehnder interferometer (MZI)-sensor was demonstrated to detect COVID-19 with the help of single-stranded nucleic acid. The fiber surface was treated with piranha solution, 3-aminopropyltriethoxylsilan, and

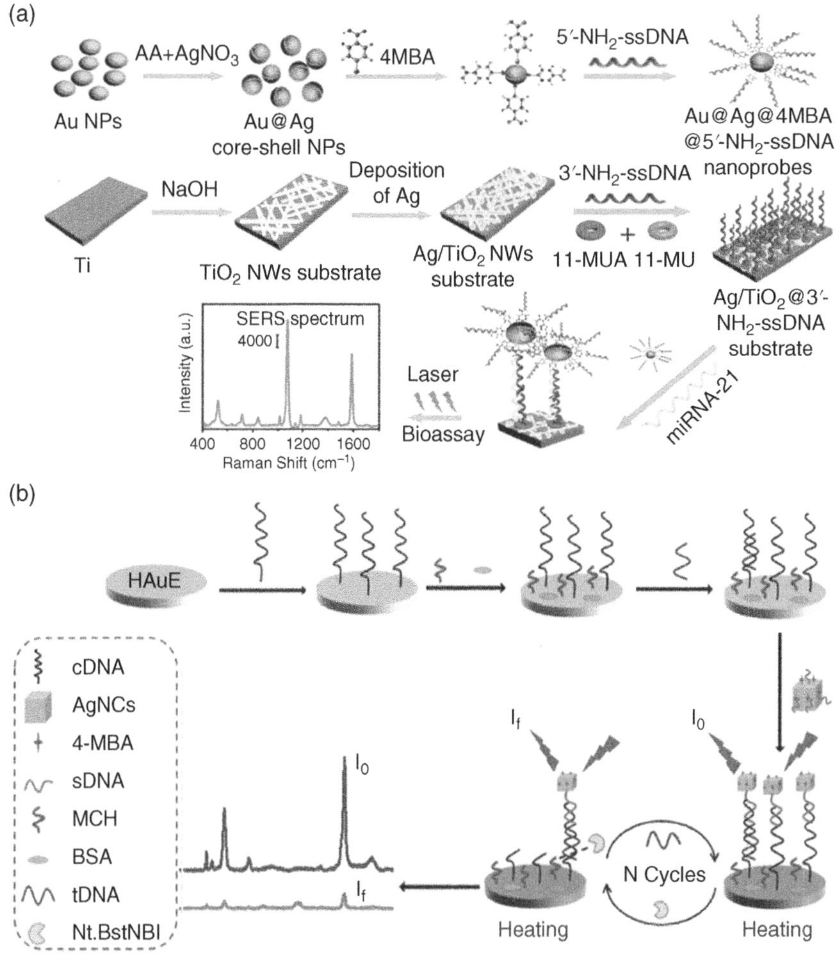

Figure 3.6 Schematic of (a) Au@Ag@4MBA@5′-NH_2-ssDNA probe-based SERS sensor. *Source:* [94]/with permission of The Royal Society of Chemistry. (b) A plasmonic Ag nanocube-based SERS sensor. *Source:* [99]/with permission of Elsevier.

glutaraldehyde to modify it that include hydroxylation, silanization, coupling, and immobilization. A sensor structure was fabricated with single mode core-offset and is illustrated in Figure 3.7a. Nucleic acid sequence can be detected with sensitivity, LOD, and concentration range of 0.175 dB/nM, 1 nM, 1–10 nM in response time of 30 seconds [100]. Figure 3.7b shows an exposed-core micro-structured based MZI sensor sandwiched between two single mode fiber to detect the DNA hybridization. The exposed-core micro-structured optical fiber used a core and clad diameter of

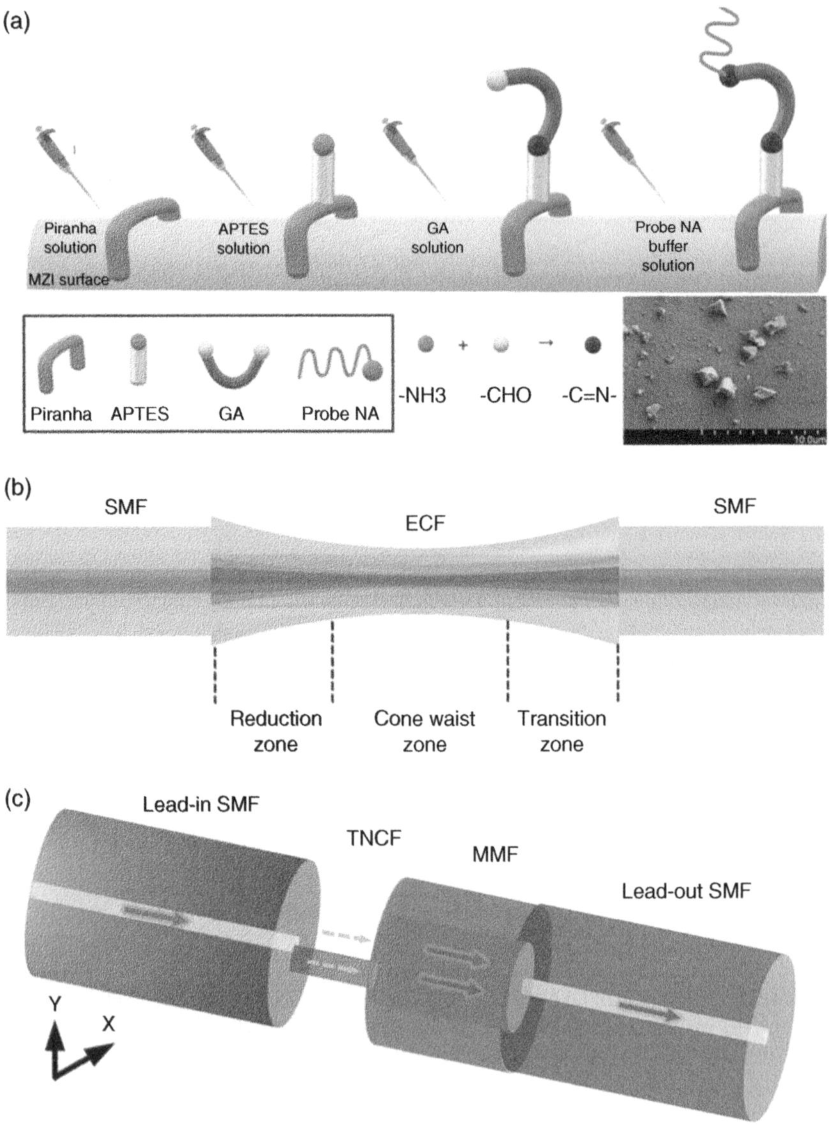

Figure 3.7 (a) Schematic diagram of the MZI fiber surface modification process that includes (i) hydroxylation; (ii) silanization; (iii) coupling; (iv) immobilization of probe NA to detect the single-stranded nucleic acid for COVID-19. *Source:* [100]/with permission of Elsevier. (b) Exposed core fiber (ECF) based interferometric sensor. *Source:* [101]/with permission of Elsevier. (c) A black phosphorus (BP) nano-interface-based MZI fiber sensor. *Source:* [102]/with permission of Elsevier.

9 and 160 μm. Analysis was done by using COMSOL simulation for target refractive index of 1.33–1.37 RIU. The target was detected using probe DNA and complementary DNA by immobilizing it on the surface of core. DNA hybridization was detected with LOD and sensitivity of 0.31 nM and 0.0618 nm/nM [101]. Another MZI fiber sensor used black phosphorus to detect deafness gene DNA with ultra-sensitivity. The sensor consists of a single-mode fiber-thin no-core fiber-multimode fiber-single-mode fiber, structure with a lateral offset, as depicted in Figure 3.7c. The sensor has a LOD, linear range, and sensitivity of 0.24 pM, 1 pM–1 M, and 0.719 nm/log M for deafness gene DNA hybridization detection [102].

3.8 Conclusions and Future Prospects

Nucleic acid–based biosensors have made significant progress in recent years for various applications. The emergence of new materials, including black phosphorus, phosphorene, silicene, MXenes, immobilization methods, synthesis methods, and gene-editing technologies, has led to a significant improvement in the sensitivity of these sensors. They offer a number of advantages over other bioreceptors due to their label-free nature, increased safety in use, and no need for specialized equipment. Nucleic acid–based biosensors also have some disadvantages, including complex sample preparation procedures, being time-consuming, requiring skilled personnel, and being expensive to produce. Additionally, the presence of interfering substances or variations in sample quality can lead to false-positive or false-negative results, impacting the accuracy of the analysis.

The future prospects of nucleic acid-based biosensors are highly promising and encompass a wide range of applications. One key area of focus is to develop a biosensor design that has high sensitivity, specificity, and multiplexing capabilities. This involves refining probe design, exploring novel recognition elements such as aptamers, and integrating signal-amplification strategies to detect even lower concentrations of target molecules. Additionally, the integration of nucleic acid–based biosensors with emerging technologies that include microfluidics, CRISPR, lab-on-a-chip devices, and wearable sensors holds great potential. These advancements will enable point-of-care testing, real-time monitoring, and personalized medicine, revolutionizing diagnostics and patient care.

References

1 Fertier, A., Montarnal, A., Truptil, S., and Bénaben, F. (2023). Electrochemical nucleic acid sensors: competent pathways for mobile molecular diagnostics. *Biosens. Bioelectron.* 115407. https://doi.org/10.1016/j.bios.2023.115407.

2 Hashem, A., Hossain, M.A.M., Marlinda, A.R. et al. (2021). Nanomaterials based electrochemical nucleic acid biosensors for environmental monitoring: a review. *Appl. Surf. Sci. Adv.* 4 (January): 100064. https://doi.org/10.1016/j.apsadv.2021.100064.

3 Huo, B., Hu, Y., Gao, Z., and Li, G. (2021). Recent advances on functional nucleic acid-based biosensors for detection of food contaminants. *Talanta* 222: https://doi.org/10.1016/j.talanta.2020.121565.

4 Kim, E.R., Joe, C., Mitchell, R.J., and Gu, M.B. (2023). Biosensors for healthcare: current and future perspectives. *Trends Biotechnol.* 41 (3): 374–395. https://doi.org/10.1016/j.tibtech.2022.12.005.

5 Yang, Q., Zhu, G., Singh, L. et al. (2020). Highly sensitive and selective sensor probe using glucose oxidase/gold nanoparticles/graphene oxide functionalized tapered optical fiber structure for detection of glucose. *Optik (Stuttg)* 208: 164536. https://doi.org/10.1016/j.ijleo.2020.164536.

6 Kumar, S. and Singh, R. (2021). Recent optical sensing technologies for the detection of various biomolecules: review. *Opt. Laser Technol.* 134: 106620. https://doi.org/10.1016/j.optlastec.2020.106620.

7 Zhang, F., Chen, G., Gao, C. et al. (2023). Updated toolkits for nucleic acid-based biosensors. *TrAC – Trends Anal. Chem.* 159: 116943. https://doi.org/10.1016/j.trac.2023.116943.

8 Kaur, B., Kumar, S., and Kaushik, B.K. (2023). Novel wearable optical sensors for vital health monitoring systems—a review. *Biosensors* 13 (2): 181.

9 Kaur, B., Kumar, S., and Kaushik, B.K. (2023). Trends, challenges, and advances in optical sensing for pathogenic bacteria detection (PathoBactD). *Biosens. Bioelectron. X* 14: 100352. https://doi.org/10.1016/j.biosx.2023.100352.

10 Kaur, B., Kumar, S., and Kaushik, B.K. (2022). Recent advancements in optical biosensors for cancer detection. *Biosens. Bioelectron.* 197: 113805.

11 Sharma, A.K., Pandey, A.K., and Kaur, B. (2018). A review of advancements (2007–2017) in plasmonics-based optical fiber sensors. *Opt. Fiber Technol.* 43: 20–34. https://doi.org/10.1016/j.yofte.2018.03.008.

12 Kaur, B., Kumar, S., and Kaushik, B.K. (2022). MXenes-based fiber-optic SPR sensor for colorectal cancer diagnosis. *IEEE Sens. J.* 22 (7): 6661–6668.

13 Kaur, B., Kumar, S., and Kumar, B. (2022). Advances in photonic crystal fiber: sensing and supercontinuum generation applications. *Opt. Fiber Technol.* 72: 102982.

14 Sahu, S.K., Reddy, S.K., Singh, M., and Avrutin, E. (2022). Hybrid plasmonic waveguide based platform for refractive index and temperature sensing. *IEEE Photonics Technol. Lett.* 34 (18): 953–956. https://doi.org/10.1109/LPT.2022.3195666.

15 Chaudhary, V.S., Kumar, D., Pandey, B.P., and Kumar, S. (2022). Advances in photonic crystal fiber-based sensor for detection of physical and biochemical parameters – a review. *IEEE Sens. J.* 23 (2): 1012–1023. https://doi.org/10.1109/JSEN.2022.3222969.

16 Kaushik, B.K., Singh, L., Singh, R. et al. (2020). Detection of collagen-IV using highly reflective metal nanoparticles-immobilized photosensitive optical fiber-based MZI structure. *IEEE Trans. Nanobiosci.* 19 (3): 477–484. https://doi.org/10.1109/TNB.2020.2998520.

17 Li, M., Singh, R., Soares, M.S. et al. (2022). Convex fiber-tapered seven core fiber-convex fiber (CTC) structure-based biosensor for creatinine detection in aquaculture. *Opt. Express* 30 (8): 13898. https://doi.org/10.1364/oe.457958.

18 Dhote, C., Singh, A., and Kumar, S. (2022). Silicon photonics sensors for biophotonic applications – a review. *IEEE Sens. J.* 22 (19): 18228–18239. https://doi.org/10.1109/JSEN.2022.3199663.

19 Singh, S.U., Chatterjee, S., Lone, S.A. et al. (2022). Advanced wearable biosensors for the detection of body fluids and exhaled breath by graphene. *Mikrochim. Acta* 189 (6). Springer Vienna: https://doi.org/10.1007/s00604-022-05317-2.

20 Pandit, S., Li, M., Chen, Y. et al. (2021). Graphene-based sensor for detection of bacterial pathogens. *Sensors* 21 (23): https://doi.org/10.3390/s21238085.

21 Kumar, S., Singh, R., Zhu, G. et al. (2020). Development of uric acid biosensor using gold nanoparticles and graphene oxide functionalized micro-ball fiber sensor probe. *IEEE Trans. Nanobiosci.* 19 (2): 173–182. https://doi.org/10.1109/TNB.2019.2958891.

22 Gong, Q., Han, H., Yang, H. et al. (2019). Sensitive electrochemical DNA sensor for the detection of HIV based on a polyaniline/graphene nanocomposite. *J. Mater.* 5 (2): 313–319. https://doi.org/10.1016/j.jmat.2019.03.004.

23 Wang, R., Chen, R., Qian, C. et al. (2021). Ultrafast visual nucleic acid detection with CRISPR/Cas12a and rapid PCR in single capillary. *Sens. Actuators, B* 326: 128618. https://doi.org/10.1016/j.snb.2020.128618.

24 Ali, Z., Aman, R., Mahas, A. et al. (2020). iSCAN: an RT-LAMP-coupled CRISPR-Cas12 module for rapid, sensitive detection of SARS-CoV-2. *Virus Res.* 288: 198129. https://doi.org/10.1016/j.virusres.2020.198129.

25 Hu, F., Liu, Y., Zhao, S. et al. (2022). A one-pot CRISPR/Cas13a-based contamination-free biosensor for low-cost and rapid nucleic acid diagnostics. *Biosens. Bioelectron.* 202: 113994. https://doi.org/10.1016/j.bios.2022.113994.

26 Zhang, Y., Huang, X., Li, W. et al. (2023). Dual-target nucleic acid sequences responsive electrochemiluminescence biosensor using single type carbon dots as probe for SARS-CoV-2 detection based on series catalytic hairpin assembly amplification. *Sens. Actuators B* 379: 133223. https://doi.org/10.1016/j.snb.2022.133223.

27 Zhang, K., Fan, Z., Ding, Y., and Xie, M. (2022). A pH-engineering regenerative DNA tetrahedron ECL biosensor for the assay of SARS-CoV-2 RdRp gene based on CRISPR/Cas12a trans-activity. *Chem. Eng. J.* 429: 132472. https://doi.org/10.1016/j.cej.2021.132472.

28 Mobed, A., Hasanzadeh, M., Hassanpour, S. et al. (2019). An innovative nucleic acid based biosensor toward detection of Legionella pneumophila using DNA immobilization and hybridization: a novel genosensor. *Microchem. J.* 148: 708–716. https://doi.org/10.1016/j.microc.2019.05.027.

29 Aly, A.H., Mohamed, D., Zaky, Z.A. et al. (2021). Novel biosensor detection of tuberculosis based on photonic band gap materials. *Mater. Res.* 24 (3): https://doi.org/10.1590/1980-5373-MR-2020-0483.

30 Prabowo, B.A., Alom, A., Secario, M.K. et al. (2016). Graphene-based portable SPR sensor for the detection of Mycobacterium tuberculosis DNA strain. *Procedia Eng.* 168: 541–545. https://doi.org/10.1016/j.proeng.2016.11.520.

31 Moccia, M., Caratelli, V., Cinti, S. et al. (2020). Paper-based electrochemical peptide nucleic acid (PNA) biosensor for detection of miRNA-492: a pancreatic ductal adenocarcinoma biomarker. *Biosens. Bioelectron.* 165 (May): 112371. https://doi.org/10.1016/j.bios.2020.112371.

32 Heo, W., Lee, K., Park, S. et al. (2022). Electrochemical biosensor for nucleic acid amplification-free and sensitive detection of severe acute respiratory syndrome coronavirus 2 (SARS-CoV-2) RNA via CRISPR/Cas13a trans-cleavage reaction. *Biosens. Bioelectron.* 201 (January): 113960. https://doi.org/10.1016/j.bios.2021.113960.

33 Pandey, R., Lu, Y., McConnell, E.M. et al. (2023). Electrochemical DNAzyme-based biosensors for disease diagnosis. *Biosens. Bioelectron.* 224 (November 2022): 114983. https://doi.org/10.1016/j.bios.2022.114983.

34 You, S., Chen, L., Li, D. et al. (2023). Construction of a novel 'self-regenerative' electrochemical biosensor based on metal–organic frameworks and its application to the detection of Mycoplasma ovine pneumonia. *Bioelectrochemistry* 152 (November 2022): 108409. https://doi.org/10.1016/j.bioelechem.2023.108409.

35 Li, Z., Ding, X., Yin, K. et al. (2021). Electric field-enhanced electrochemical CRISPR biosensor for DNA detection. *Biosens. Bioelectron.* 192 (June): 113498. https://doi.org/10.1016/j.bios.2021.113498.

36 Hu, Z., Zhao, B., Miao, P. et al. (2021). Three-way junction DNA based electrochemical biosensor for microRNAs detection with distinguishable locked nucleic acid recognition and redox cycling signal amplification. *J. Electroanal. Chem.* 880: 114861. https://doi.org/10.1016/j.jelechem.2020.114861.

37 Qu, D., Gu, Z., Wu, J. et al. (2023). An unique DNA junction scaffold-based electrochemical sensing platform achieving multilevel signal responses for amplified multiplexed nucleic acid analysis and logic operation. *Sens. Actuators B* 390 (April): 133956. https://doi.org/10.1016/j.snb.2023.133956.

38 Li, C., Liu, C., Liu, R. et al. (2023). A novel CRISPR/Cas14a-based electrochemical biosensor for ultrasensitive detection of *Burkholderia* *pseudomallei* with PtPd@PCN-224 nanoenzymes for signal amplification. *Biosens. Bioelectron.* 225 (November 2022): 115098. https://doi.org/10.1016/j.bios.2023.115098.

39 Kashefi-Kheyrabadi, L., Nguyen, H.V., Go, A. et al. (2022). Rapid, multiplexed, and nucleic acid amplification-free detection of SARS-CoV-2 RNA using an electrochemical biosensor. *Biosens. Bioelectron.* 195 (August 2021): 113649. https://doi.org/10.1016/j.bios.2021.113649.

40 Fu, P., Xing, S., Xu, M. et al. (2020). Peptide nucleic acid-based electrochemical biosensor for simultaneous detection of multiple microRNAs from cancer cells with catalytic hairpin assembly amplification. *Sens. Actuators, B* 305 (August 2019): 127545. https://doi.org/10.1016/j.snb.2019.127545.

41 Zhou, K. and Dai, J. (2023). A duplex-specific nuclease based electrochemical biosensor for the assay of SARS-CoV-2 RdRp RNA. *Anal. Biochem.* 661 (November 2022): 114983. https://doi.org/10.1016/j.ab.2022.114983.

42 Zhong, Y., Hu, X.G., Zuo, S.Y. et al. (2023). A microscale electrochemical DNA biosensor based on sandwich structure and enzyme-mediated electrocatalysis for sensitive determination of hand, foot and mouth disease-related gene. *Microchem. J.* 191 (May): 108837. https://doi.org/10.1016/j.microc.2023.108837.

43 Shawky, S.M., Awad, A.M., Allam, W. et al. (2017). Gold aggregating gold: a novel nanoparticle biosensor approach for the direct quantification of hepatitis C virus RNA in clinical samples. *Biosens. Bioelectron.* 92: 349–356. https://doi.org/10.1016/j.bios.2016.11.001.

44 Zou, L., Li, R., Zhang, M. et al. (2017). A colorimetric sensing platform based upon recognizing hybridization chain reaction products with oligonucleotide modified gold nanoparticles through triplex formation. *Nanoscale* 9 (5): 1986–1992. https://doi.org/10.1039/c6nr09089c.

45 Ma, X., Gao, L., Tang, Y., and Miao, P. (2018). Gold nanoparticles-based DNA logic gate for miRNA inputs analysis coupling strand displacement reaction and hybridization chain reaction. *Part. Part. Syst. Charact.* 35: 1700326.

46 Li, S., Shang, X., Liu, J. et al. (2017). A universal colorimetry for nucleic acids and aptamer-specific ligands detection based on DNA hybridization amplification. *Anal. Biochem.* 528: 47–52. https://doi.org/10.1016/j.ab.2017.04.013.

47 Wang, Y., Guo, J., Guo, Y. et al. (2018). Enzymatically driven formation of palindromic DNA-Au nanoparticles for snowball assembly and colorimetric biosensing. *Sens. Actuators, B* 267: 328–335. https://doi.org/10.1016/j.snb.2018.04.062.

48 Teengam, P., Siangproh, W., Tuantranont, A. et al. (2017). Multiplex paper-based colorimetric DNA sensor using pyrrolidinyl peptide nucleic acid-induced AgNPs aggregation for detecting MERS-CoV, MTB, and HPV oligonucleotides. *Anal. Chem.* 89 (10): 5428–5435. https://doi.org/10.1021/acs.analchem.7b00255.

49 Huang, Z., Chen, J., Luo, Z. et al. (2019). Label-free and enzyme-free colorimetric detection of Pb^{2+} based on RNA cleavage and annealing-accelerated hybridization chain reaction. *Anal. Chem.* 91 (7): 4806–4813. https://doi.org/10.1021/acs.analchem.9b00410.

50 Kumar, N., Bhatia, S., Pateriya, A.K. et al. (2020). Label-free peptide nucleic acid biosensor for visual detection of multiple strains of influenza A virus suitable for field applications. *Anal. Chim. Acta* 1093: 123–130. https://doi.org/10.1016/j.aca.2019.09.060.

51 Wang, W., Wang, W., Liu, J. et al. (2022). CRISPR/Cas12a-based biosensor for colorimetric detection of serum prostate-specific antigen by taking nonenzymatic and isothermal amplification. *Sens. Actuators B* 354: 131228. https://doi.org/10.1016/j.snb.2021.131228.

52 Kim, D., Han, S., Ji, Y. et al. (2022). RNA polymerization actuating nucleic acid membrane (RANAM)-based biosensing for universal RNA virus detection. *Biosens. Bioelectron.* 199 (December 2021): 113880. https://doi.org/10.1016/j.bios.2021.113880.

53 Wang, Y., Peng, Y., Li, S. et al. (2023). The development of a fluorescence/colorimetric biosensor based on the cleavage activity of CRISPR-Cas12a for the detection of non-nucleic acid targets. *J. Hazard. Mater.* 449: 131044. https://doi.org/10.1016/j.jhazmat.2023.131044.

54 Kitto, R.Z., Christiansen, K.E., and Hammond, M.C. (2021). RNA-based fluorescent biosensors for live cell detection of bacterial sRNA. *Biopolymers* 112 (1): e23394. https://doi.org/10.1002/bip.23394.

55 Liu, J., Zhou, X., and Shi, H. (2018). An optical biosensor-based quantification of the microcystin synthetase a gene: early warning of toxic cyanobacterial blooming. *Anal. Chem.* 90 (3): 2362–2368. https://doi.org/10.1021/acs.analchem.7b04933.

56 Wang, R., Zhu, X., Xing, Y. et al. (2019). Multitag-regulated cascade reaction: a generalizable ultrasensitive microRNA biosensing approach for cancer prognosis. *ACS Appl. Mater. Interfaces* 11 (40): 36444–36448. https://doi.org/10.1021/acsami.9b14452.

57 Wu, H., Qian, C., Wu, C. et al. (2020). End-point dual specific detection of nucleic acids using CRISPR/Cas12a based portable biosensor. *Biosens. Bioelectron.* 157: 112153. https://doi.org/10.1016/j.bios.2020.112153.

58 Chen, L.L., Huang, H., Wang, Z. et al. (2022). Sensitive fluorescence detection of pathogens based on target nucleic acid sequence-triggered transcription. *Talanta* 243: 123352. https://doi.org/10.1016/j.talanta.2022.123352.

59 Wei, Y., Tao, Z., Wan, L. et al. (2022). Aptamer-based Cas14a1 biosensor for amplification-free live pathogenic detection. *Biosens. Bioelectron.* 211 (December 2021): 114282. https://doi.org/10.1016/j.bios.2022.114282.

60 Ma, J.Y., Liu, B., Raza, S. et al. (2023). CRISPR/Cas12a-based hypochlorous acid and myeloperoxidase biosensors designed on RESET effect. *Sens. Actuators B* 376 (PA): 133000. https://doi.org/10.1016/j.snb.2022.133000.

61 Duan, M., Li, B., Zhao, Y. et al. (2023). A CRISPR/Cas12a-mediated, DNA extraction and amplification-free, highly direct and rapid biosensor for Salmonella Typhimurium. *Biosens. Bioelectron.* 219: 114823. https://doi.org/10.1016/j.bios.2022.114823.

62 Song, D., Xu, W., Han, X. et al. (2023). CRISPR/Cas12a-powered evanescent wave fluorescence nanobiosensing platform for nucleic acid amplification-free detection of Staphylococcus aureus with multiple signal enhancements. *Biosens. Bioelectron.* 225 (January): 115109. https://doi.org/10.1016/j.bios.2023.115109.

63 Zhu, Y., Zheng, X., Zhu, R. et al. (2023). CRISPR-Cas12a powered multifunctional DNA nanodumbbell lock biosensor for multiple molecular detection. *Chem. Eng. J.* 468: 143494. https://doi.org/10.1016/j.cej.2023.143494.

64 Diao, W., Tang, M., Ding, S. et al. (2018). Highly sensitive surface plasmon resonance biosensor for the detection of HIV-related DNA based on dynamic and structural DNA nanodevices. *Biosens. Bioelectron.* 100: 228–234. https://doi.org/10.1016/j.bios.2017.08.042.

65 Hossain, M.B. and Rana, M.M. (2016). DNA hybridization detection based on resonance frequency readout in graphene on Au SPR biosensor. *J. Sensors* 2016: 6070742. https://doi.org/10.1155/2016/6070742.

66 Rahman, M.S., Anower, M.S., Rahman, M.K. et al. (2017). Modeling of a highly sensitive MoS_2-graphene hybrid based fiber optic SPR biosensor for sensing DNA hybridization. *Optik (Stuttg)* 140: 989–997. https://doi.org/10.1016/j.ijleo.2017.05.001.

67 Zou, R., Ma, Y., Li, C. et al. (2020). A label-free resonance light scattering biosensor for nucleic acids using triple-helix molecular switch and G-quadruplex nanowires. *Microchem. J.* 156: 104764. https://doi.org/10.1016/j.microc.2020.104764.

68 Roether, J., Chu, K.Y., Willenbacher, N. et al. (2019). Real-time monitoring of DNA immobilization and detection of DNA polymerase activity by a microfluidic nanoplasmonic platform. *Biosens. Bioelectron.* 142: 111528. https://doi.org/10.1016/j.bios.2019.111528.

69 Yang, W., Yan, J., Liu, R. et al. (2023). Ultra-sensitive specific detection of nucleic acids in pathogenic infections by Ta2C-MXene sensitization-based ultrafine plasmon spectroscopy combs. *Sens. Actuators B* 387: 133785. https://doi.org/10.1016/j.snb.2023.133785.

70 Vasimalla, Y., Shekhar Pradhan, H., and Jashvantbhai Pandya, R. (2020). SPR performance enhancement for DNA hybridization employing black phosphorus, silver, and silicon. *Appl. Opt.* 59 (24): 7299. https://doi.org/10.1364/ao.397452.

71 Yi, Z., Zhou, Y., Ren, Y. et al. (2022). A novel sensitive DNAzyme-based optical fiber evanescent wave biosensor for rapid detection of Pb^{2+} in human serum. *Analyst* 147 (7): 1467–1477. https://doi.org/10.1039/d2an00043a.

72 Li, L., Zhang, Y.n., Zheng, W. et al. (2022). Optical fiber SPR biosensor based on gold nanoparticle amplification for DNA hybridization detection. *Talanta* 247: 123599. https://doi.org/10.1016/j.talanta.2022.123599.

73 Cheng, R., Li, L.T., Huang, M. et al. (2023). Highly sensitive plasmonic biosensor for hepatitis B virus DNA based on the surface etching of the active helical gold nanorods. *Chem. Eng. J.* 468: 143627. https://doi.org/10.1016/j.cej.2023.143627.

74 Xu, S., Jiang, S., Zhang, C. et al. (2018). Ultrasensitive label-free detection of DNA hybridization by sapphire-based graphene field-effect transistor biosensor. *Appl. Surf. Sci.* 427: 1114–1119. https://doi.org/10.1016/j.apsusc.2017.09.113.

75 Liu, Y.H., Deng, H.H., Li, H.N. et al. (2018). A DNA electrochemical biosensor based on homogeneous hybridization for the determination of Cryptococcus neoformans. *J. Electroanal. Chem.* 827: 27–33. https://doi.org/10.1016/j.jelechem.2018.09.001.

76 Mohammadian, N. and Faridbod, F. (2018). ALS genosensing using DNA-hybridization electrochemical biosensor based on label-free immobilization of ssDNA on Sm2O3 NPs-rGO/PANI composite. *Sens. Actuators, B* 275: 432–438. https://doi.org/10.1016/j.snb.2018.07.103.

77 Wang, R., Wang, L., Xu, X., and Jiang, W. (2018). An enzyme-free and label-free fluorescence biosensor for microRNA detection based on cascade amplification of DNAzyme-powered three-dimensional DNA walker and hybridization chain reaction. *Sens. Actuators, B* 268: 287–292. https://doi.org/10.1016/j.snb.2018.04.109.

78 He, Y. and Fan, Z. (2018). A novel biosensor based on DNA hybridization for ultrasensitive detection of NOS terminator gene sequences. *Sens. Actuators, B* 257: 538–544. https://doi.org/10.1016/j.snb.2017.10.183.

79 Rahman, M.S., Hasan, M.R., Rikta, K.A., and Anower, M.S. (2018). A novel graphene coated surface plasmon resonance biosensor with tungsten disulfide (WS_2) for sensing DNA hybridization. *Opt. Mater. (Amst).* 75: 567–573. https://doi.org/10.1016/j.optmat.2017.11.013.

80 Xu, C., Lan, L., Yao, Y. et al. (2018). An unmodified gold nanorods-based DNA colorimetric biosensor with enzyme-free hybridization chain reaction amplification. *Sens. Actuators, B* 273: 642–648. https://doi.org/10.1016/j.snb.2018.06.035.

81 Ebrahimi, M., Raoof, J.B., and Ojani, R. (2018). Design of an electrochemical DNA-based biosensor for selective determination of cadmium ions using a DNA hybridization indicator. *Int. J. Biol. Macromol.* 108: 1237–1241. https://doi.org/10.1016/j.ijbiomac.2017.11.023.

82 Subak, H. and Ozkan-Ariksoysal, D. (2018). Label-free electrochemical biosensor for the detection of influenza genes and the solution of guanine-based displaying problem of DNA hybridization. *Sens. Actuators, B* 263: 196–207. https://doi.org/10.1016/j.snb.2018.02.089.

83 Zhou, L., Wang, Y., Yang, C. et al. (2019). A label-free electrochemical biosensor for microRNAs detection based on DNA nanomaterial by coupling with Y-shaped DNA structure and non-linear hybridization chain reaction. *Biosens. Bioelectron.* 126 (November 2018): 657–663. https://doi.org/10.1016/j.bios.2018.11.028.

84 Su, Y., Liang, Y., Wu, H. et al. (2019). A three-dimensional cloth-based microfluidic label-free proximity hybridization-electrochemiluminescence biosensor for ultrasensitive detection of K-ras gene. *Sens. Actuators, B* 296: 126654. https://doi.org/10.1016/j.snb.2019.126654.

85 Can, F., Ökten, H.E., Ergön-Can, T. et al. (2020). Thermodynamically designed target-specific DNA probe as an electrochemical hybridization biosensor. *Bioelectrochemistry* 135: 107553. https://doi.org/10.1016/j.bioelechem.2020.107553.

86 Wu, H., Su, Y., Jiang, J. et al. (2020). Ultrasensitive electrochemiluminescence detection of p53 gene by a novel cloth-based microfluidic biosensor with luminol-gold nanoparticles and hybridization chain reaction amplification. *J. Lumin.* 226 (April): 117485. https://doi.org/10.1016/j.jlumin.2020.117485.

87 Miti, A., Thamm, S., Müller, P. et al. (2020). A miRNA biosensor based on localized surface plasmon resonance enhanced by surface-bound hybridization chain reaction. *Biosens. Bioelectron.* 167 (112465): https://doi.org/10.1016/j.bios.2020.112465.

88 Manohar Raju, V., Bhavana, V., Gayathri, G.K. et al. (2020). A novel disposable electrochemical DNA biosensor for the rapid detection of Bacillus thuringiensis. *Microchem. J.* 159 (May): 105434. https://doi.org/10.1016/j.microc.2020.105434.

89 Rizi, K.S., Hatamluyi, B., Rezayi, M. et al. (122099, 2021). Response surface methodology optimized electrochemical DNA biosensor based on HAPNPTs/PPY/MWCNTs nanocomposite for detecting Mycobacterium tuberculosis. *Talanta* 226 (December 2020): https://doi.org/10.1016/j.talanta.2021.122099.

90 Wang, H.B., Zhong, Z.T., Zhang, T., and Di Zhao, Y. (2020). Development of dual strip biosensors based on hybridization chain reaction and microplate strategies for signal amplification of HBV-DNA detection. *Sens. Actuators, B* 310: 127829. https://doi.org/10.1016/j.snb.2020.127829.

91 Liu, T., Li, Z., Chen, M. et al. (2021). Sensitive electrochemical biosensor for Uracil-DNA glycosylase detection based on self-linkable hollow Mn/Ni layered doubled hydroxides as oxidase-like nanozyme for cascade signal amplification. *Biosens. Bioelectron.* 194: 113607. https://doi.org/10.1016/j.bios.2021.113607.

92 Fertier, A., Montarnal, A., Truptil, S., and Bénaben, F. (2020). Design of a rapid electrochemical biosensor based on MXene/Pt/C nanocomposite and DNA/RNA hybridization for the detection of COVID-19. *Decis. Support Syst.* 265 (January): 113260. https://doi.org/10.1016/j.talanta.2023.124804.

93 Bao, J., Ding, K., and Zhu, Y. (2023). An electrochemical biosensor for detecting DNA methylation based on AuNPs/rGO/g-C3N4 nanocomposite. *Anal. Biochem.* 673: 115180. https://doi.org/10.1016/j.ab.2023.115180.

94 Peng, L., Zhou, J., Liang, Z. et al. (2019). SERS-based sandwich bioassay protocol of miRNA-21 using Au@Ag core–shell nanoparticles and a Ag/TiO_2 nanowires substrate. *Anal. Methods* 11 (23): 2960–2968. https://doi.org/10.1039/C9AY00573K.

95 Cui, Y., Wang, H., Liu, S. et al. (2020). Target-activated DNA nanomachines for the ATP detection based on the SERS of plasmonic coupling from gold nanoparticle aggregation. *Analyst* 145 (2): 445–452. https://doi.org/10.1039/c9an02051a.

96 Ge, S., Ran, M., Mao, Y. et al. (2021). A novel DNA biosensor for the ultrasensitive detection of DNA methyltransferase activity based on a high-density 'hot spot' SERS substrate and rolling circle amplification strategy. *Analyst* 146 (17): 5326–5336. https://doi.org/10.1039/d1an01034d.

97 Zhou, X., Ge, S., Sun, Y. et al. (2021). Highly sensitive SERS assay of genetically modified organisms in maize: via a nanoflower substrate coupled with hybridization chain reaction amplification. *New J. Chem.* 45 (44): 20586–20595. https://doi.org/10.1039/d1nj03913j.

98 Matanfack, G.A., Pistiki, A., Rösch, P., and Popp, J. (2021). Raman ^{18}O labeling of bacteria in visible and deep UV-ranges. *J. Biophotonics* 14: e202100013.

99 Liu, Y., Wu, S.H., Du, X.Y., and Sun, J.J. (2021). Plasmonic Ag nanocube enhanced SERS biosensor for sensitive detection of oral cancer DNA based on nicking endonuclease signal amplification and heated electrode. *Sens. Actuators, B* 338: 129854. https://doi.org/10.1016/j.snb.2021.129854.

100 Shen, C., Chen, X., Huang, Z. et al. (2022). High sensitivity and fast response optical fiber nucleic acid sensor. *Opt. Laser Technol.* 154: 108271. https://doi.org/10.1016/j.optlastec.2022.108271.

101 Li, X., Chen, N., Zhou, X. et al. (2022). In-situ DNA detection with an interferometric-type optical sensor based on tapered exposed core microstructured optical fiber. *Sens. Actuators B* 351: 130942. https://doi.org/10.1016/j.snb.2021.130942.

102 Wang, L., Yi, D., Geng, Y. et al. (2023). Ultrasensitive deafness gene DNA hybridization detection employing a fiber optic Mach-Zehnder interferometer: enabled by a black phosphorus nanointerface. *Biosens. Bioelectron.* 222: 1–9. https://doi.org/10.1016/j.bios.2022.114952.

4

Antibody-Based Biosensors

4.1 Polyclonal Antibody and Monoclonal Antibody

Antibodies, or immunosensors, employ antibodies as bioreceptors to detect specific targets such as microorganisms, gases, pollutants, chemicals, and biomolecules. The antibodies are immobilized on a sensing surface and fabricated using different materials that include glass, metals, or plastic [1–4]. As a target molecule binds to the antibody, it triggers a signal that is transduced into a measurable output signal via various mechanisms, providing a quantitative measurement of the target's concentration. Antibodies are globular heterodimeric blood proteins that are Y-shaped in the immune system. Plasma cells generate these antibodies as unwanted substances enter the human body and interact with external particles or molecules [5].

Polypeptide chains are the basic components of an antibody that consists of two heavy (H) chains and two light (L) chains coupled to disulfide bonds, as shown in Figure 4.1 [6]. The molecular weights of heavy and light chains are 50 and 25 kDa made of constant (C) and variable (V) regions. A heavy chain variable region (V_H) with three constant regions (C_{H1}, C_{H2}, and C_{H3}), light chain with variable region (V_L) and constant region (C_L) bind the antigen and various other functions. Antibodies can be classified into five isotypes that have different functions in the body due to five types of heavy chains (α, γ, μ, δ, ε) and perform different role in the body: IgM, IgG, IgA, IgD, and IgE [7].

IgM is the largest antibody with 10 antigen binding sites that consists of five protein sub-units, i.e. pentamer. IgG is found in abundance in the blood plasma, with two binding sites for antigen, and is almost 80% of the total antibody content.

Biosensors: Nanomaterials, Approaches, and Performance-Enhancement Strategies,
First Edition. Baljinder Kaur, Santosh Kumar, and Brajesh Kumar Kaushik.

Published 2025 by John Wiley & Sons, Inc.
Companion website: www.wiley.com/go/kaur

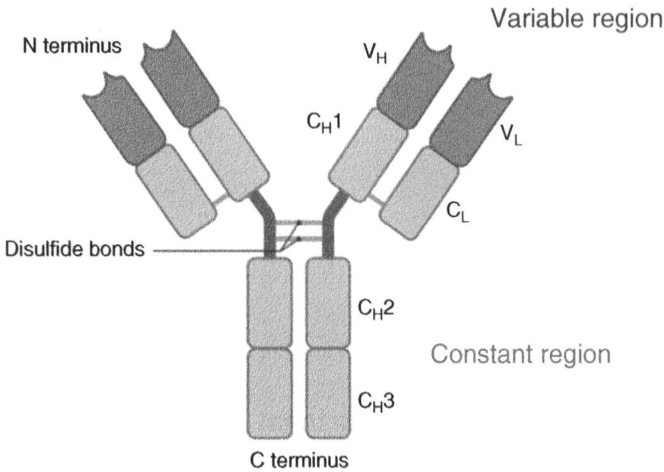

Figure 4.1 Schematic of immunoglobulin with heavy and light chains, variable and constant regions linked connected through noncovalent as well as disulfide bonds.

The function of IgG is to detoxify harmful substances that enters the body by binding to the antigen. It is further divided into four categories in order of decreasing abundance (IgG1, IgG2, IgG3, and IgG4), with different structures and numbers of interchain-disulfide bonds [8]. IgA occurs in two forms, i.e. monomeric and dimeric. It is of two types, IgA1 and IgA2, having different properties (glycosylation patterns) and five to six binding sites, and is present in the serum, breast milk, saliva, and intestinal fluids [9]. IgD is available in monomer form with two binding sites and a concentration of less than 1% of the total immunoglobulin content. IgE is present in a minimum amount of 0.02% of the total immunoglobulin content in monomer form with two antigen-antibody binding sites [10]. Immunosensors or assays exhibit several advantages as compared to conventional detection methods such as specificity toward target, sensitivity, multianalyte, and selectivity [11]. These biosensors have been explored in the bio-medical field, environmental monitoring, and the food industry [12–19]. For example, in medical diagnosis, they are used to detect biomarkers for diseases such as cancer and infectious diseases [20]. In environmental monitoring, they are used to detect pollutants in water and air [21–23]. In food safety, they are used to detect contaminants such as bacteria and toxins [24].

Antibodies are monoclonal and polyclonal in nature that depend on number of epitopes an antibody can bind to itself [8]. Monoclonal antibodies are clones of a single type of immune B cell that bind to the same type antigen that the antibody recognizes [25]. Monoclonal antibodies are highly specific and have a well-defined structure, making them useful in applications where specificity is critical. Polyclonal antibodies are antibodies produced by multiple types of B cells, contains different type of antibodies, and can bind to different antigens. As compared to monoclonal antibody, polyclonal is less specific but it can be used to detect the multiple analytes [26].

Recombinant antibodies are antibodies that are produced by recombinant DNA technology, using genetic engineering to create antibodies with specific properties. Recombinant antibodies can be produced by inserting the genes that code for the antibody into bacteria, yeast, or mammalian cells, allowing for large-scale production of the antibody. Recombinant antibodies can be engineered to have specific properties, such as increased affinity for a target antigen, reduced immunogenicity, or modified effector functions [26, 27]. Recombinant antibodies are becoming increasingly important in therapeutic applications due to their specificity, potency, and reduced immunogenicity [28]. The selection of an appropriate antibody for a particular application is a critical step in any research, diagnostic, or therapeutic program. There are three key factors to consider during the selection of antibodies:

1) The binding between the target antigen and antibody should be specific with minimum cross-reactivity [29]. This can be determined by various methods such as Western blot, enzyme-linked immunosorbent assay (ELISA), or immunohistochemistry.
2) The sensitivity of an antibody should be as high as possible and with lowest concentration while producing minimal background signal. The source and quality of the antibody can affect its performance. Antibodies from reputable manufacturers or those with published validation data are preferred. The format of the antibody should be appropriate for the application, such as monoclonal or polyclonal, purified or crude, conjugated or unconjugated, and suitable for the chosen detection method. The cost and availability of the antibody should also be considered, as some antibodies may be more expensive or difficult to obtain than others.
3) The antibody should be validated for reactivity with the species of interest, as some antibodies may cross-react with other species. By considering these factors, researchers can select an antibody that is most suitable for their specific application, leading to more accurate and reliable results [30]. Despite their advantages, antibody-based biosensors also have several drawbacks that include specialist trainers, cost, and the potential for cross-reactivity with other molecules that have similar structures [31–34]. However, current research is focused on improving the performance of antibody-based biosensors by developing new immobilization strategies and enhancing the sensitivity and selectivity of the detection mechanisms.

4.2 Cardiovascular Biomarker, Autoimmune Disorder, and Cholesterol Biomarker

ECL, optical, and mass-based biosensors are all promising technologies for cancer detection. Table 4.1 shows cardiovascular, autoimmune disorder, and cholesterol biomarkers. Among cardiovascular biomarkers, myoglobin is a nonspecific old biomarker and creatine kinase is widely explored but limited after the emergence of Troponin biomarker and is not used for cardiovascular diseases detection. Troponin I and troponin T proteins are currently the most common biomarkers used for diagnosis. Out of creatine kinase, troponin I, troponin T, myoglobin, troponin I is highly specific to detect myocardial infarctions as compared to less specificity of troponin T. Low-density lipoprotein is a less commonly used biomarker because it lacks the specificity and accuracy of troponin T and troponin I. Brain-type natriuretic peptide is also considered a good indicator for detecting heart failure, dialysis, and end-stage renal diseases.

Common antibody-based biomarkers in different disease are described in this section (Table 4.1). Section 4.2.4 specifically discusses autoimmune diseases such as psoriasis, rheumatoid arthritis, lupus, diabetes, Crohn's disease, and thyroiditis diseases. In case of commonly observed rheumatoid arthritis disease, an autoantibody called rheumatoid factor targets the Fc region of IgG antibodies. Among all reported biomarkers, anti-cyclic citrullinated peptide antibodies target are commonly used due to their high specificity [30]. Systemic lupus erythematosus is a chronic disease reported in the different part of skin, kidneys, joints, and brain. Anti-double-stranded DNA, antinuclear antibodies, and anti-Smith antibody-based biomarkers are commonly used to detect this disease.

4.2.1 Cancer Detection

Immunosensors have been explored to detect various diseases that include thyroid, cancer, infection, and heart-related diseases. These sensors work by using antibodies that are specific to certain biomarkers that are indicative of the presence of cancer [18, 42–44]. Antibody-based sensors have excellent sensitivity and specificity, making them useful tools for early cancer detection [45]. Microfluidic technology has been applied in various antibody-based sensor for cancer detection [46, 47]. A fiber sensor that consists of multi-core, AuNPs, GO, and copper oxide nano-flowers uses localized surface plasmon resonance (LSPR) effect to detect the cancerous cells lines (hepatoblastoma cell line: HepG2, Hepa 1–6, Michigan cancer foundation-7 (MCF-7), and A549). Cores have been arranged in terms of a hexagon to construct the sensor structure and are depicted in Figure 4.2a. AuNPs supports surface plasmons, GO enhances sensitivity due to its good conductivity and other properties, and copper oxide nano-flowers provide

Table 4.1 Cardiovascular, autoimmune disorder, and cholesterol biomarkers.

Disease type	Diseases details	Biomarkers	Refs.
Cardiovascular biomarkers	Myocardial infarction	Creatine kinase, cardiovascular protein, glycogen phosphorylase isoenzyme BB, troponin I, troponin T, Myoglobin	[35–37]
	Inflammation for stroke	Lipoprotein-associated phospholipase A2	
	Atherosclerotic plaque	Interleukin-1	
	Plaque	Low-density lipoprotein	
	Inflammation, coronary artery disease, plaque	Myeloperoxidase,	
	Inflammation, cardiovascular	TnF-alpha	
	Coronary syndrome, ventricular ejection	Brain-type natriuretic peptide, atrial natriuretic peptide	
	Myocardial necrosis	Heart fatty acid binding protein, fatty-acid-binding protein, Ischemia-modified albumin	
Autoimmune disorder	Systemic lupus erythematosus	Anti-double stranded DNA, Contactin-1, anti-Smith antibodies, Chitinase-3-like protein 1	[38–40]
	Celiac disease	Tissue transglutaminase, gliadin, human leukocyte antigen, anti-deamidated, gliadin peptide, gluten	
	Rheumatoid arthritis	Rheumatoid factor, multi-biomarker disease activity, Anti-citrullinated peptide, Dickkopf-1, C-reactive protein, cyclic citrullinated peptide and proteins, Erythrocyte sedimentation rate, Tumor necrosis factor -α,	
	Psoriasis	Interleukin-17, Interleukin-23, Anti-cyclic citrullinated peptide	

(*Continued*)

Table 4.1 (Continued)

Disease type	Diseases details	Biomarkers	Refs.
	Multiple sclerosis	Cytokines, Cystatin C, myelin basic protein antibodies, aquaporin-4 antibodies, Glial fibrillary acidic protein, Lipocalin 2, Anti-CSF114	
	Crohn's disease	Fecal calprotectin antibodies, erythrocyte sedimentation rate, anti-neutrophil cytoplasmic antibodies	
	Antiphospholipid syndrome	Anti-phospholipid, glycoprotein-I, anti-cardiolipin IgA, anti-cardiolipin, anti-annexin V	
	Hashimoto thyroiditis	Thyroid-stimulating hormone, free thyroxine, anti–thyroid peroxidase, thyroglobulin	
	Diabetes	Glucose, oxytocin, anti-glutamic acid decarboxylase, nesfatin-1, insulin, omentin, hepatocyte growth factor	
	Sjogren syndrome	Anti-ribonucleoprotein, CD163, anti-Sjogren's syndrome, MicroRNAs:	
	Chronic autoimmune hepatitis	Anti-soluble liver antigen, gamma-glutamyl transferase	
	Thyroid	Anti-thyroid-stimulating hormone	
Cholesterol biomarker	Heart related diseases	Low-density lipoprotein, high-density lipoprotein, triglycerides, total cholesterol	[41]

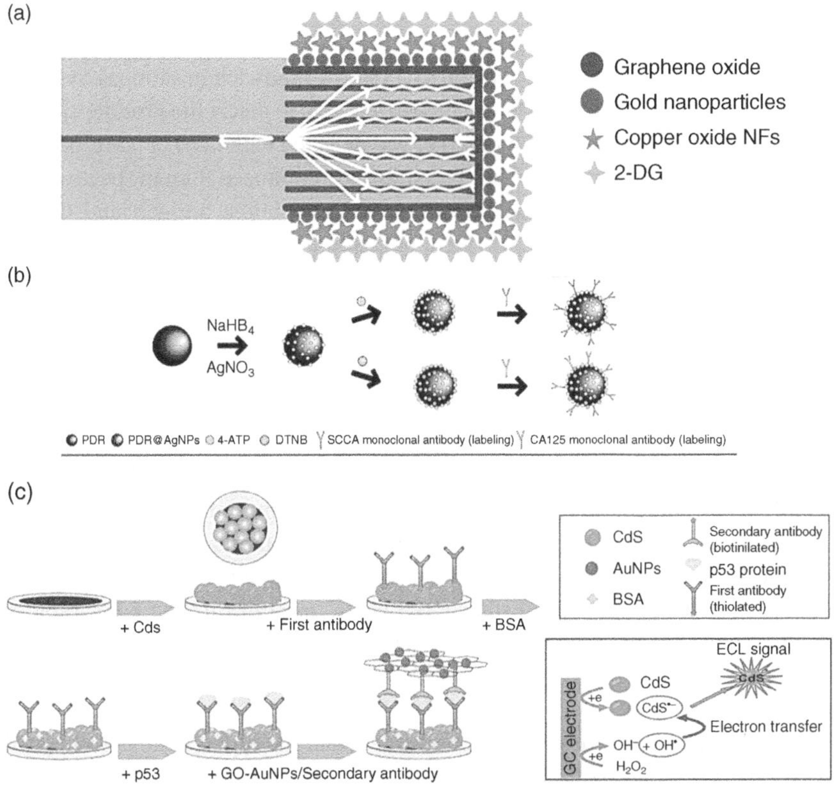

Figure 4.2 Schematic of (a) antibody-based multicore fiber LSPR sensor. *Source:* [4]/with permission of Elsevier. (b) Nitrocellulose membrane-based SERS-biosensor CA125 cancer detection. *Source:* [48]/with permission of The Royal Society of Chemistry. (c) CdS QDs, AuNPs and antibody-based ECL immunosensor. *Source:* [49]/with permission of Elsevier.

large surface area and biocompatibility. Etching removes the coating from the core and improves the coupling between evanescent waves and electromagnetic fields that have strong affinity toward cancer cells. Various cancerous cell lines that include HepG2 were detected with limit of detection (LoD) of 3 cells/ml, Hepal 6, A549, MCF-7 of 2 cells/ml, LO2, and normal canine fibroblasts (NCF) cell lines 4, 10 cells/ml in concentration span of 10^2–10^6 cells/ml [4]. An Au-fused silica and titanium dioxide (TiO_2)-coated photonic crystal fiber (PCF) SPR sensor was investigated to detect various cancerous cells using COMSOL software. The cell lines are breast cancer cell line (MDAMB-231 and MCF-7), adrenal glands cancer (PC12), cervical cancer cell line (HeLa), and blood cancer (Jurkat). The resolution, LOD, and linear RI range was 10^{-5} RIU, 0.014–0.024, and 1.385–1.390 RIU for all cell lines. Sensitivity value of cancer cell lines lies in the range of 5500–10 714.28 nm/RIU for cell lines. It is maximum in case of MCF-7 (10 714 nm/RIU) and minimum for HeLa was 5500 nm/RIU [50]. A sandwich immunoassay made up of Ag nanorods, SiO_2 and 4-mercaptobenzoic acid to detect the prostate-specific antigen (PSA) biomarker. PSA biomarker was detected with LOD of 0.3 fg/ml [51].

Figure 4.2b depicts a nanosphere-based surface-enhanced Raman spectroscopy (SERS)-biosensor to detect the squamous cell carcinoma antigen and CA125 simultaneously. Two SERS probes were prepared in one probe. A polydopamine with Ag nanospheres with Raman reporter (4-aminothiophenol and 5,5-dithiobis-[2-nitrobenzoic acid]) and antibody was used to fabricate the sensor. Squamous cell carcinoma antigen and CA125 were detected with LOD of 7.156, 7.182 pg/ml and 8.093, 7.370 pg/ml in phosphate buffer and human serum solution [48]. Heidari et al. reported an AuNPs and cadmium sulfide QDs-based ECL immunosensor to detect the protein biomarker p53 for cancer detection. Figure 4.2c shows that the sensor was designed using a glassy carbon electrode with cadmium sulfide QDs and AuNPs formed a sandwich-type immuno-complex between antibodies and protein biomarkers. QDs and H_2O_2 are used as luminophores and co-reactants, while AuNPs can play dual roles one as quencher and the other as enhancer, depending on the distance. GO is also used during the fabrication of sensors that attract a large number of AuNPs that enhance ECL signal intensity. The linear range of 20–1000 fg/ml and p53 biomarker of concentration of 4 fg/ml can be detected [49].

Table 4.2 summarized various platform to detect the different analytes related with cancer diseases that involve 2D materials, QDs and various nanomaterials.

4.2.2 Tuberculosis Detection

Tuberculosis is a bacterial infection that primarily affects the lungs and is caused by the bacteria *Mycobacterium Tuberculosis* (*M. Tuberculosis*). Early detection of tuberculosis (TB) is crucial for effective treatment and the prevention of transmission. Biosensors are analytical devices that can detect specific biological molecules and have the potential for early and accurate TB diagnosis [96]. The Au nanotube array has a higher electron transfer capacity as compared to bare Au electrodes due to its high surface area-based ECL sensor to detect the *M. Tuberculosis* bacteria. A DNA probe was immobilized on the Au nanotube array surface, and complementary DNA was hybridized on it. In the process, the electron transfers of the redox indicator $[Fe\ (CN)6]^{3-/4-}$ were monitored using cyclic voltammetry. The target DNA concentration in the linear range of 0.01–100 ng/μl can be detected [97]. Tufa et al. demonstrated an antigen-antibody-based immunosensor based on the interaction for tuberculosis detection. The structure consists of three monolayers consisting of graphene quantum dot-coated Fe_3O_4@Ag core-shell

Table 4.2 Recent optical, ECL and mass-based biosensors to detect the cancer.

Sensing technology		Linear range	LoD	Refs.
Cadmium sulfide QDs, AuNPs and streptavidin-based ECL biosensor for p53 cancer biomarker		20–1000 fg/ml	4 fg/ml	[49]
Au metal and aptamer coated on fiber-based breast cancer SPR sensor	Without labeling	8 fM–8 nM	9.3 ng/ml	[52]
GO–AuNPs hybrids-based SPR sensor for miRNA-141 detection		1 pM–1 fM	1 fM	[53]
Metal-insulator-metal nano-disk-based LSPR sensor for A549 cancer cells		1.28–1.40 RIU	n.r.[a]	[54]
ZnO nanowires-AuNPs-based LSPR sensor PSA biomarker		0.001 pg/ml–1 ng/ml	0.51 pg/ml	[55]
U-shaped fiber LSPR cyto-sensor		10^2–10^6 cells/ml	30 cells/ml	[56]
CdSe-CdS QDs and nanodots and Au-based sensor for cancer		1.0–2.0 RIU	n.r.[a]	[57]
Silicon on insulator nano-cavity-based PCF biosensor		1.34–1.40 RIU	n.r.[a]	[58]
Silica with dual core PCF RI sensor for cancer detection		1.36–1.399 RIU	0.014 nm	[59]
Titanium-coated SPR PCF biosensor with bowl-shape for cancer		1.36–1.39 RIU	0.014–0.024	[60]
Fused silica with double-core PCF biosensor for blood cancer detection		n.r.[a]	n.r.[a]	[61]
Infiltration method and SiO_2-Ag nano composite material coated PCF biosensor		1.36–1.39 RIU	n.r.[a]	[62]
SiO_2 GaAs layer-based 1D PCF biosensor		1.35–1.401 RIU	10^{-7} RIU	[63]
2D photonic crystal waveguide biosensor		1.34–1.351 RIU	99.765	[64]
Taper interferometer and fiber Bragg grating (FBG) biosensor to detect HER2 for breast cancer		1.335–1.362 RIU	2 ng/ml	[65]

(*Continued*)

Table 4.2 (Continued)

Sensing technology	Linear range	LoD	Refs.
Mach-Zehnder interferometer (MZI) biosensor to detect brain tumor	n.r.[a]	n.r.[a]	[66]
Si and Si_3N_4-based MZI biosensor to detect bladder cancer miRNA let-7	1 pmol/µl–100 fmol/µl	1 nM	[67]
Silica-based Sagnac interfeometer PCF biosensor for different cancer cells	1.376–1.399 RIU	0.014 nm	[68]
Au coated Fabry-Perot interferometric biosensor for PSA	1.343–1.348 RIU	n.r.[a]	[69]
Atactic polystyrene and thyroglobulin long period grating sensor for thyroid cancer	0–4 ng/ml	sub ng/ml	[70]
Au coated tilted FBG biosensor for lung cancer biomarker cytokeratin-17	10^{-12}–10^{-6} g/ml	1 pM	[71]
AuNPs-based LPG biosensor for carbonic anhydrase-IX biomarker in hypoxia condition	10^5–10^4 cells/ml	n.r.[a]	[72]
Multilayered Au and aluminum 1-D grating-based SPR biosensor for lung cancer biomarker carcinoembryonic antigen and EGFR	1.32–1.37 RIU	n.r.[a]	[73]
Silica microfiber interferometry sensor for breast cancer HER2 biomarker	1.332–1.34 RIU	n.r.[a]	[74]
Metal-insulator-metal-based grating biosensor for cancer cells	n.r.[a]	n.r.[a]	[75]
Anti-PSA coated LPG biosensor PSA detection	5–500 ng/ml	9.9 ng/ml	[76]
Optical backscatter reflectometry-based ball resonator to detect the thrombin	0.4–100 pM	1.56 pM	[77]
Au/Bi_2Se_3 nanosheets-based colorimetric CEA biosensor	10 ng/ml–5 µg/ml	10.25 c/ng/ml	[78]

Head-flocked Au nanopillar-based miRNAs (miR-10b, miR-21, and miR-373) sensor		1 μM–100 aM	3.53 fM – miR-10b, 2.17 fM – miR-21, 2.16 fM – miR-373	[79]
Label-free platinum-doped CdTe QDs, magnetic framework and AuNPs-based biosensor for breast cancer	Breast cancer	1 pg/mL-l0^2 ng/mL	0.175 pg/ml	[80]
Fibrous nano-silica and folate receptor-based sensor for colorectal cancer	Label-free	50–10^4 cells/ml	50 cells/ml	[81]
Aptamer-based fluorescence sensor for HEPG2 cancer cell	With labeling	0–375 nM	100 cells/ml	[82]
Biotinylated anti-PSA antibody and AuNPs-based switchable linkers PSA bioassay	Without labeling	15–40 μg/ml	100 fg/ml	[83]
Glucose oxidase-based biosensor for different cancer cells platelet-derived growth factor-BB biomarker	With labeling	0–500 pM	0.94 pM	[84]
Rectangular core-based PCF biosensor for breast cancer		n.r.[a]	n.r.[a]	[85]
Graphene-based iterative process for breast cancer		n.r.[a]	n.r.[a]	[86]
Graphene, anti-epithelial cell adhesion molecule and Au-based paper sensor for breast cancer		n.r.[a]	600 cells	[87]
Ag nanorod array-hairpin-shaped molecular beacons-based SERS sensor for miRNA-21, miRNA-486, and miRNA-375		n.r.[a]	393 aM – miRNA-21 176 aM – miRNA-486 144 aM – miRNA-375	[88]
Au-NPs and Au-coated paramagnetic NPs for miR-141		200 nM–200 pM	100 fM	[89]
Au-Ag alloy nano-boxes and nano-yeast-based sensor for cancer biomarker detection		1–10 ng/ml	0.68 pg/ml	[90]
SERS nano-probes with plasmonic receptor and EGFR-targeting peptides for breast cancer		n.r.[a]	n.r.[a]	[91]

(Continued)

Table 4.2 (Continued)

Sensing technology	Linear range	LoD	Refs.
Au on carbon electrode and molecularly-imprinted polymers-based SERS colon cancer sensor	1–000 ng/ml	1 ng/ml	[92]
Au-4-Mercaptoben-zonitrile-Ag Tryptophan aptamer-based sensor for CEA biomarker	3.125–625 ng/ml	0.278 ng/ml	[93]
Thyroid stimulant hormone -oxalyl diimidazole chemiluminescent enzyme-based thyroid cancer sensor	0.013–12 mU/l	0.005 mU/l	[94]
TiO_2 meso-crystalline and reduced GO hybrid ovarian cancer sensor	10^{-5}–1000 ng/ml	3.3×10^{-6} ng/ml	[95]

[a] not reported.

nanostructure (Fe_3O_4@Ag/GQD). The culture filtrate protein antibody conjugated with AuNPs enhances the signal intensity. Fe_3O_4 has high surface energy, low mass transfer resistance, and a large surface area [98, 99]. A biosensor that uses gold nanoparticles functionalized with thiolated DNA probes for the detection of *M. Tuberculosis* was reported. The biosensor is highly sensitive and selective, and it can detect *M. Tuberculosis* DNA even in the presence of another bacterial DNA. A colorimetric biosensor was reported for the detection of *M. Tuberculosis* based on the ELISA method. The biosensor uses gold nanoparticles functionalized with anti-*M. Tuberculosis* antibodies and provides results in less than 2 hours [100]. A study by Azmi et al. utilized aptamer-antibody specific to detect the *M. Tuberculosis* biomarker CFP10-ESAT6 using Fe_3O_4/Au MNPs and graphene/polyaniline nanocomposite on Au electrode. In this case, magnetic nanoparticles (MNPs) are used for labeling purpose and nanocomposite amplifies the signal. The biosensor was able to detect as few as 1.52 ng/ml of the CFP10-ESAT6 with relative standard deviation (RSD) of 2.5% [101]. Another study by Sepulveda et al. (2020) reported the development of a bio-ECL immunosensor using polyclonal antibody-functionalized Au electrode with self-assembled monolayer (SAM) of 4-aminothiophenol and a polyclonal antibody to detect the tuberculosis using 6 kDa early secretory antigen target-6 (ESAT-6). This sensor is fabricated on printed circuit board using 40 independent ECL sensors. The biosensor was able to detect the antigen ESAT-6 concentrations of 0.5 μg/ml [102]. Additionally, a study by Owens et al. reported a SERS biosensor using Au surface functionalized with polyclonal rabbit antibody for the detection of the tuberculosis biomarker Mannose-capped lipoarabinomannan. The biosensor showed high sensitivity and specificity, and LOD of 1.1 ng/ml in the concentration range of 0–50 ng/ml [103]. An immune-ECL biosensor using $[Fe\ (CN)6]^{3-}/^{4-}$ redox probe-based square wave voltammetry method was reported for tuberculosis detection as shown in Figure 4.3. An anti-early secreted antigenic target-6 kDa protein monoclonal antibody was used as a bioreceptor to detect the *Mycobacterium tuberculosis*. LOD of 7 ng/ml was achieved with ECL biosensor [104].

Antibody-based biosensors offer several advantages for tuberculosis detection, but they also have some limitations that need to be addressed. One major limitation is the potential for cross-reactivity with other antigens or bacteria, which can result in false positives or false negatives. Another limitation is the potential for antibody degradation or denaturation during storage or handling, which can affect the biosensor's sensitivity and specificity [105]. Additionally, antibody-based biosensors may require careful optimization of the antibody immobilization and detection strategies to ensure optimal performance, which can be time-consuming and challenging [106]. Furthermore, antibodies may not be readily available or affordable in resource-limited settings, which can limit the widespread adoption of antibody-based biosensors for tuberculosis detection. Finally, antibody-based

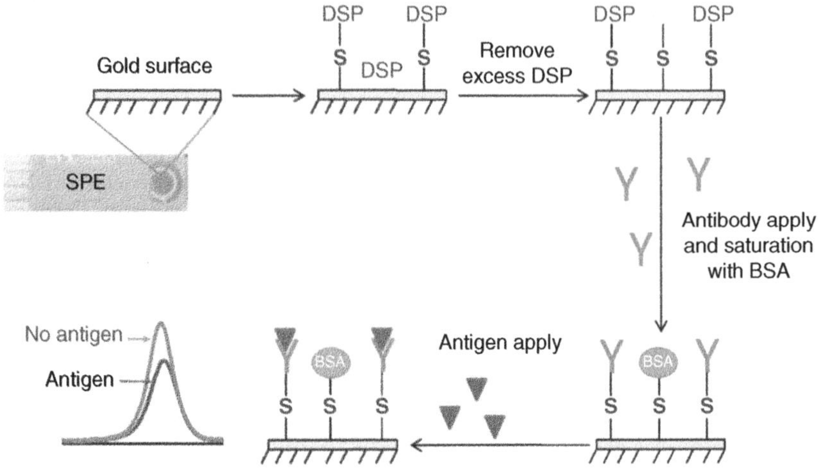

Figure 4.3 Schematic illustration of an Au screen-printed electrode and an anti-early secreted antigenic target-6 kDa protein monoclonal antibody-based ECL sensor for *M. Tuberculosis* detection. *Source:* [104]/with permission of Elsevier.

biosensors may face regulatory or logistical challenges for commercialization and deployment in clinical settings. Nonetheless, continued research and development of antibody-based biosensors for tuberculosis detection could help address these limitations and potentially improve the diagnosis and management of this global health challenge [107]. Table 4.3 lists antibody-based biosensors designed for tuberculosis detection.

4.2.3 Cardiovascular Disease

Cardiovascular biomarkers indicate the condition of heart diseases and stresses and are available inside the bloodstream [113, 114]. Tables 4.1 and 4.4 show the various biomarkers and biosensor designs related to cardiovascular diseases and their cutoff values. Troponin I is a type of protein found in muscle cells, specifically in the thin filament of skeletal and cardiovascular muscle cells. It is one of the three subunits of the troponin complex, which plays a crucial role in regulating muscle contraction. In cardiovascular muscle cells, an increase in the concentration of troponin I in the blood is a sensitive and specific marker of myocardial damage, which is why it is widely used in the diagnosis of acute myocardial infarction (heart attack). A graphene quantum dots-polyamidoamine nanohybrid-Au screen-printed electrode-based ECL sensor to detect troponin-I is shown in Figure 4.4. In this case, 4-aminothiophenol was used as a linker molecule to functionalize the Au electrode. A monoclonal anti-troponin I antibody was used for the specific detection of the analyte by measuring the change in current using

Table 4.3 Biosensor for tuberculosis detection.

Biosensor devices	LOD/Linear range	Refs.
Fe_3O_4@Ag/graphene QD-based ECL sensor	0.33 ng/ml/0.005–500 μ/ml	[98]
Graphene-and Au nano urchin-based SPR sensor	28 fM/0–10^9 fM	[108]
Ni-rGO-PANI electrode-based immunosensor	1.25 ng/ml/1–100 ng/ml	[100]
Aluminum, Polydimethylsiloxane (PDMS)-based amperometric biosensor	100 CFU/ml/10^2–10^5 CFU/ml	[109]
Padlock probes-based lateral flow nucleic acid biosensors (LFNAB)	3 ng	[110]
Au nanotubes and DNA hybridization-based ECL biosensor	0.05 ng/ml/0.01–100 ng/μl	[97]
Peptide nucleic acid, NH_2-GO, CdS QDs on carbon electrode-based ECL sensor	8.95×10^{-13} M/10^{-11}–10^{-7} M	[111]
Early secretory antigen target-6-based sensor	500 μg/ml	[112]

cyclic voltammetry and differential pulse voltammetry. A high sensitivity of 109.23 μA/cm/μg and LoD of 20 fg/ml was obtained [126].

4.2.4 Autoimmune Disease

This section discusses various reported biosensors to detect autoimmune diseases, using autoantibodies as bio-recognition elements [39]. This can lead to chronic inflammation, tissue damage, and dysfunction in various organs and systems of the body. Autoimmune diseases can affect virtually any part of the body, including the skin, joints, muscles, organs, and nerves. There are more than 80 types of autoimmune diseases, including rheumatoid arthritis, lupus, multiple sclerosis, thyroid diseases, myasthenia gravis, pernicious anemia, reactive arthritis, inflammatory bowel disease, rheumatoid arthritis, Sjogren syndrome, systemic lupus erythematosus, and type I diabetes [127]. Due to the malfunctioning of the immune system, an autoimmune disease mistakenly attacks healthy cells, tissues, and organs [4]. Platforms to detect autoimmune diseases are summarized in Table 4.5.

4.2.5 Detection of Stress Biomarkers

Stress biomarkers are measurable indicators of the physiological changes that occur in the body in response to stress. Several stress biomarkers can be detected through various methods, such as blood tests, saliva tests, and urine tests [26]. Cortisol is a hormone produced by the adrenal glands in response to stress. Cortisol levels can be measured through a blood or saliva test [138]. Adrenaline and

Table 4.4 Recently reported biosensor designs to detect the cardiovascular disease detection.

Technology	LOD	Linear range	Refs.
Graphene sheet and antibody-based ECL sensor for D-dimer detection	0.3 pg/ml	10^{-6}–10^{-3} μg/l	[115]
Peroxidase-labeled B-type natriuretic peptide antibodies on AuNPs on carbon electrodes-based ECL biosensor for B-type natriuretic peptide detection	4 pg/mL	0.014–15 ng/ml	[116]
Au-anti-cardiovascular troponin I monoclonal antibody-based SPR sensor for cardiac troponin I detection	0.12 pg/ml	0.001–8 ng/ml	[117]
Au sensor with molecularly imprinted Polymer (MIP) receptor SPR sensor for troponin T	14.8 nM	n.r.[a]	[118]
SAM of conjugated polymers and AuNPs LSPR sensor for troponin T detection	100 ng/ml	1–50 μg/ml	[119]
AuNPs self-assembled layer SPR sandwich assay for troponin T detection	0.5 ng/ml	5–400 ng/ml	[120]
GO-AuNPs and magnetic beads-based sensor for Cardiovascular troponin I detection	5 pg/ml	0.01–1000 ng/ml	[121]
Core-shell nanoparticles of Au-Ag and magnetic beads for Cardiovascular troponin I and heart-type fatty acid–binding protein detection using SERS sensor	0.6396 ng/ml 0.0044 ng/ml	0–100 ng/ml	[122]
Au@Ag core-shell NPs with MGITC Raman reporter for creatine kinase-MB and cardiac troponin I	8.9 pg/ml Troponin I 9.7 pg/ml Creatine kinase	0–100 ng/ml	[123]
Imprinted Au and fluoro-micro beads with 3–3′-dithiobis-propionic acid N-hydroxy-succinimide ester fluorescence sensor	1.4 pM	3.4 pM–3.4 nM	[124]
QD beads@SiO_2-COOH based lateral-flow immunoassay for creatine kinase-MB and cardiac troponin I	36 pg/ml	0.12–125 ng/ml	[125]

[a] not reported.

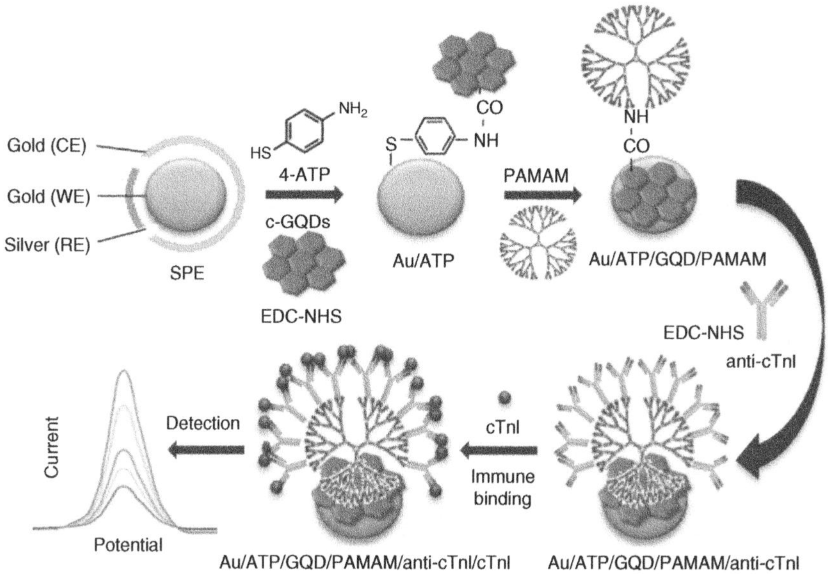

Figure 4.4 Illustration of a graphene quantum dots (GQD)-polyamidoamine nanohybrid (PAMAM)-Au screen-printed electrode-based ECL sensor to detect Troponin-I. CE, WE, and RE indicate counter, working, and reference electrodes. *Source:* [126]/with permission of Elsevier.

noradrenaline are hormones produced by the adrenal glands and the sympathetic nervous system, respectively, in response to stress. They can be detected through blood tests. C-reactive protein (CRP) is a protein that increases in the blood in response to inflammation, which can be caused by stress. CRP levels can be measured through a blood test.

Heart rate variability is a measure of the variability in the time between heartbeats, which can be affected by stress. Heart rate variation (HRV) (HRV) can be measured through an electrocardiogram (ECG) or a heart rate monitor [139, 140]. Alpha-amylase is an enzyme that is released by the salivary glands in response to stress [141, 142]. Alpha-amylase levels can be measured through a saliva test. Immunoglobulin A (IgA) is an antibody that helps protect the body against infections. Stress can lower IgA levels, which can be detected through a saliva test [143, 144]. Table 4.6 summarizes recently reported immunosensors for stress related diseases.

4.2.6 Cholesterol Disease

Cholesterol is a type of lipid that is important for the normal functioning of the body. However, high levels of cholesterol in the blood can increase the risk of cardiovascular disease. Therefore, the accurate measurement of cholesterol levels

Table 4.5 Biosensor designs to detect the autoimmune diseases.

Sensor details	LOD	Linear range	Refs.
Graphene QDs-anti-tissue transglutaminase on AuNPs with multiwalled-CNT-based ECL sensor	20 fg/ml	0–10 pg/ml	[128]
Si-TiO_2-SiO_2-Au nanostructure-based plasmonic sensor	n.r.[a]	1.45–1.49 RIU	[23]
Anti-dsDNA-based ECL sensor for α-dsDNA detection	0.8 μg/ml	0–2.5 μg/ml	[129]
GO/trimethylolpropane tris [poly (propylene glycol)]/anti-myelin basic protein/anti-tau proteins ECL nano-immuno-sensor to detect the myelin basic protein and Tau proteins	0.30 nM Myelin basic protein 0.15 nM Tau proteins	58–227 nM 0.5–15.1 nM	[130]
Nafion-film-palladium NPs on carbon electrode ECL biosensor for L-cysteine	0.15 μM	0.5–10 μM	[131]
Oxytocin-monolayer based ECL biosensor to detect the zinc and copper ions	500 fM – Copper Ions 100 fM – Zinc Ions	n.r.[a]	[132]
Cystamine SAM with fluorine-doped tin oxide electrode-based ECL biosensor to detect the α-synuclein	1130 pg/ml	10^3–10^6 pg/ml	[133]
Glycopeptide antigen CSF114-based SPR sensor for rheumatoid arthritis	n.r.[a]	31.25 nM	[134]
BK7-Cr-Au deposited with Fe_3O_4 NPs-antibody-based SPR sensor for Parkinson's α-Synuclein	5.6 fg/ml	0.01–100 pg/ml	[135]
RNA-based fluorescent biosensor to detect the cyclic guanosine monophosphate-adenosine monophosphate	0.95 μM	2.5–7.5 nM	[127]
Type 1 diabetes mellitus biomarker glutamate decarboxylase antibody and insulin autoantibody using AgNPs SERS sensor	6.5×10^{-10} g/ml 4.9×10^{-10} g/ml	10^{-9}–10^{-5} g/ml 10^{-9}–10^{-7} g/ml	[136]
Silicon photonic micro-ring resonators with antibody for miR-21 detection	10 pM	10 pM–40 nM	[137]

[a] not reported.

Table 4.6 Recently reported immunosensors for stress related diseases.

Sensor details	Stress biomarker	LOD/Linear range	Refs.
MoS_2 nanosheet with cortisol antibody-based ECL sensor	Cortisol	1 ng/ml/1–500 ng/ml	[141]
Au labeled-anti-cortisol-based fluorescent SPR sensor	Cortisol	0.02 μg/ml/0.03–0.2 μg/ml	[145]
Ferrocene tags labeled antibody, indium tin oxide.	Cortisol	1.03 pg/ml – Cortisol	[146]
(ITO) electrode-based ECL sensor	Cortisone	0.68 pg/ml – Cortisone/0–50 ng/ml	
Uncladded plastic fiber SPR sensor with Au-palladium plasmonic layer	Cortisol	1 pg/ml/0.005–10 ng/ml	[147]
AuNPs–multiwalled CNTs–PDMS-antibody-based ECL sensor	Cortisol	10^{-15} g/ml/10^{-15}–10^{-6} g/ml	[148]
MnO_2 cacti-like nanostructures on carbon electrode and antibody-based ECL sensor	Cortisol	0.023 pM/0.1–1500 pg/ml	[149]
Interleukin-6-antibody Au electrode-based ECL sensor	Interleukin-6	1.63 pg/ml/10 pg/ml–10 ng/ml	[150]
Antibody-based label free ECL immunosensor	Interleukin-6	0.088 pg/ml/1–20 pg/ml	[151]
Au electrode on needle-shaped substrate ECL immunosensor	Interleukin-6	20 pg/ml/0–25 pg/ml	[152]
3,3′-dithiobis (sulfosuccinimidyl-propionate) on screen-printed Au-electrode ECL immunosensor	Adrenocorticotropic hormone	100 fg/ml/10 pg/ml–10 fg/ml	[153]
Silica nanoparticles, glucose dehydrogenase with pyrroloquinoline quinone enzyme fluorescent biosensor	α-amylase	2 pM/0.11–0.55 μg/ml	[154]
Cysteamine SAM on Au electrodes disposable ECL sensor	α-amylase	10^{-4} mg/ml/10^{-4}–10^{-2} mg/ml	[155]
Carbon electrodes-based salivary ECL biosensor	α-amylase	1.1 U/ml/100–1200 U/ml	[156]
Zinc oxide nanocrystals with copper- and antibody-based ECL sensor	α-amylase	0.00196 U/ml	[157]
AuNP/MoS_2/AuNP and polyethylene glycol SAM on screen-printed electrode-based ECL sensor	Cortisol	0.11 nM/0.5–200 nM	[158, 159]
ZnO nanorod on flexible carbon membrane-based ECL sensor	Cortisol	10^{-15} g/ml/0^{-15}–10^{-6} g/ml	[160]

is important for the diagnosis and management of cardiovascular disease [161–163]. Despite these advancements, there are still some challenges associated with cholesterol detection using biosensors. Some of the difficulties in detection include cholesterol biosensors require a clean and well-prepared sample, which can be time-consuming and requires specialized training. The presence of other compounds in the sample, such as triglycerides or other lipids, can interfere with cholesterol detection and lead to false readings. Biosensors must be stable and reproducible over time in order to provide reliable results, which can be a challenge in some applications [41]. Cholesterol is sterol synthesized in the human cells that acts as a precursor for steroid vitamin D, hormones, and bile acids. It is important to note that these ranges may vary depending on factors such as age, sex, and other medical conditions [41]. Table 4.7 lists the details of biosensor designs for cholesterol detection.

4.2.7 Glucose Measurement

Glucose monitoring using biosensors is a widely used method for monitoring blood glucose levels in individuals with diabetes. Biosensors are devices that combine a biological component (e.g. an enzyme) with a transducer that converts the biological signal into a measurable signal (e.g. electrical or optical) [173]. There are several types of glucose biosensors available, including invasive and noninvasive options. Invasive biosensors require a small sample of blood to be taken from the patient, typically by pricking the finger with a lancet. Noninvasive biosensors use other bodily fluids, such as saliva or tears, to measure glucose levels. Glucose biosensors are an important tool for individuals with diabetes to manage their blood glucose levels and prevent complications associated with high or low blood sugar. They are also used in clinical research to study the effects of diet and exercise on glucose levels, as well as to develop new treatments for diabetes [174]. Glucose biosensors typically use an enzyme called glucose oxidase and antibodies, which react with glucose to produce hydrogen peroxide and gluconic acid. The hydrogen peroxide can then be detected using a transducer, such as a glucose meter, which measures the electrical or optical signal generated by the reaction. One type of antibody-based glucose monitoring biosensor is a competitive binding assay. In this type of biosensor, a labeled glucose molecule competes with glucose in the sample for binding to the immobilized antibody. The amount of labeled glucose that binds to the antibody is inversely proportional to the amount of glucose in the sample. The label can be detected using a transducer, such as an optical or ECL sensor [175].

Another type of antibody-based glucose monitoring biosensor is a sandwich assay. In this type of biosensor, two antibodies are used to bind glucose between them, creating a "sandwich." One antibody is immobilized on the sensor surface,

Table 4.7 Antibody-based biosensor designs for cholesterol detection.

Structure	LOD	Linear range	Refs.
CdTe/CdSe/ZnSe QDs-poly (propylene imine)-cholesterol oxidase-based ECL sensor to detect cholesterol	0.075 mM	0.1–10 mM	[164]
Fiber optic sensor to detect cholesterol	n.r.[a]	140–250 mg/dl	[163]
TiO_2-NPs and cholesterol oxidase-based ECL biosensor to detect cholesterol	4.4829 mM	3–10 mM	[165]
Streptavidin, cholesterol oxidase to detect cholesterol	n.r.[a]	125–2000 nM	[166]
3,3′,5,5′-tetramethylbenzidine hydrochloride substrate, cholesterol oxidase and chitosan nanofibers-based colorimetric sensor to detect cholesterol	50 mg/dl	50–300 mg/dl	[167]
MoS_2 nanosheets, tetramethylbenzidine cholesterol oxidase colorimetric sensor to detect cholesterol	0.76 μmol/l	2–200 μmol/l	[168]
Gallium-doped ZnO-based long-range SPR sensor to detect cholesterol	n.r.[a]	1.32–1.34 RIU	[169]
A poly(*N*-isopropylacrylamide)-co-acrylamide, glucose oxidase-based fiber sensor to detect cholesterol	11.8 mg/dl	25–250 mg/dl	[170]
AuNPs, TiO_2 nanotubes and CdS QDs to detect cholesterol	0.012 μM	0.024–1.2 mM	[171]
Au electrode, 4-aminothiophenol, B-100 antibody-based ECL sensor to detect low-density lipoprotein	0.31 ng/ml	0.01–1.0 ng/ml	[172]

[a] not reported.

while the other antibody is labeled and detects the glucose molecule. The label can be detected using a transducer, such as an optical or ECL sensor. Antibody-based glucose monitoring biosensors have several advantages over enzyme-based biosensors. They are less prone to interference from other substances in the sample, and they can detect glucose levels over a wider range. However, they are typically more expensive and require more complex fabrication than enzyme-based biosensors [176]. Table 4.8 summarizes the biosensors design for glucose detection.

4.2.8 Microbe Detection: Viruses, Bacteria, Archaea, Fungi, and Protists

Pathogenic bacteria have a small length in μm and are single-celled living microorganisms with an average diameter of 0.5–2.0 μm. These bacteria have different shapes, such as rods (bacillus), spirals (twisted), and spheres (coccus), and the ability to survive in any environment [187]. The most common pathogenic bacteria are *Mycobacterium tuberculosis, Escherichia coli (E. coli), Vibrio cholera (V. cholera), Clostridium botulinum, Streptococcus pneumonia (S. pneumonia),* and *Staphylococcus aureus (S. aureus),* which cause tuberculosis, bloody diarrhea, cholera, botulism poisoning, paralysis, pneumonia, meningitis, and skin infections [188]. Bacterial infection is classified into two categories: (i) Gram-positive (Gram+) and (ii) Gram-negative (Gram−) that depend on its cell wall structure's interaction with a purple-colored dye, known as Gram staining. Gram+ retains the purple color of the dye as it is absorbed by the outermost thick cell wall of thickness in the range of 30–100 nm made of peptidoglycan [189]. Gram− bacteria turns red or pink after interaction with dye as they contain a thin layer (less than 4 nm) of peptidoglycan protected by additional lipoproteins, phospholipids, and lipopolysaccharides. The thick peptidoglycan layer of Gram+ bacteria can absorb foreign substances such as dye and toxin easily, making it easier to kill Gram+ bacteria, but Gram− bacteria are more resistant and do not absorb external substances [190]. An antibody coated on AuNPs and SERS chips is used to detect the *L. innocua* bacteria and utilizes a neodymium magnet for the concentration of the beads. The magnet also reduces the stabilization time of the sample and can improve it by up to 35% [191]. Table 4.9 details the detection of different bacteria with various optical, ECL, and quartz crystal microbalance (QCM) sensing schemes.

4.2.9 Toxins Detection

Immuno-biosensors use antibodies to detect specific molecules, such as toxins, in a sample. Toxins are harmful substances produced by living organisms, such as bacteria, fungi, or plants, and can cause various diseases and health problems in

Table 4.8 Performance study of biosensors for glucose detection.

Sensor	Range	LOD	Refs.
Poly (toluidine blue O) and glucose oxidase-based tear ECL sensor	0.075–7.5 mmol/l	22.2 μM	[177]
Au nanowires having mushroom like structure-based ECL wearable sensor to detect the strain and glucose	0–1.15 mM	10 μM	[178]
PMMA-Au nanostructure- glucose oxidase-based ECL sensor to detect hyperglycemia/hypoglycemia	n.r.[a]	n.r.[a]	[179]
6-(ferrocenyl)hexanethiol-glucose oxidase-Au-graphene monolayer oxidase-based ECL sensor	0.0005–5000 μM	0.0001 μM	[180]
Glucose oxidase/reduced GO/Au nanorod-based ECL sensor	0.01–7 mM	3 μM	[181]
Graphene-multiwalled CNTs-AuNPs-glucose oxidase-based ECL sensor	10 μM–2 mM	4.1 μM	[182]
Au platinum NPs-reduced GO-enzyme-naflon-based ECL sensor	0–2.4 mM	5 pathobacts M	[183]
Glucose oxidase on polypyrrole-$(AuNPs\text{-}GOD)_4$-based ECL sensor	0.2–8 mM	5.6 μM	[184]
Glucose oxidase/AuNPs/graphene-based ECL sensor	0–40 mg/dl	0.3 mg/dl	[185]
Glucose oxidase-GO–SH–Au-based ECL sensor	3–9 mM	0.3194 mM	[186]

[a] not reported.

Table 4.9 Detection of different bacteria with various sensing schemes.

Biosensor structure	Analyte	Linear range	LoD	Refs.
AuNPs-antibody based SERS-sensor	*L. innocua*	10^6–10^8 CFU/ml	10^5 CFU/ml	[191]
Reduced GO-NiO antibody-based electrochemical impedance spectrum (EIS) sensor	Low density lipoprotein	0–130 mg/dl	5 mg/dl	[192]
Electro-catalytic peroxide reduction, with insulin concentration ECL sensor	Insulin	0.01–100 ng/ml	3.0 pg/ml	[193]
Au NPs nano-molecularly imprinted-based SPR sensor	Vancomycin	10–125 ng/ml	17.7 ng/ml	[194]
Tungsten oxide-vancomycin-based LSPR sensor	*S. aureus*	10^2–10^7 CFU/ml	10^2 CFU/ml	[195]
An Ag -black phosphorus-based prism SPR sensor	*Pseudomonas*	1.33–1.34 RIU	n.r.[a]	[196]
AuNPs and MoS_2 multi-core fiber LSPR-based sensor	*Shigella*	1–10^9 CFU/ml	2.30 CFU/ml	[13]
Au-based evanescent wave-based biosensor	*E. coli*	10^2 CFU/ml	10^5 CFU/ml	[197]
Aptamer-based in-line Mach-Zehnder interferometer biosensor	*E. coli*	17 000 nm/RIU	10–70 CFU/25 g	[198]
AuNPs and sialic acid-based LSPR biosensor	*S. aureus* *P. aeruginosa*	n.r.[a]	10^5 CFUμ/l	[199]
Omega-shaped polyadenine-tailed aptamer and AuNPs-based fiber-LSPR sensor	*S. typhimurium*	10^1–10^7 CFU/ml	7.4 CFU/ml	[200]
CdSe/ZnS QDs-antibodies-based fluorescent biosensor	*E. coli* *L. monocytogenes* *S. typhimurium*	n.r.[a]	10^2 CFU/ml 10^3 CFU/ml 10^3 CFU/ml	[201]
AuNPs -magnetic NPs-dithiothreitol-based fluorescence sensor	*V. cholera*	10–250 ng/ml	2.34 ng/ml	[202]
Peptide-based fluorescent biosensor	*E. coli*	n.r.[a]	10^7 CFU/ml	[203]

AuNPs and iron NPs with Sulfosuccinimidyl 4-Nmaleimidomethyl cyclohexane-1-carboxylate-based fluorescence DNA sensor	*Shigella*	10^2–10^7 CFU/ml	90 CFU/ml	[204]
Carbon QDs doping with nitrogen-doped-based fluorescence sensor	*Acinetobacter baumannii*	n.r.[a]	3.0×10^2 CFU/ml	[205]
A fluorescent biosensor using photonic crystals and DNA nano machine	*Shigella* Mercury ions *DNA*	10–10^7 CFU/ml	9 CFU/ml 22.1 ppt 31.6 fM	[206]
An integrated SERS biosensor using 4-mercaptophenylboronic acid and Ag dendrites	*S. enterica*	n.r.[a]	10^3 CFU/ml	[207]
Magnetic nanobead and peptide-based colorimetric sensor	*S. aureus*	10^5–4.1 CFU/ml	7 CFU/ml	[208]
$ZnFe_2O_4$ with reduced graphene oxide-based colorimetric aptasensor	*S. typhimurium*	11–1.10×10^5 CFU/ml	11 CFU/ml	[209]
Au and aptamer-based colorimetric aptasensor	*Cronobacter sakazakii*	10^3–10^7 CFU/ml	7.1×10^3 CFU/ml	[210]
Two-staged-colorimetric aptasensor	*C. jejuni* *C. coli*	80.0%	1.1×10^5 CFU/ml 5.6×10^5 CFU/ml	[211]
M13 phage-based colorimetric sensor	*E. coli* *P. aeruginosa* *V. cholera*, *X. campestris*	n.r.[a]	100 cells	[212]
AuNPs and CRISPR technology-based colorimetric sensor	*P. aeruginosa, Staphylococcus* *S. aureus typhimurium, L. monocytogene, Nencephalitis*	n.r.[a]	25 ng/μl	[213]
CRISPR-Cas12a and AuNPs-based colorimetric sensor	*Salmonella*	n.r.[a]	1 CFU/ml	[214]

(*Continued*)

Table 4.9 (Continued)

Biosensor structure	Analyte	Linear range	LoD	Refs.
Quadruplex structure and CRISPR-Cas12a-based colorimetric sensor	*Salmonella*	1 CFU/ml	1 CFU/ml	[215]
Two stage SELEX colorimetric aptasensor	*B. carboniphilus*	n.r.[a]	5×10^3 CFU/ml	[216]
Cascaded chirped long-period gratings interferometry immunosensor	*E. coli*	10 CFU/ml	7 CFU/ml	[217]
Long-period fiber grating interferometry-based sensor	*S. aureus*	0.478 nm/log (CFU/ml)	224 CFU/ml	[218]
Peptide aptamer-based MZI interferometry sensor	*E. coli*	17 000 nm/RIU	10 CFU/ml	[198]
Double-taper microfiber-based MZI biosensor	*S. aureus*	2731.1 nm/RIU	11 CFU/ml	[219]
Graphene nanostructure-based ECL sensor	*E. coli*	4 pF	$10–10^2$ cells/ml	[220]
Automatic microfluidic channel-based ECL sensor	*E. coli*	n.r.[a]	50 CFU/ml	[221]
Mannose/11-mercapto eleven acid-mercapto hexanol/Au-based ECL sensor	*S. typhimurium*	n.r.[a]	50 CFU/ml	[222]
Metal-organic framework (MOF) nanozyme-based sensor	*S. aureus*	n.r.[a]	6 CFU/ml	[223]
Silica NPs on polyelectrolyte multilayer on Au electrode	*E. coli*	18 μA/CFU/mL	2×10^3 CFU/ml	[224]

[a] not reported.

humans and animals. Immuno-biosensors offer a rapid, sensitive, and specific way to detect toxins in various types of samples, including food, water, and environmental samples [225].

To detect toxins using an immuno-biosensor, specific antibodies are immobilized on the surface of a transducer, such as a quartz crystal microbalance or an ECL sensor, as shown in Table 4.10. When the sample containing the toxin is introduced to the sensor, the toxin binds to the antibody, resulting in a change in the transducer signal. The magnitude of the signal change is proportional to the concentration of the toxin in the sample, allowing for quantitative detection of the toxin. There are several advantages to using immuno-biosensors for toxin detection [225]. They offer high sensitivity and specificity, allowing for the detection of toxins at low concentrations. They are also rapid and can provide results in minutes, making them useful for on-site testing. Additionally, immuno-biosensors can be easily miniaturized, making them portable and cost-effective. Immuno-biosensors have been developed to detect mycotoxins, bacterial toxins, and marine toxins. They have potential applications in food safety, environmental monitoring, and clinical diagnostics [225].

Table 4.10 Nanomaterials integrated with ECL and optical biosensors for AFB_1 detection.

Nanomaterial type	LOD	Linear range	Refs.
Single walled CNTs/CS-based ECL sensor	$0.0035\,ng^{-1}\,ml$	$0.01–100\,ng^{-1}\,ml$	[226]
PEDOT/AuNPs/ITO-based ECL sensor	$0.0045\,ng^{-1}\,ml$	$1–25\,ng^{-1}\,ml$	[227]
CS-AuNPs/Au-based ECL sensor	$0.12\,ng^{-1}\,ml$	$0.2–2.0\,ng^{-1}\,ml$	[228]
ZnS/APTES/ITO-based ECL sensor	$0.02\,ng^{-1}\,ml$	$0.25–2.0\,ng^{-1}\,ml$	[229]
GQDs/ITO-based ECL sensor	$0.003\,ng^{-1}\,ml$	$0.1–2.0\,ng^{-1}\,ml$	[226]
AuNPs/GCE-based ECL sensor	$87\,ng^{-1}\,kg$	$0.1–5.0\,\mu g^{-1}\,kg$	[230]
Au chip-based SPR sensor	2.5 ppb	16–200 ppb	[231]
AuNPs beta cyclo-dextrin-based SPR sensor	$1\,pg^{-1}\,ml$	$0.001–23.6\,ng^{-1}\,ml$	[149]
QDs-AuNPs-based SPR sensor	3.4 nM	10–400 nM	[150]
Polymer dots-AgNPs-based fluorescence sensor	0.3 pg/ml	5 pg/ml ng/ml	[151]
GO-aptamers-QDs-based fluorescence sensor	1 nM	3.2 nM–320 μM	[152]

4.3 Conclusions and Future Directions

Antibody-based biosensors have the potential to revolutionize disease detection by providing highly specific and sensitive methods for detecting disease biomarkers. The development of biosensors that can detect multiple disease biomarkers simultaneously and can provide a more comprehensive picture of a patient's health status. This can lead to earlier detection and more effective treatment of diseases. The miniaturization of biosensors can lead to the development of portable and point-of-care devices that can be used for rapid and accurate diagnosis of diseases in remote or resource-limited settings. Integration of biosensors with other technologies, such as microfluidics and nanotechnology, can further enhance their sensitivity and specificity. Antibody-based biosensors can take various forms, such as ECL, optical, and piezoelectric biosensors. Each type of biosensor has its own unique advantages and challenges associated with antibody-based biosensors. The selection of appropriate antibodies for a particular target biomarker is crucial for the sensitivity and specificity of the biosensor. However, identifying the most suitable antibody can be a challenging and time-consuming process. Antibodies can be sensitive to environmental factors such as temperature, pH, and humidity, which can affect their stability and shelf life. Maintaining the stability of antibodies is essential for the accuracy and reproducibility of the biosensor. The presence of other substances in the sample can interfere with the detection of the target biomarker and lead to false-positive or false-negative results. Sample preparation can be a time-consuming and labor-intensive process, particularly for biosensors that require extraction or purification of the target biomarker. The production and use of antibody-based biosensors can be expensive, which can limit their widespread adoption and use in resource-limited settings.

References

1 Wei, L., Luo, L., Wang, B.Z. et al. (2023). Biosensors for detection of paralytic shellfish toxins: recognition elements and transduction technologies. *Trends Food Sci. Technol.* 133 (February): 205–218. https://doi.org/10.1016/j.tifs.2023.02.012.

2 Sharma, S., Byrne, H., and O'Kennedy, R.J. (2016). Antibodies and antibody-derived analytical biosensors. *Essays Biochem.* 60 (1): 9–18. https://doi.org/10.1042/EBC20150002.

3 Pandey, P.S., Raghuwanshi, S.K., and Kumar, S. (2022). Recent advances in two-dimensional materials-based Kretschmann configuration for SPR sensors: a review. *IEEE Sens. J.* 22 (2): 1069–1080. https://doi.org/10.1109/JSEN.2021.3133007.

4 Singh, R., Kumar, S., Liu, F.Z. et al. (2020). Etched multicore fiber sensor using copper oxide and gold nanoparticles decorated graphene oxide structure for cancer cells detection. *Biosens. Bioelectron.* 168: 112557. https://doi.org/10.1016/j.bios.2020.112557.

5 Hillman, Y., Gershberg, J., Lustiger, D. et al. (2021). Monoclonal antibody-based biosensor for point-of-care detection of type III secretion system expressing pathogens. *Anal. Chem.* 93 (2): 928–935. https://doi.org/10.1021/acs.analchem.0c03621.

6 Safari, M., Moghaddam, A., Moghaddam, A.S. et al. (2022). Carbon-based biosensors from graphene family to carbon dots: a viewpoint in cancer detection. *Talanta* 258 (November): 2023. https://doi.org/10.1016/j.talanta.2023.124399.

7 Ma, C., Lu, D., Gan, H. et al. (2023). The critical experimental aspects for developing pathogen electrochemical biosensors: a lesson during the COVID-19 pandemic. *Talanta* 253 (June 2022): 124009. https://doi.org/10.1016/j.talanta.2022.124009.

8 Chiu, M.L., Goulet, D.R., Teplyakov, A., and Gilliland, G.L. (2019). Antibody structure and function: the basis for engineering therapeutics. *Antibodies* 8 (4): 55. https://doi.org/10.3390/antib8040055.

9 Steffen, U., Koeleman, C.A., Sokolova, M.V. et al. (2020). IgA subclasses have different effector functions associated with distinct glycosylation profiles. *Nat. Commun.* 11 (1): 120. https://doi.org/10.1038/s41467-019-13992-8.

10 Vidarsson, G., Dekkers, G., and Rispens, T. (2014). IgG subclasses and allotypes: from structure to effector functions. *Front. Immunol.* 5 (October): 1–17. https://doi.org/10.3389/fimmu.2014.00520.

11 Conroy, P.J., Hearty, S., Leonard, P., and O'Kennedy, R.J. (2009). Antibody production, design and use for biosensor-based applications. *Semin. Cell Dev. Biol.* 20 (1): 10–26. https://doi.org/10.1016/j.semcdb.2009.01.010.

12 Kaur, B., Kumar, S., and Kumar, B. (2022). Advances in photonic crystal fiber: sensing and supercontinuum generation applications. *Opt. Fiber Technol.* 72: 102982.

13 Kumar, S., Guo, Z., Singh, R. et al. (2021). MoS_2 Functionalized multicore fiber probes for selective detection of Shigella bacteria based on localized plasmon. *J. Lightwave Technol.* 39 (12): 4069–4081. https://doi.org/10.1109/JLT.2020.3036610.

14 Kumar, S., Wang, Z., Zhang, W. et al. (2023). Optically active nanomaterials and its biosensing applications—a review. *Biosensors* 13 (1): 85. https://doi.org/10.3390/bios13010085.

15 Kumar, R., Pal, S., Prajapati, Y.K. et al. (2022). Sensitivity improvement of a MXene- immobilized SPR sensor with Ga-doped-ZnO for biomolecules detection. *IEEE Sens. J.* 22 (7): 6536–6543. https://doi.org/10.1109/jsen.2022.3154099.

16 Kumar, V., Raghuwanshi, S.K., and Kumar, S. (2022). Advances in nanocomposite thin-film-based optical fiber sensors for environmental health monitoring – a review. *IEEE Sens. J.* 22 (15): 14696–14707. https://doi.org/10.1109/JSEN.2022.3185004.

17 Zhu, G., Wang, Y., Wang, Z. et al. (2022). Localized plasmon-based multicore fiber biosensor for acetylcholine detection. *IEEE Trans. Instrum. Meas.* 71: https://doi.org/10.1109/TIM.2021.3133335.
18 Singh, R. and Kumar, S. (2022). Cancer targeting and diagnosis: recent trends with carbon nanotubes. *Nanomaterials* 12: 2283. https://doi.org/10.3390/nano12132283.
19 Chaudhary, V.S., Kumar, D., and Kumar, S. (2021). SPR-Assisted photonic crystal fiber-based dual-wavelength single polarizing filter with improved performance. *IEEE Trans. Plasma Sci.* 49 (12): 3803–3810. https://doi.org/10.1109/TPS.2021.3126671.
20 Khatami, S.H., Karami, S., Siahkouhi, H.R. et al. (2022). Aptamer-based biosensors for Pseudomonas aeruginosa detection. *Mol. Cell. Probes* 66 (June): 101865. https://doi.org/10.1016/j.mcp.2022.101865.
21 Kaur, B., Kumar, S., and Kaushik, B.K. (2021). 2D Materials based fiber optic SPR biosensor for cancer detection at 1550 nm. *IEEE Sens. J.* 21 (21): 23957–23964.
22 Kaur, B., Kumar, S., and Kaushik, B.K. (2021). Recent advancements in optical biosensors for cancer detection. *Biosens. Bioelectron.* 197 (August 2021): 113805.
23 Sahu, S.K., Reddy, S.K., Singh, M., and Avrutin, E. (2022). Hybrid plasmonic waveguide based platform for refractive index and temperature sensing. *IEEE Photonics Technol. Lett.* 34 (18): 953–956. https://doi.org/10.1109/LPT.2022.3195666.
24 Cao, X., Chen, C., and Zhu, Q. (2023). Biosensors based on functional nucleic acids and isothermal amplification techniques. *Talanta* 253 (September 2022): 123977. https://doi.org/10.1016/j.talanta.2022.123977.
25 Byrne, B., Stack, E., Gilmartin, N., and O'Kennedy, R. (2009). Antibody-based sensors: principles, problems and potential for detection of pathogens and associated toxins. *Sensors* 9 (6): 4407–4445. https://doi.org/10.3390/s90604407.
26 Rudenko, N., Fursova, K., Shepelyakovskaya, A. et al. (2021). Antibodies as biosensors' key components: state-of-the-art in Russia 2020–2021. *Sensors* 21 (22): https://doi.org/10.3390/s21227614.
27 Singh, A., Chaudhary, S., Agarwal, A., and Verma, A.S. (2013). *Antibodies: Monoclonal and Polyclonal*. Elsevier https://doi.org/10.1016/B978-0-12-416002-6.00015-8.
28 Basu, K., Green, E.M., Cheng, Y. et al. (2019). Why recombinant antibodies—benefits and applications. *Curr. Opin. Biotechnol.* 60: 153–158. https://doi.org/10.1016/j.copbio.2019.01.012.
29 Peltomaa, R., Barderas, R., Benito-Peña, E., and Moreno-Bondi, M.C. (2022). Recombinant antibodies and their use for food immunoanalysis. *Anal. Bioanal. Chem.* 414 (1): 193–217. https://doi.org/10.1007/s00216-021-03619-7.
30 Gopalakrishnakone, P., Balali-Mood, M., Llewellyn, L., and Singh, B.R. (2015). *Biological Toxins and Bioterrorism*, 1–604. https://doi.org/10.1007/978-94-007-5869-8.

31 Kumar, S., Singh, R., Zhu, G. et al. (2020). Development of uric acid biosensor using gold nanoparticles and graphene oxide functionalized micro-ball fiber sensor probe. *IEEE Trans. Nanobiosci.* 19 (2): 173–182. https://doi.org/10.1109/TNB.2019.2958891.

32 Gangwar, R.K., Min, R., Kumar, S., and Li, X. (2021). GeO_2 doped optical fiber plasmonic sensor for refractive index detection. *Front. Phys.* 9 (October): 1–7. https://doi.org/10.3389/fphy.2021.707113.

33 Kaur, B., Kumar, S., and Kaushik, B.K. (2022). MXenes-based fiber-optic SPR sensor for colorectal cancer diagnosis. *IEEE Sens. J.* 22 (7): 6661–6668.

34 Kaushik, B.K., Singh, L., Singh, R. et al. (2020). Detection of collagen-IV using highly reflective metal nanoparticles-immobilized photosensitive optical fiber-based MZI structure. *IEEE Trans. Nanobiosci.* 19 (3): 477–484. https://doi.org/10.1109/TNB.2020.2998520.

35 Campu, A., Muresan, I., Craciun, A. et al. (2022). Cardiovascular troponin biosensor designs: current developments and remaining challenges. *Int. J. Mol. Sci.* 23: 7728.

36 Dasgupta, A. and Wahed, A. (2014). *Clinical Chemistry, Immunology and Laboratory Quality Control*. New York: Elsevier https://doi.org/10.1016/c2012-0-06507-6.

37 Maxson & Mitchell (2016). Cardiovascular biomarkers: what is and what can be. *Indian J. Cardiovasc. Dis. Women WINCARS* 176 (1): 139–148. https://doi.org/10.1055/s-0039-1679104.

38 Imas, J., Zamarreño, C.R., Zubiate, P. et al. (2020). Optical biosensors for the detection of rheumatoid arthritis (RA) biomarkers: a comprehensive review. *Sensors* 20: 6289.

39 Ghorbani, F., Abbaszadeh, H., Mehdizadeh, A., and Ebrahimi-warkiani, M. (2019). Biosensors and nanobiosensors for rapid detection of autoimmune diseases: a review. *Microchim. Acta* 186: 838.

40 Paul, A., Comabella, M., and Gandhi, R. (2019). Biomarkers in multiple sclerosis. *Cold Spring Harb. Perspect. Med.* 9 (3): 1–22. https://doi.org/10.1101/cshperspect.a029058.

41 Domínguez-Renedo, O., Navarro-Cuñado, A.M., and Alonso-Lomillo, M.A. (2023). Electrochemical devices for cholesterol detection. *J. Pharm. Biomed. Anal.* 224: 115195. https://doi.org/10.1016/j.jpba.2022.115195.

42 Singh, R., Cheng, S., Zeng, Q. et al. (2022). Synergistic anti-tumor effect of Palmitoylcarnitine and Dasatinib in liver cancer. *Livers* 2 (4): 344–360. https://doi.org/10.3390/livers2040026.

43 Sajan, S.C., Singh, A., Sharma, P.K., and Kumar, S. (2023). Silicon photonics biosensors for cancer cells detection – a review. *IEEE Sens. J.* 23 (4): 3366–3377. https://doi.org/10.1109/JSEN.2023.3235920.

44 Pollap, A. and Świt, P. (2022). Recent Advances in Sandwich SERS Immunosensors for Cancer Detection. *International Journal of Molecular Sciences* 23 (9): 4740. https://doi.org/10.3390/ijms23094740.

45 Ghosh, G. (2020). Early detection of cancer: focus on antibody coated metal and magnetic nanoparticle-based biosensors. *Sens. Int.* 1 (June): 100050. https://doi.org/10.1016/j.sintl.2020.100050.

46 Sempionatto, J.R., Lasalde-Ramírez, J.A., Mahato, K. et al. (2022). Wearable chemical sensors for biomarker discovery in the omics era. *Nat. Rev. Chem.* 6: 899–915. https://doi.org/10.1038/s41570-022-00439-w.

47 Wang, Q., Zou, L., Yang, X. et al. (2019). Direct quantification of cancerous exosomes via surface plasmon resonance with dual gold nanoparticle-assisted signal amplification. *Biosens. Bioelectron.* 135: 129–136.

48 Xia, J., Liu, Y., Ran, M. et al. (2020). The simultaneous detection of the squamous cell carcinoma antigen and cancer antigen 125 in the cervical cancer serum using nano-Ag polydopamine nanospheres in an SERS-based lateral flow immunoassay. *RSC Adv.* 10 (49): 29156–29170. https://doi.org/10.1039/d0ra05207h.

49 Heidari, R., Rashidiani, J., Abkar, M. et al. (2019). CdS nanocrystals/graphene oxide-AuNPs based electrochemiluminescence immunosensor in sensitive quantification of a cancer biomarker: p53. *Biosens. Bioelectron.* 126: 7–14. https://doi.org/10.1016/j.bios.2018.10.031.

50 Chaudhary, V.S., Kumar, D., and Kumar, S. (2023). Au-TiO_2 coated photonic crystal fiber based SPR refractometric sensor for detection of cancerous cells. *IEEE Trans. Nanobiosci.* 22 (3): 562–569. https://doi.org/10.1109/TNB.2022.3219104.

51 Lai, W., Zhou, J., Liu, Y. et al. (2015). 4MBA-labeled Ag-nanorod aggregates coated with SiO_2: synthesis, SERS activity, and biosensing applications. *Anal. Methods* 7 (20): 8832–8838. https://doi.org/10.1039/c5ay01886b.

52 Loyez, M., Lobry, M., Hassan, E.M. et al. (2021). HER2 breast cancer biomarker detection using a sandwich optical fiber assay. *Talanta* 221: 121452. https://doi.org/10.1016/j.talanta.2020.121452.

53 Wang, Q., Li, Q., Yang, X. et al. (2016). Graphene oxide-gold nanoparticles hybrids-based surface plasmon resonance for sensitive detection of microRNA. *Biosens. Bioelectron.* 77: 1001–1007. https://doi.org/10.1016/j.bios.2015.10.091.

54 Chang, C.Y., Lin, H.T., Lai, M.S. et al. (2018). Flexible localized surface plasmon resonance sensor with metal–insulator–metal nanodisks on PDMS substrate. *Sci. Rep.* 8: 11812. https://doi.org/10.1038/s41598-018-30180-8.

55 Kim, H.M., Park, J.H., and Lee, S.K. (2019). Fiber optic sensor based on ZnO nanowires decorated by Au nanoparticles for improved plasmonic biosensor. *Sci. Rep.* 9 (1): 1–9. https://doi.org/10.1038/s41598-019-52056-1.

56 Luo, Z., Wang, Y., Xu, Y. et al. (2019). Ultrasensitive U-shaped fiber optic LSPR cytosensing for label-free and in situ evaluation of cell surface N-glycan expression. *Sens. Actuators, B* 284: 582–588. https://doi.org/10.1016/j.snb.2019.01.015.

57 Sasi, S., Francis, S.M., Jacob, J., and Thomas, V.I. (2021). A tunable plasmonic refractive index sensor with ultrabroad sensing range for cancer detection. *Plasmonics* 1–13. https://doi.org/10.1007/s11468-021-01418-5.

58 Jindal, S., Sobti, S., Kumar, M. et al. (2016). Nanocavity-coupled photonic crystal waveguide as highly sensitive platform for cancer detection. *IEEE Sens. J.* 16 (10): 3705–3710. https://doi.org/10.1109/JSEN.2016.2536105.

59 Ayyanar, N., Thavasi Raja, G., Sharma, M., and Sriram Kumar, D. (2018). Photonic crystal fiber-based refractive index sensor for early detection of cancer. *IEEE Sens. J.* 18 (17): 7093–7099. https://doi.org/10.1109/JSEN.2018.2854375.

60 Jabin, M.A., Ahmed, K., Rana, M.J. et al. (2019). Surface plasmon resonance based titanium coated biosensor for cancer cell detection. *IEEE Photonics J.* 11 (4): 1. https://doi.org/10.1109/JPHOT.2019.2924825.

61 Mollah, M.A., Yousufali, M., Ankan, I.M. et al. (2020). Twin core photonic crystal fiber refractive index sensor for early detection of blood cancer. *Sens. Bio-Sens. Res.* 29: 100344. https://doi.org/10.1016/j.sbsr.2020.100344.

62 Ramanujam, N.R., Amiri, I.S., Taya, S.A. et al. (2019). Enhanced sensitivity of cancer cell using one dimensional nano composite material coated photonic crystal. *Microsyst. Technol.* 25 (1): 189–196. https://doi.org/10.1007/s00542-018-3947-6.

63 Aly, A.H. and Zaky, Z.A. (2019). Ultra-sensitive photonic crystal cancer cells sensor with a high-quality factor. *Cryogenics (Guildf)* 104: 102991. https://doi.org/10.1016/j.cryogenics.2019.102991.

64 Panda, A. and Devi, P. (2020). Photonic crystal biosensor for refractive index based cancerous cell detection. *Opt. Fiber Technol.* 54: 102123. https://doi.org/10.1016/j.yofte.2019.102123.

65 Sun, D., Ran, Y., and Wang, G. (2017). Label-free detection of cancer biomarkers using an in-line taper fiber-optic interferometer and a fiber Bragg grating. *Sensors* 17 (11): 2559. https://doi.org/10.3390/s17112559.

66 Hosseinzadeh, M., Salmani, S., and Ara, M.H.M. (2019). Interferometric optical testing to discriminate benign and malignant brain tumors. *J. Photochem. Photobiol., B* 199: 111590. https://doi.org/10.1016/j.jphotobiol.2019.111590.

67 Liu, Q., Shin, Y., Kee, J.S. et al. (2015). Mach-Zehnder interferometer (MZI) point-of-care system for rapid multiplexed detection of microRNAs in human urine specimens. *Biosens. Bioelectron.* 71: 365–372. https://doi.org/10.1016/j.bios.2015.04.052.

68 Mollah, M.A., Usha, R.J., Tasnim, S., and Ahmed, K. (2020). Detection of cancer affected cell using Sagnac interferometer based photonic crystal fiber refractive index sensor. *Opt. Quantum Electron.* 52 (9): 1–12.

69 Viphavakit, C., O'Keeffe, S., Andersson-Engels, S., and Lewis, E. (2017). Gold-coated Fabry-Perot based optical fiber sensor for monitoring hypoxic state of the tumor from the change of refractive index in red blood cells. *Proc. IEEE Sensors* 1–3. https://doi.org/10.1109/ICSENS.2017.8234124.

70 Quero, G., Consales, M., Severino, R. et al. (2016). Long period fiber grating nano-optrode for cancer biomarker detection. *Biosens. Bioelectron.* 80: 590–600. https://doi.org/10.1016/j.bios.2016.02.021.

71 Ribaut, C., Loyez, M., Larrieu, J.C. et al. (2017). Cancer biomarker sensing using packaged plasmonic optical fiber gratings: towards in vivo diagnosis. *Biosens. Bioelectron.* 92: 449–456. https://doi.org/10.1016/j.bios.2016.10.081.

72 Tyagi, D., Mishra, S.K., Zou, B. et al. (2018). Nano-functionalized long-period fiber grating probe for disease-specific protein detection. *J. Mater. Chem. B* 6 (3): 386–392. https://doi.org/10.1039/c7tb02406a.

73 Teotia, P.K. and Kaler, R.S. (2018). 1-D grating based SPR biosensor for the detection of lung cancer biomarkers using Vroman effect. *Opt. Commun.* 406: 188–191. https://doi.org/10.1016/j.optcom.2017.03.079.

74 Sun, D., Fu, Y., and Yang, Y. (2020). Label-free detection of breast cancer biomarker using silica microfiber interferometry. *Opt. Commun.* 463: 125375. https://doi.org/10.1016/j.optcom.2020.125375.

75 Nejat, M. and Nozhat, N. (2020). Multi-band MIM refractive index biosensor based on Ag-air grating with equivalent circuit and T-matrix methods in near-infrared region. *Sci. Rep.* 10 (1): 1–12. https://doi.org/10.1038/s41598-020-63459-w.

76 Xiao, P., Sun, Z., Huang, Y. et al. (2020). Development of an optical microfiber immunosensor for prostate specific antigen analysis using a high-order-diffraction long period grating. *Opt. Express* 28 (11): 15783. https://doi.org/10.1364/oe.391889.

77 Ayupova, T., Shaimerdenova, M., and Sypabekova, M. (2021). Picomolar detection of thrombin with fiber-optic ball resonator sensor using optical backscatter reflectometry. *Optik (Stuttg)* 241: 166969. https://doi.org/10.1016/j.ijleo.2021.166969.

78 Ahirwar, R. and Nahar, P. (2016). Development of a label-free gold nanoparticle-based colorimetric aptasensor for detection of human estrogen receptor alpha. *Anal. Bioanal. Chem.* 408 (1): 327–332. https://doi.org/10.1007/s00216-015-9090-7.

79 Kim, W., Lee, J., Song, S. et al. (2019). Label-free, ultra-highly sensitive and multiplexed SERS nanoplasmonic biosensor for miRNA detection using head-flocked gold nanopillar. *Analyst* 144 (5): 1768–1776. https://doi.org/10.1039/C8AN01745J.

80 Ehzari, H. and Safari, M. (2022). A sandwich-type electrochemical immunosensor using antibody-conjugated Pt-doped CdTe QDs as enzyme-free labels for sensitive HER2 detection based on a magnetic framework. *Front. Chem.* 10: 1–12. https://doi.org/10.3389/fchem.2022.881960.

81 Soleymani, J., Hasanzadeh, M., Somi, M.H. et al. (2019). Highly sensitive and specific cytosensing of HT 29 colorectal cancer cells using folic acid functionalized-KCC-1 nanoparticles. *Biosens. Bioelectron.* 132: 122–131. https://doi.org/10.1016/j.bios.2019.02.052.

82 Lai, Z., Tan, J., Wan, R. et al. (2017). An activatable aptamer-based fluorescence probe for the detection of HepG2 cells. *Oncol. Rep.* 37: 2688–2694.

83 Hahn, J., Kim, E., You, Y., and Choi, Y.J. (2019). Colorimetric switchable linker-based bioassay for ultrasensitive detection of prostate-specific antigen as a cancer biomarker. *Analyst* 144 (14): 4439–4446.

84 Miao, X., Zhu, Z., Jia, H. et al. (2020). Colorimetric detection of cancer biomarker based on enzyme enrichment and pH sensing. *Sens. Actuators, B* 320: 128435.

85 Bulbul, A.A.M., Rahaman, H., Biswas, S. et al. (2020). Design and numerical analysis of a PCF-based bio-sensor for breast cancer cell detection in the THz regime. *Sens. Bio-Sens. Res.* 30: 100388. https://doi.org/10.1016/j.sbsr.2020.100388.

86 Hlali, A., Oueslati, A., and Zairi, H. (2021). Numerical simulation of tunable terahertz graphene-based sensor for breast tumor detection. *IEEE Sens. J.* 21 (8): 9844–9851. https://doi.org/10.1109/JSEN.2021.3060326.

87 Zhou, J., Zheng, Y., Liu, J. et al. (2016). A paper-based detection method of cancer cells using the photo-thermal effect of nanocomposite. *J. Pharm. Biomed. Anal.* 117: 333–337. https://doi.org/10.1016/j.jpba.2015.09.017.

88 Song, C.Y., Yang, Y.J., Yang, B.Y. et al. (2016). An ultrasensitive SERS sensor for simultaneous detection of multiple cancer-related miRNAs. *Nanoscale* 8 (39): 17365–17373. https://doi.org/10.1039/c6nr05504d.

89 Zhang, H., Yi, Y., Zhou, C. et al. (2017). SERS detection of microRNA biomarkers for cancer diagnosis using gold-coated paramagnetic nanoparticles to capture SERS-active gold nanoparticles. *RSC Adv.* 7 (83): 52782–52793. https://doi.org/10.1039/c7ra10918k.

90 Li, J., Wang, J., Grewal, Y.S. et al. (2018). Multiplexed SERS detection of soluble cancer protein biomarkers with gold-silver alloy nanoboxes and nanoyeast single-chain variable fragments. *Anal. Chem.* 90 (17): 10377–10384. https://doi.org/10.1021/acs.analchem.8b02216.

91 Li, M., Liao, Y., Chen, B.S., and Li, M. (2019). Surface-enhanced Raman spectroscopy (SERS) nanoprobes for ratiometric detection of cancer cells. *J. Mater. Chem. B* 7 (5): 815–822. https://doi.org/10.1039/c8tb02828a.

92 Carneiro, M.C.C.G., Sousa-Castillo, A., Correa-Duarte, M.A., and Sales, M.G.F. (2019). Dual biorecognition by combining molecularly-imprinted polymer and antibody in SERS detection. Application to carcinoembryonic antigen. *Biosens. Bioelectron.* 146: 111761.

93 Fan, M., She, Q., You, R. et al. (2021). 'On-off' SERS sensor triggered by IDO for non-interference and ultrasensitive quantitative detection of IDO. *Sens. Actuators, B* 344: 130166.

94 Choi, G., Kim, E., Park, E., and Lee, J.H. (2017). A cost-effective chemiluminescent biosensor capable of early diagnosing cancer using a combination of magnetic beads and platinum nanoparticles. *Talanta* 162: 38–45. https://doi.org/10.1016/j.talanta.2016.09.061.

95 Fang, D., Pan, M., Yi, H. et al. (2019). Enhanced electrochemiluminescence of luminol-DBAE system based on self-assembled mesocrystalline hybrid for the detection of ovarian cancer marker. *Sens. Actuators, B* 286: 608–615. https://doi.org/10.1016/j.snb.2019.01.151.

96 Kaur, B., Kumar, S., and Kaushik, B.K. (2022). Antimonene, CNT and MoS_2 based SPR-fiber-optic probe for tuberculosis detection. *IEEE Sens. J.* 22 (15): 14903–14910.

97 Ramulu, S., Reddy, V., Soo, S., and Kim, C. (2016). Electrochemical biosensor for Mycobacterium tuberculosis DNA detection based on gold nanotubes array electrode platform. *Biosens. Bioelectron.* 78: 483–488. https://doi.org/10.1016/j.bios.2015.11.098.

98 Teshome, L., Oh, S., Kim, J. et al. (2018). Electrochemical immunosensor using nanotriplex of graphene quantum dots, Fe_3O_4, and Ag nanoparticles for tuberculosis. *Electrochim. Acta* 290: 369–377.

99 Aly, A.H., Mohamed, D., Zaky, Z.A. et al. (2021). Novel biosensor detection of tuberculosis based on photonic band gap materials. *Mater. Res.* 24 (3): https://doi.org/10.1590/1980-5373-MR-2020-0483.

100 Omar, R.A., Verma, N., and Arora, P.K. (2021). Development of ESAT-6 based immunosensor for the detection of Mycobacterium tuberculosis. *Front. Immunol.* 12: 1–12. https://doi.org/10.3389/fimmu.2021.653853.

101 Azmi, U.Z.M., Yusof, N.A., Abdullah, J. et al. (2021). Aptasensor for the detection of mycobacterium tuberculosis in sputum utilising cfp10-esat6 protein as a selective biomarker. *Nanomaterials* 11 (9): 1–14. https://doi.org/10.3390/nano11092446.

102 Uhuo, O.V., Waryo, T.T., Douman, S.F. et al. (2022). Bioanalytical methods encompassing label-free and labeled tuberculosis aptasensors: a review. *Anal. Chim. Acta* 1234: 340326. https://doi.org/10.1016/j.aca.2022.340326.

103 Owens, N.A., Pinter, A., and Porter, M.D. (2019). Surface-enhanced resonance Raman scattering for the sensitive detection of a tuberculosis biomarker in human serum. *J. Raman Spectrosc.* 50 (1): 15–25. https://doi.org/10.1002/jrs.5500.

104 Diouani, M.F., Ouerghi, O., Refai, A. et al. (2017). Detection of ESAT-6 by a label free miniature immuno-electrochemical biosensor as a diagnostic tool for tuberculosis. *Mater. Sci. Eng., C* 74: 465–470. https://doi.org/10.1016/j.msec.2016.12.051.

105 Arshavsky-Graham Sofia, S.E., Christopher, H., and Xin, J. (2022). Engineering in Life Sciences - 2022 - Arshavsky-Graham - Aptasensors versus immunosensors Which will prevail.pdf. [Online]. https://doi.org/10.1002/elsc.202100148

106 Sin, M.L., Mach, K.E., Wong, P.K., and Liao, J.C. (2014). Advances and challenges in biosensor-based diagnosis of infectious diseases. *Expert Rev. Mol. Diagn.* 14 (2): 225–244. https://doi.org/10.1586/14737159.2014.888313.

107 Joshi, H., Kandari, D., Maitra, S.S., and Bhatnagar, R. (2022). Biosensors for the detection of Mycobacterium tuberculosis: a comprehensive overview. *Crit. Rev. Microbiol.* 48 (6): 784–812. https://doi.org/10.1080/1040841X.2022.2035314.

108 Prabowo, B.A., Alom, A., Secario, M.K. et al. (2016). Graphene-based portable SPR sensor for the detection of Mycobacterium tuberculosis DNA strain. *Procedia Eng.* 168: 541–545. https://doi.org/10.1016/j.proeng.2016.11.520.

109 Hiraiwa, M., Kim, J.H., Lee, H.B. et al. (2015). Amperometric immunosensor for rapid detection of Mycobacterium tuberculosis. *J. Micromech. Microeng.* 25 (5): https://doi.org/10.1088/0960-1317/25/5/055013.

110 Pavankumar, A.R., Engström, A., Liu, J. et al. (2016). Proficient detection of multi-drug-resistant mycobacterium tuberculosis by padlock probes and lateral flow nucleic acid biosensors. *Anal. Chem.* 88 (8): 4277–4284. https://doi.org/10.1021/acs.analchem.5b04312.

111 Mat Zaid, M.H., Abdullah, J., Yusof, N.A. et al. (2017). PNA biosensor based on reduced graphene oxide/water soluble quantum dots for the detection of Mycobacterium tuberculosis. *Sens. Actuators, B* 241: 1024–1034. https://doi.org/10.1016/j.snb.2016.10.045.

112 Sepulveda, D., Aroca, M.A., Varela, A. et al. (2017). Bioelectrochemical detection of mycobacterium tuberculosis ESAT-6 in an antibody-based biomicrosystem. *Sensors* 17 (10): 2178. https://doi.org/10.3390/s17102178.

113 Vuillaume, L.A., Frija-Masson, J., Hadjiat, M. et al. (2022). Biosensors for the rapid detection of cardiovascular biomarkers of vital interest: needs, analysis and perspectives. *J. Pers. Med.* 12: 1942.

114 Szunerits, S., Mishyn, V., Grabowska, I., and Boukherroub, R. (2019). Electrochemical cardiovascular platforms: current state of the art and beyond. *Biosens. Bioelectron.* 131: 287–298. https://doi.org/10.1016/j.bios.2019.02.010.

115 Nikoleli, G.P., Nikolelis, D.P., Tzamtzis, N., and Psaroudakis, N. (2014). A selective immunosensor for D-dimer based on antibody immobilized on a graphene electrode with incorporated lipid films. *Electroanalysis* 26 (7): 1522–1527. https://doi.org/10.1002/elan.201400161.

116 Serafín, V., Torrente-Rodríguez, R.M., González-Cortés, A. et al. (2018). An electrochemical immunosensor for brain natriuretic peptide prepared with screen-printed carbon electrodes nanostructured with gold nanoparticles grafted through aryl diazonium salt chemistry. *Talanta* 179: 131–138. https://doi.org/10.1016/j.talanta.2017.10.063.

117 Çimen, D., Bereli, N., Günaydın, S., and Denizli, A. (2020). Detection of cardiovascular troponin-I by optic biosensors with immobilized anti-cardiovascular troponin-I monoclonal antibody. *Talanta* 219: 121259. https://doi.org/10.1016/j.talanta.2020.121259.

118 Palladino, P., Minunni, M., and Scarano, S. (2018). Cardiovascular troponin T capture and detection in real-time via epitope-imprinted polymer and optical biosensing. *Biosens. Bioelectron.* 106: 93–98. https://doi.org/10.1016/j.bios.2018.01.068.

119 Tsai, J., Chen, C.J., Ikoma, T. et al. (2011). Surface plasmon resonance biosensor with high anti-fouling ability for the detection of cardiovascular marker troponin T. *Anal. Chim. Acta* 703 (1): 80–86. https://doi.org/10.1016/j.aca.2011.07.019.

120 Pawula, M., Altintas, Z., and Tothill, I.E. (2016). SPR detection of cardiovascular troponin T for acute myocardial infarction. *Talanta* 146: 823–830. https://doi.org/10.1016/j.talanta.2015.06.006.

121 Fu, X., Wang, Y., Liu, Y. et al. (2019). A graphene oxide/gold nanoparticle-based amplification method for SERS immunoassay of cardiovascular troponin I. *Analyst* 144: 1582–1589. https://doi.org/10.1039/c8an02022a.

122 Cunming, H., Ma, L., Guan, M. et al. (2020). SERS-based magnetic immunoassay for simultaneous detection of cTnI and H-FABP using. *Anal. Methods* 5442–5449. https://doi.org/10.1039/d0ay01564d.

123 Cheng, Z., Wang, R., Xing, Y., and Fabiao, Y. (2019). SERS-based immunoassay using gold-patterned array chips for rapid and sensitive detection of dual cardiovascular biomarkers. *Analyst* 144 (22): 6533. https://doi.org/10.1039/c9an01260e.

124 Yeon, S., Duk, Y., Kim, K. et al. (2011). A fluoro-microbead guiding chip for simple and quantifiable immunoassay of cardiovascular troponin I (cTnI). *Biosens. Bioelectron.* 26 (9): 3818–3824. https://doi.org/10.1016/j.bios.2011.02.036.

125 Li, J., Lv, Y., Li, N. et al. (2021). Chemical dual protecting encapsulation synthesis of ultrastable quantum-dot nanobeads for sensitive and accurate detection of cardiovascular biomarkers. *Sens. Actuators, B* 344: 130275. https://doi.org/10.1016/j.snb.2021.130275.

126 Bhatnagar, D., Kaur, I., and Kumar, A. (2017). Ultrasensitive cardiovascular troponin I antibody based nanohybrid sensor for rapid detection of human heart attack. *Int. J. Biol. Macromol.* 95: 505–510. https://doi.org/10.1016/j.ijbiomac.2016.11.037.

127 Bose, D., Su, Y., Marcus, A. et al. (2016). An RNA-based fluorescent biosensor for high-throughput analysis of the cGAS-cGAMP-STING pathway. *Cell Chem. Biol.* 23 (12): 1539–1549. https://doi.org/10.1016/j.chembiol.2016.10.014.

128 Gupta, S., Kaushal, A., Kumar, A., and Kumar, D. (2017). Ultrasensitive transglutaminase based nanosensor for early detection of celiac disease in human. *Int. J. Biol. Macromol.* 105: 905–911. https://doi.org/10.1016/j.ijbiomac.2017.07.126.

129 Fagúndez, P., Brañas, G., Cairoli, E. et al. (2018). An electrochemical biosensor for rapid detection of anti-dsDNA antibodies in absolute scale. *Analyst* 143 (16): 3874–3882. https://doi.org/10.1039/c8an00020d.

130 Derkus, B., Acar Bozkurt, P., Tulu, M. et al. (2017). Simultaneous quantification of myelin basic protein and Tau proteins in cerebrospinal fluid and serum of multiple sclerosis patients using nanoimmunosensor. *Biosens. Bioelectron.* 89: 781–788. https://doi.org/10.1016/j.bios.2016.10.019.

131 Yusoff, N., Rameshkumar, P., Mohamed Noor, A., and Huang, N.M. (2018). Amperometric determination of L-cysteine using a glassy carbon electrode modified with palladium nanoparticles grown on reduced graphene oxide in a

Nafion matrix. *Microchim. Acta* 185 (4): 246. https://doi.org/10.1007/s00604-018-2782-x.

132 Tadi, K.K., Alshanski, I., Mervinetsky, E. et al. (2017). Oxytocin-monolayer-based impedimetric biosensor for zinc and copper ions. *ACS Omega* 2 (12): 8770–8778. https://doi.org/10.1021/acsomega.7b01404.

133 Ge, C.-Y., Rahman, M.M., Zhang, W. et al. (2020). An electrochemical immunosensor based on a self-assembled monolayer modified electrode for label-free detection of α-Synuclein. *Sensors* 20: 317.

134 Real-fernández, F., Passalacqua, I., Peroni, E. et al. (2012). Glycopeptide-based antibody detection in multiple sclerosis by surface plasmon resonance. *Sensors* 114: 5596–5607. https://doi.org/10.3390/s120505596.

135 Husin, S., Liu, T.J., Chen, C.M. et al. (2021). Enhanced plasmonic biosensor utilizing paired antibody and label-free Fe_3O_4 nanoparticles for highly sensitive and selective detection of Parkinson's α -synuclein in serum. *Biosensors* 11 (402): 1–17.

136 Wang, J., Zhao, J., Liu, Y. et al. (2023). SERS-based detection of early Type 1 diabetes mellitus biomarkers: glutamate decarboxylase antibody and insulin autoantibody. *Sens. Actuators, B* 381: 133456. https://doi.org/10.1016/j.snb.2023.133456.

137 Qavi, A.J., Kindt, J.T., Gleeson, M.A., and Bailey, R.C. (2011). Anti-DNA:RNA antibodies and silicon photonic microring resonators: increased sensitivity for multiplexed microRNA detection. *Anal. Chem.* 83 (15): 5949–5956. https://doi.org/10.1021/ac201340s.

138 Mugo, S.M. and Alberkant, J. (2020). Flexible molecularly imprinted electrochemical sensor for cortisol monitoring in sweat. *Anal. Bioanal. Chem.* 412 (8): 1825–1833. https://doi.org/10.1007/s00216-020-02430-0.

139 Parlak, O., Keene, S.T., Marais, A. et al. (2018). Molecularly selective nanoporous membrane-based wearable organic electrochemical device for noninvasive cortisol sensing. *Sci. Adv.* 4 (7): eaar2904. https://doi.org/10.1126/sciadv.aar2904.

140 Bhardwaj, V., Srinivasan, S., Dua, R., and McGoron, A.J. (2013). SERS biosensor for label free monitoring of environmental stress. *Proc. - 29th South. Biomed. Eng. Conf. SBEC 2013*, 79–80. http://dx.doi.org/10.1109/SBEC.2013.48.

141 Kinnamon, D., Ghanta, R., Lin, K.C. et al. (2017). Portable biosensor for monitoring cortisol in low-volume perspired human sweat. *Sci. Rep.* 7 (1): 1–13. https://doi.org/10.1038/s41598-017-13684-7.

142 Singh, S.A., Kumar Gupta, P., Rajeshwari, M., and Janumala, T. (2018). Detection of stress using biosensors. *Mater. Today Proc.* 5 (10): 21003–21010. https://doi.org/10.1016/j.matpr.2018.06.492.

143 Samson, C. and Koh, A. (2020). Stress monitoring and recent advancements in wearable biosensors. *Front. Bioeng. Biotechnol.* 8 (September): 1–8. https://doi.org/10.3389/fbioe.2020.01037.

144 Wu, J.Y., Ching, C.T.S., Wang, H.M.D., and De Liao, L. (2022). Emerging wearable biosensor technologies for stress monitoring and their real-world applications. *Biosensors* 12 (12): https://doi.org/10.3390/bios12121097.

145 Safarian, S.M., Kusov, P.A., Kosolobov, S.S. et al. (2021). Surface-specific washing-free immunosensor for time-resolved cortisol monitoring. *Talanta* 225: 122070. https://doi.org/10.1016/j.talanta.2020.122070.

146 Abdulsattar, J.O., Greenway, G.M., and Wadhawan, J.D. (2020). Electrochemical immunoassay for the detection of stress biomarkers. *Heliyon* 6 (3): e03558. https://doi.org/10.1016/j.heliyon.2020.e03558.

147 Leitão, C., Leal-Junior, A., Almeida, A.R. et al. (2021). Cortisol AuPd plasmonic unclad POF biosensor. *Biotechnol. Rep.* 29: e00587. https://doi.org/10.1016/j.btre.2021.e00587.

148 Liu, Q., Shi, W., Tian, L. et al. (2021). Preparation of nanostructured PDMS film as flexible immunosensor for cortisol analysis in human sweat. *Anal. Chim. Acta* 1184: 339010. https://doi.org/10.1016/j.aca.2021.339010.

149 Zhou, Q., Kannan, P., Natarajan, B. et al. (2020). MnO_2 cacti-like nanostructured platform powers the enhanced electrochemical immunobiosensing of cortisol. *Sens. Actuators, B* 317: 128134. https://doi.org/10.1016/j.snb.2020.128134.

150 Oh, C., Park, B., Li, C. et al. (2021). Electrochemical immunosensing of Interleukin-6 in human cerebrospinal fluid and human serum as an early biomarker for traumatic brain injury. *ACS Meas. Sci. Au* 1 (2): 65–73. https://doi.org/10.1021/acsmeasuresciau.1c00013.

151 Cruz, A., Vieira, M., Mesquita, A.R. et al. (2022). Non-invasive diagnosis and monitoring tool of children's mental health: a point-of-care immunosensor for IL-6 quantification in saliva samples. *Front. Neurosci.* 16: 1–10. https://doi.org/10.3389/fnins.2022.919551.

152 Russell, C., Ward, A.C., Vezza, V. et al. (2019). Development of a needle shaped microelectrode for electrochemical detection of the sepsis biomarker interleukin-6 (IL-6) in real time. *Biosens. Bioelectron.* 126: 806–814. https://doi.org/10.1016/j.bios.2018.11.053.

153 Li, N., Larin, E.M., and Kerman, K. (2017). A miniaturized impedimetric immunosensor for the competitive detection of adrenocorticotropic hormone. *Sensors* 17: 2836.

154 Wells, P.K., Smutok, O., Guo, Z. et al. (2023). Fluorometric biosensing of α-amylase using an artificial allosteric biosensor immobilized on nanostructured interface. *Talanta* 255: 124215. https://doi.org/10.1016/j.talanta.2022.124215.

155 Rebelo, T.S.C.R., Miranda, I.M., Brandão, A.T. et al. (2021). A disposable saliva electrochemical MIP-based biosensor for detection of the stress biomarker α-amylase in point-of-care applications. *Electrochem* 2 (3): 427–438. https://doi.org/10.3390/electrochem2030028.

156 Garcia, P.T., Guimarães, L.N., Dias, A.A. et al. (2018). Amperometric detection of salivary A-amylase on screen-printed carbon electrodes as a simple and inexpensive alternative for point-of-care testing. *Sens. Actuators, B* 258: 342–348. https://doi.org/10.1016/j.snb.2017.11.068.

157 Martins, B.R., Sampaio, T.M., de Farias, A.K.S.R. et al. (2021). Immunosensor based on zinc oxide nanocrystals decorated with copper for the electrochemical detection of human salivary alpha-amylase. *Micromachines* 12 (6): 657. https://doi.org/10.3390/mi12060657.

158 Ronkainen, N.J. and Okon, S.L. (2014). Nanomaterial-based electrochemical immunosensors for clinically significant biomarkers. *Materials* 4669–4709. https://doi.org/10.3390/ma7064669.

159 Liu, J., Xu, N., Men, H. et al. (2020). Salivary cortisol determination on smartphone-based differential pulse. *Sensors* 20 (5): 1422.

160 Madhu, S., Anthuuvan, A.J., Ramasamy, S. et al. (2020). ZnO Nanorod integrated flexible carbon fibers for sweat cortisol detection. *ACS Appl. Electron. Mater.* 2 (2): 499–509. https://doi.org/10.1021/acsaelm.9b00730.

161 Alagappan, M., Immanuel, S., Sivasubramanian, R., and Kandaswamy, A. (2020). Development of cholesterol biosensor using Au nanoparticles decorated f-MWCNT covered with polypyrrole network. *Arabian J. Chem.* 13 (1): 2001–2010. https://doi.org/10.1016/j.arabjc.2018.02.018.

162 Batra, B., Narwal, V., Sumit, J.A., and Sharma, M. (2021). An amperometric cholesterol biosensor based on immobilization of cholesterol oxidase onto titanium dioxide nanoparticles. *Sens. Int.* 2 (June): 100111. https://doi.org/10.1016/j.sintl.2021.100111.

163 Kane, S.N., Mishra, A., and Dutta, A.K. (2016). Preface: international conference on recent trends in physics (ICRTP 2016). *J. Phys. Conf. Ser.* 755 (1): https://doi.org/10.1088/1742-6596/755/1/011001.

164 Mokwebo, K.V., Oluwafemi, O.S., and Arotiba, O.A. (2018). An electrochemical cholesterol biosensor based on a CdTe/CdSe/znse quantum dots-poly (propylene imine) dendrimer nanocomposite immobilisation layer. *Sensors* 18 (10): 1–16. https://doi.org/10.3390/s18103368.

165 Narwal, V., Batra, B., Kalra, V. et al. (2021). An amperometric cholesterol biosensor based on immobilization of cholesterol oxidase onto titanium dioxide nanoparticles. *Sens. Bio-Sens. Res.* 33: 100436. https://doi.org/10.1016/j.sbsr.2021.100436.

166 He, P., Faris, S., Sagabala, R.S. et al. (2022). Cholesterol chip for the study of cholesterol–protein interactions using SPR. *Biosensors* 12 (10): 1–9. https://doi.org/10.3390/bios12100788.

167 Dhawane, M., Deshpande, A., Jain, R., and Dandekar, P. (2019). Colorimetric point-of-care detection of cholesterol using chitosan nanofibers. *Sens. Actuators, B* 281 (April 2018): 72–79. https://doi.org/10.1016/j.snb.2018.10.060.

168 Lin, T., Zhong, L., Chen, H. et al. (2017). A sensitive colorimetric assay for cholesterol based on the peroxidase-like activity of MoS_2 nanosheets. *Microchim. Acta* 184 (4): 1233–1237. https://doi.org/10.1007/s00604-017-2147-x.

169 Ruan, B., You, Q., Zhu, J. et al. (2018). Improving the performance of an SPR biosensor using long-range surface plasmon of ga-doped zinc oxide. *Sensors* 18 (7): https://doi.org/10.3390/s18072098.

170 Huang, J., Liu, Y., Zhang, P. et al. (2017). A temperature-triggered fiber optic biosensor based on hydrogel-magnetic immobilized enzyme complex for sequential determination of cholesterol and glucose. *Biochem. Eng. J.* 125: 123–128. https://doi.org/10.1016/j.bej.2017.06.002.

171 Khaliq, N., Rasheed, M.A., Khan, M. et al. (2021). Voltage-switchable biosensor with gold nanoparticles on TiO_2 nanotubes decorated with CdS quantum dots for the detection of cholesterol and H_2O_2. *ACS Appl. Mater. Interfaces* 13 (3): 3653–3668. https://doi.org/10.1021/acsami.0c19979.

172 Rudewicz-Kowalczyk, D. and Grabowska, I. (2021). Detection of low density lipoprotein—comparison of electrochemical immuno-and aptasensor. *Sensors* 21 (22): 7733. https://doi.org/10.3390/s21227733.

173 Tang, L., Chang, S.J., Chen, C.J., and Liu, J.T. (2020). Non-invasive blood glucose monitoring technology: a review. *Sensors (Switzerland)* 20 (23): 1–32. https://doi.org/10.3390/s20236925.

174 Li, D. (2015). Comparison of cultural backgrounds of Chinese and western cyberliterature. *Theory Pract. Lang. Stud.* 5 (2): 421. https://doi.org/10.17507/tpls.0502.25.

175 Mohammadpour-Haratbar, A., Mohammadpour-Haratbar, S., Zare, Y. et al. (2022). A review on non-enzymatic electrochemical biosensors of glucose using carbon nanofiber nanocomposites. *Biosensors* 12 (11): https://doi.org/10.3390/bios12111004.

176 Peng, Z., Xie, X., Tan, Q. et al. (2022). Blood glucose sensors and recent advances: a review. *J. Innovative Opt. Health Sci.* 15 (2): https://doi.org/10.1142/S1793545822300038.

177 Agustini, D., Bergamini, M.F., and Marcolino-Junior, L.H. (2017). Tear glucose detection combining microfluidic thread based device, amperometric biosensor and microflow injection analysis. *Biosens. Bioelectron.* 98: 161–167. https://doi.org/10.1016/j.bios.2017.06.035.

178 Zhai, Q., Gong, S., Wang, Y. et al. (2019). Enokitake mushroom-like standing gold nanowires toward wearable noninvasive bimodal glucose and strain sensing. *ACS Appl. Mater. Interfaces* 11 (10): 9724–9729. https://doi.org/10.1021/acsami.8b19383.

179 Chen, Y., Lu, S., Zhang, S. et al. (2017). Skin-like biosensor system via electrochemical channels for noninvasive blood glucose monitoring. *Sci. Adv.* 3 (12): 1–8. https://doi.org/10.1126/sciadv.1701629.

180 Yuan, Y., Wang, Y., Wang, H., and Hou, S. (2019). Gold nanoparticles decorated on single layer graphene applied for electrochemical ultrasensitive glucose biosensor. *J. Electroanal. Chem.* 855: 113495. https://doi.org/10.1016/j.jelechem.2019.113495.

181 Mazaheri, M., Simchi, A., and Aashuri, H. (2018). Enzymatic biosensing by covalent conjugation of enzymes to 3D-networks of graphene nanosheets on arrays of vertically aligned gold nanorods: application to voltammetric glucose sensing. *Microchim. Acta* 185 (3): https://doi.org/10.1007/s00604-018-2722-9.

182 Devasenathipathy, R., Mani, V., Chen, S.M. et al. (2015). Glucose biosensor based on glucose oxidase immobilized at gold nanoparticles decorated graphene-carbon nanotubes. *Enzyme Microb. Technol.* 78: 40–45. https://doi.org/10.1016/j.enzmictec.2015.06.006.

183 Xuan, X., Yoon, H.S., and Park, J.Y. (2018). A wearable electrochemical glucose sensor based on simple and low-cost fabrication supported micro-patterned reduced graphene oxide nanocomposite electrode on flexible substrate. *Biosens. Bioelectron.* 109: 75–82. https://doi.org/10.1016/j.bios.2018.02.054.

184 Wu, B., Hou, S., Xue, Y., and Chen, Z. (2018). Electrodeposition–assisted assembled multilayer films of gold nanoparticles and glucose oxidase onto polypyrrole-reduced graphene oxide matrix and their electrocatalytic activity toward glucose. *Nanomaterials* 8 (12): https://doi.org/10.3390/nano8120993.

185 Pu, Z., Wang, R., Xu, K. et al. (2015). *A Flexible Electrochemical Sensor Modified by Graphene and AuNPs for Continuous Glucose Monitoring*, 1–4. *IEEE SENSORS – Proc* https://doi.org/10.1109/ICSENS.2015.7370301.

186 Akhtar, M.A., Batool, R., Hayat, A. et al. (2019). Functionalized graphene oxide bridging between enzyme and Au-sputtered screen-printed interface for glucose detection. *ACS Appl. Nano Mater.* 2 (3): 1589–1596. https://doi.org/10.1021/acsanm.9b00041.

187 Samota, S., Rani, R., Chakraverty, S., and Kaushik, A. (2022). Biosensors for simplistic detection of pathogenic bacteria: a review with special focus on field-effect transistors. *Mater. Sci. Semicond. Process.* 141 (August 2021): 106404. https://doi.org/10.1016/j.mssp.2021.106404.

188 Ali, Q., Zheng, H., Rao, M.J. et al. (2022). Advances, limitations, and prospects of biosensing technology for detecting phytopathogenic bacteria. *Chemosphere* 296: 133773. https://doi.org/10.1016/j.chemosphere.2022.133773.

189 Silhavy, T.J., Kahne, D., and Walker, S. (2010). The bacterial cell envelope. *Cold Spring Harb Perspect Biol* 2: 1–16. https://www.ncbi.nlm.nih.gov/pmc/articles/PMC2857177/pdf/cshperspect-PRK-a000414.pdf.

190 Cani, P.D. (2018). Human gut microbiome: hopes, threats and promises. *Gut* 67 (9): 1716–1725. https://doi.org/10.1136/gutjnl-2018-316723.

191 Uusitalo, S., Kögler, M., Välimaa, A.L. et al. (2017). Stability optimization of microbial surface-enhanced Raman spectroscopy detection with immunomagnetic separation beads. *Opt. Eng.* 56 (3): 037102. https://doi.org/10.1117/1.oe.56.3.037102.

192 Ali, M.A., Singh, C., Mondal, K. et al. (2016). Mesoporous few-layer graphene platform for affinity biosensing application. *ACS Appl. Mater. Interfaces* 8 (12): 7646–7656. https://doi.org/10.1021/acsami.5b12460.

193 Gao, Z., Li, Y., Zhang, C. et al. (2019). Label-free electrochemical immunosensor for insulin detection by high-efficiency synergy strategy of Pd NPs@3D MoS_x towards H_2O_2. *Biosens. Bioelectron.* 126: 108–114. https://doi.org/10.1016/j.bios.2018.10.017.

194 Altintas, Z. (2018). Surface plasmon resonance based sensor for the detection of glycopeptide antibiotics in milk using rationally designed nanoMIPs. *Sci. Rep.* 8 (1): 1–12. https://doi.org/10.1038/s41598-018-29585-2.

195 Singh, S., Moudgil, N., Mishra, N. et al. (2019). Vancomycin functionalized WO_3 thin film-based impedance sensor for efficient capture and highly selective detection of gram-positive bacteria. *Biosens. Bioelectron.* 136: 23–30.

196 Vasimalla, Y., Pradhan, H.S., and Pandya, R.J. (2021). Sensitivity enhancement of the SPR biosensor for Pseudomonas bacterial detection employing a silicon-barium titanate structure. *Appl. Opt.* 60 (19): 5588. https://doi.org/10.1364/ao.427499.

197 Petrovszki, D., Valkai, S., Gora, E. et al. (2021). An integrated electro-optical biosensor system for rapid, low-cost detection of bacteria. *Microelectron. Eng.* 239: 111523. https://doi.org/10.1016/j.mee.2021.111523.

198 Janik, M., Brzozowska, E., Czyszczoń, P. et al. (2021). Optical fiber aptasensor for label-free bacteria detection in small volumes. *Sens. Actuators, B* 330: 129316. https://doi.org/10.1016/j.snb.2020.129316.

199 Landa, G., Miranda-Calderon, L.G., Sebastian, V. et al. (2021). Selective point-of-care detection of pathogenic bacteria using sialic acid functionalized gold nanoparticles. *Talanta* 234: 122644. https://doi.org/10.1016/j.talanta.2021.122644.

200 Li, Y., Wang, X., Ning, W. et al. (2022). Sandwich method-based sensitivity enhancement of Ω-shaped fiber optic LSPR for time-flexible bacterial detection. *Biosens. Bioelectron.* 201: 113911. https://doi.org/10.1016/j.bios.2021.113911.

201 Xu, L., Lu, Z., Cao, L. et al. (2017). In-field detection of multiple pathogenic bacteria in food products using a portable fluorescent biosensing system. *Food Control* 75: 21–28. https://doi.org/10.1016/j.foodcont.2016.12.018.

202 Narmani, A., Kamali, M., Amini, B. et al. (2018). Highly sensitive and accurate detection of Vibrio cholera O1 OmpW gene by fluorescence DNA biosensor based on gold and magnetic nanoparticles. *Process Biochem.* 65: 46–54. https://doi.org/10.1016/j.procbio.2017.10.009.

203 Jeong, W.j., Choi, S.H., Lee, H.s., and Lim, Y.b. (2019). A fluorescent supramolecular biosensor for bacterial detection via binding-induced changes in coiled-coil molecular assembly. *Sens. Actuators, B* 290: 93–99. https://doi.org/10.1016/j.snb.2019.03.112.

204 Elahi, N., Kamali, M., Baghersad, M.H., and Amini, B. (2019). A fluorescence Nano-biosensors immobilization on iron (MNPs) and gold (AuNPs) nanoparticles for detection of Shigella spp. *Mater. Sci. Eng., C* 105: 110113. https://doi.org/10.1016/j.msec.2019.110113.

205 Bahari, D., Babamiri, B., Salimi, A., and Salimizand, H. (2021). Ratiometric fluorescence resonance energy transfer aptasensor for highly sensitive and selective detection of Acinetobacter baumannii bacteria in urine sample using carbon dots as optical nanoprobes. *Talanta* 221 (June 2020): 121619. https://doi.org/10.1016/j.talanta.2020.121619.

206 Wu, M., Zhang, C., Tian, Z. et al. (2022). A universal array platform for ultrasensitive, high-throughput and microvolume detection of heavy metal, nucleic acid and bacteria based on photonic crystals combined with DNA nanomachine. *Biosens. Bioelectron.* 197: 113731. https://doi.org/10.1016/j.bios.2021.113731.

207 Panxue, W., Pang, S., Pearson, B. et al. (2017). Rapid concentration detection and differentiation of bacteria in skimmed milk using surface enhanced Raman scattering mapping on 4-mercaptophenylboronic acid functionalized silver dendrites. *Anal. Bioanal. Chem.* 409 (8): 2229–2238. https://doi.org/10.1007/s00216-016-0167-8.

208 Suaifan, G.A.R.Y., Alhogail, S., and Zourob, M. (2017). Rapid and low-cost biosensor for the detection of Staphylococcus aureus. *Biosens. Bioelectron.* 90: 230–237. https://doi.org/10.1016/j.bios.2016.11.047.

209 Wu, S., Duan, N., Qiu, Y. et al. (2017). Colorimetric aptasensor for the detection of Salmonella enterica serovar typhimurium using $ZnFe_2O_4$-reduced graphene oxide nanostructures as an effective peroxidase mimetics. *Int. J. Food Microbiol.* 261: 42–48. https://doi.org/10.1016/j.ijfoodmicro.2017.09.002.

210 Kim, H.S., Kim, Y.J., Chon, J.W. et al. (2017). Two-stage label-free aptasensing platform for rapid detection of Cronobacter sakazakii in powdered infant formula. *Sens. Actuators, B* 239: 94–99. https://doi.org/10.1016/j.snb.2016.07.173.

211 Kim, Y.J., Kim, H.S., Chon, J.W. et al. (2018). New colorimetric aptasensor for rapid on-site detection of Campylobacter jejuni and Campylobacter coli in chicken carcass samples. *Anal. Chim. Acta* 1029: 78–85. https://doi.org/10.1016/j.aca.2018.04.059.

212 Peng, H. and Chen, I.A. (2019). Rapid colorimetric detection of bacterial species through the capture of gold nanoparticles by chimeric phages. *ACS Nano* 13 (2): 1244–1252. https://doi.org/10.1021/acsnano.8b06395.

213 Yuan, C., Tian, T., Sun, J. et al. (2020). Universal and naked-eye gene detection platform based on the clustered regularly interspaced short palindromic repeats/Cas12a/13a system. *Anal. Chem.* 92 (5): 4029–4037. https://doi.org/10.1021/acs.analchem.9b05597.

214 Ma, L., Peng, L., Yin, L. et al. (2021). CRISPR-Cas12a-powered dual-mode biosensor for ultrasensitive and cross-validating detection of pathogenic bacteria. *ACS Sens.* 6 (8): 2920–2927. https://doi.org/10.1021/acssensors.1c00686.

215 Yin, L., Duan, N., Chen, S. et al. (2021). Ultrasensitive pathogenic bacteria detection by a smartphone-read G-quadruplex-based CRISPR-Cas12a bioassay. *Sens. Actuators, B* 347: 130586. https://doi.org/10.1016/j.snb.2021.130586.

216 Kim, H.K., Kim, H.R., Yoon, S.J. et al. (2021). Colorimetric aptasensor for detecting bacillus carboniphilus using aptamer isolated with a non-selex-based method. *Chemosensors* 9 (6): 121. https://doi.org/10.3390/chemosensors9060121.

217 Kaushik, S., Tiwari, U., Nilima, S. et al. (2019). Label-free detection of Escherichia coli bacteria by cascaded chirped long period gratings immunosensor. *Rev. Sci. Instrum.* 90 (2): https://doi.org/10.1063/1.5036693.

218 Yang, F., Chang, T.L., Liu, T. et al. (2019). Label-free detection of Staphylococcus aureus bacteria using long-period fiber gratings with functional polyelectrolyte coatings. *Biosens. Bioelectron.* 133: 147–153. https://doi.org/10.1016/j.bios.2019.03.024.

219 Li, H.C., Leng, Y.K., Liao, Y.C. et al. (2022). Tapered microfiber MZI biosensor for highly sensitive detection of staphylococcus aureus. *IEEE Sens. J.* 22 (6): 5531–5539. https://doi.org/10.1109/JSEN.2022.3149004.

220 Pandey, A., Gurbuz, Y., Ozguz, V. et al. (2017). Graphene-interfaced electrical biosensor for label-free and sensitive detection of foodborne pathogenic E. coli O157:H7. *Biosens. Bioelectron.* 91: 225–231. https://doi.org/10.1016/j.bios.2016.12.041.

221 Luis, F. and Moncayo, G. (2018). A fully automated microfluidic-based electrochemical sensor for real-time bacteria detection. *Biosens. Bioelectron.* 100: 541–548.

222 Cui, F., Xu, Y., Wang, R. et al. (2018). Label-free impedimetric glycan biosensor for quantitative evaluation interactions between pathogenic bacteria and mannose. *Biosens. Bioelectron.* 103: 94–98. https://doi.org/10.1016/j.bios.2017.11.068.

223 Hu, W.C., Pang, J., Biswas, S. et al. (2021). Ultrasensitive detection of bacteria using a 2D MOF Nanozyme-amplified electrochemical detector. *Anal. Chem.* 93 (24): 8544–8552. https://doi.org/10.1021/acs.analchem.1c01261.

224 Mathelié-Guinlet, M., Cohen-Bouhacina, T., Gammoudi, I. et al. (2019). Silica nanoparticles-assisted electrochemical biosensor for the rapid, sensitive and specific detection of *Escherichia coli*. *Sens. Actuators, B* 292 (April): 314–320. https://doi.org/10.1016/j.snb.2019.03.144.

225 Bhardwaj, H., Rajesh, and Sumana, G. (2022). Recent advances in nanomaterials integrated immunosensors for food toxin detection. *J. Food Sci. Technol.* 59 (1): 12–33. https://doi.org/10.1007/s13197-021-04999-5.

226 Zhang, X. et al. (2016). A novel electrochemical immunosensor for highly sensitive detection of aflatoxin B1 in corn using single-walled carbon nanotubes/chitosan. *Food Chem.* 192: 197–202. https://doi.org/10.1016/j.foodchem.2015.06.044.

227 Sharma, A., Kumar, A., and Khan, R. (2017). Electrochemical immunosensor based on poly (3,4-ethylenedioxythiophene) modified with gold nanoparticle to detect aflatoxin B1. *Mater. Sci. Eng., C* 76: 802–809. https://doi.org/10.1016/j.msec.2017.03.146.

228 Ma, H., Sun, J., Zhang, Y. et al. (2016). Label-free immunosensor based on one-step electrodeposition of chitosan-gold nanoparticles biocompatible film on Au microelectrode for determination of aflatoxin B1 in maize. *Biosens. Bioelectron.* 80: 222–229. https://doi.org/10.1016/j.bios.2016.01.063.

229 Bhardwaj, H., Singh, C., Pandey, M.K., and Sumana, G. (2016). Star shaped zinc sulphide quantum dots self-assembled monolayers: preparation and applications in food toxin detection. *Sens. Actuators, B* 231: 624–633. https://doi.org/10.1016/j.snb.2016.03.064.

230 Li, Q., Lv, S., Lu, M. et al. (2016). Potentiometric competitive immunoassay for determination of aflatoxin B1 in food by using antibody-labeled gold nanoparticles. *Microchim. Acta* 183 (10): 2815–2822. https://doi.org/10.1007/s00604-016-1929-x.

231 Moon, J., Byun, J., Kim, H. et al. (2018). On-site detection of aflatoxin B1 in grains by a palm-sized surface plasmon resonance sensor. *Sensors (Switzerland)* 18 (2): https://doi.org/10.3390/s18020598.

5

Aptamer-Based Biosensors

5.1 Introduction

Aptamers are another type of 3D bioreceptor molecule that are produced synthetically. They can be single-stranded DNA or RNA molecules. The molecular weight of aptamers lies in the range of 6–30 kDa and a small size of nearly 2 nm as compared to bulky antibodies (10 times larger than aptamers) with a weight of 150–180 kDa and a size of about 15 nm [1]. The process of recognizing target using aptamer involves the different intermolecular forces that include hydrogen bonding, Van der Waals forces, electrostatic interactions, and π–π stacking. Aptamer structure can fold into secondary structures that include a stem, loop, bulge, hairpin, G-quadruplex, and kissing complex [2]. Aptamers dissociation constant is in the pM–μM range indicating high affinity between target and aptamer, stability in harsh conditions, low cost, the ability to bind smaller and wider molecules (ions, peptides, viruses, proteins, nucleic acids [NA], toxins, whole cells, small molecules), do not require secondary reagents, and have high specificity [3].

There are SELEX technology and non-SELEX methods to synthesize the aptamers as shown in Figure 5.1a. Aptamers are synthesized using a family of test-tube experiments from a library of nucleic acids, and NA that could not bind is washed away. Steps are repeated to ensure the most suitable aptamer from the NA sequences. SELEX involves the scanning of random NA that can be bound to a specific target, the nonspecific aptamers are isolated from target specific molecule via affinity method. After isolation, aptamers molecules are amplified using polymerase chain reaction (PCR) and stepwise detail of the method is shown in

Biosensors: Nanomaterials, Approaches, and Performance-Enhancement Strategies,
First Edition. Baljinder Kaur, Santosh Kumar, and Brajesh Kumar Kaushik.

Published 2025 by John Wiley & Sons, Inc.
Companion website: www.wiley.com/go/kaur

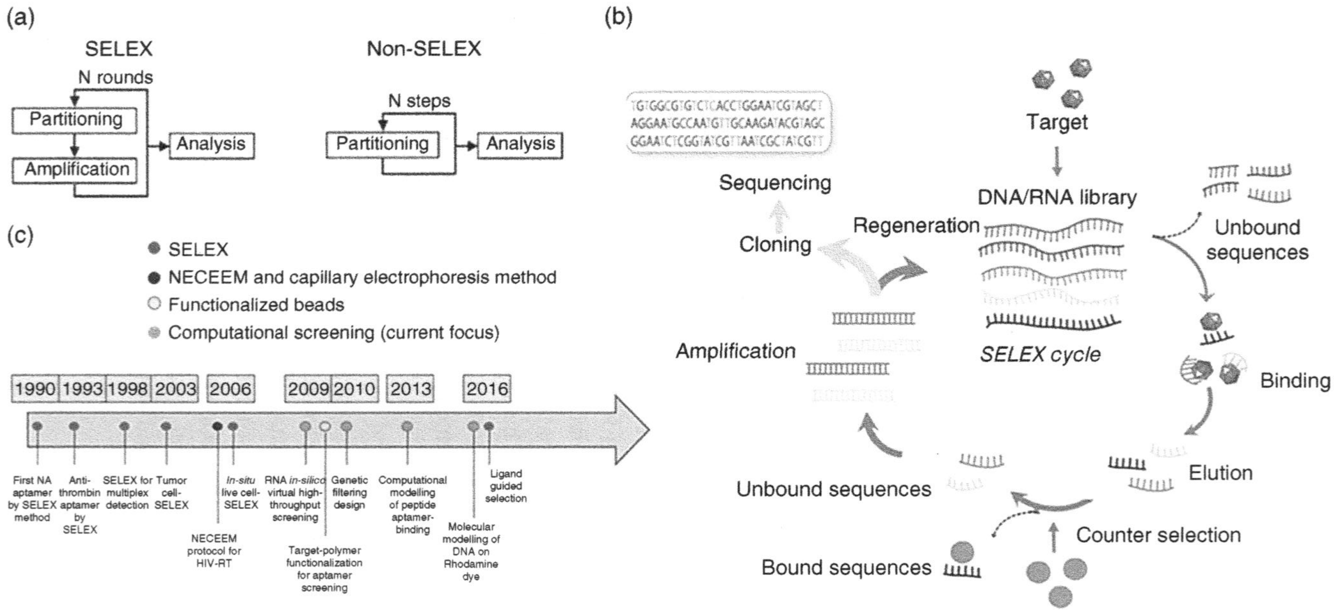

Figure 5.1 Schematic diagram of (a) SELEX and non-SELEX methods to select the aptamer. *Source:* [4]/with permission of American Chemical Society. (b) step-wise process for the SELEX technique. *Source:* [5]/with permission of Elsevier. (c) Year-wise progress made in SELEX technologies. *Source:* [6]/with permission of Elsevier.

Figure 5.1b [4]. Non-SELEX and competitive non-SELEX for aptamers have also been reported that include repetitive steps of separation without amplification steps for various applications [7, 8]. Figure 5.1c shows the year-wise progress made in SELEX technology. Researchers have explored using aptamer-based biosensors on different sensing platforms for various applications [9]. The biosensors are classified depending on the number of bioreceptors to detect a target (i) competitive (ii) sandwich. More specifically, affinity-binding based biosensors include sandwich, exonuclease, competitive, and split-aptamer biosensors.

Sandwich biosensors involve two bioreceptors (one on sensor surface and other on biomarker used for detection) molecules, either antibodies or aptamers simultaneously due to two different binding sites available for a target (e.g. proteins). It is difficult to detect small and low-molecular-weight biomolecules using sandwich biosensors due to some part of epitope or single epitope. In competitive biosensors, a labeled bioreceptor and an unlabeled competitor molecule are used to bind the target. Small and low-molecular-weight molecules can be effectively detected using single-stranded nucleic acids called split aptamers [10]. Split aptamers involve two fragments that are nonfunctional; these two fragments combine in the presence of target molecule to generate a measurable signal. In case of exonuclease biosensors, a fluorophore-labeled hairpin-shaped aptamer and a quencher are used to bind the target and bioreceptor used to detect the NA. The hairpin structure that separates the fluorophore and quencher for signal emission is destabilized. Split-aptamer biosensors involve a split aptamer made up of two separate fragments, each one labeled with a detection molecule, such as a fluorescent or enzyme tag. As the target molecule and both fragments bind to each other, the reconstitution of the aptamer structure generates an output signal [5]. Aptamers possess various advantages over other bioreceptors as they can be chemically synthesized *in vitro*, whereas antibodies used for different applications are found in animals. Aptamers can be produced rapidly and cost-effectively over 2–6 weeks. And they can be produced with low batch-to-batch variation, highly tunable binding profile, high purity, and high chemical stability. Aptamers have high specificity toward targets with minimal cross-reactivity to other molecules [3, 11, 12]. This high specificity is due to the ability to incorporate non-natural nucleotides, which can interact with the target molecule in unique ways.

Aptamers have a high affinity for targets as they easily form secondary structures that are complex but offer multiple attaching sites with the target. Aptamers have high stability and can easily be modified to change their properties suffering from disadvantages of complex, time-consuming selection process and degradation by nucleases, that limit their stability in different biological environments. It is a challenging task to isolate the aptamers toward some targets, as these are not effective toward each target [13].

5.2 Selection of Aptamers and Design Strategies

The selection and synthesis of aptamers are done through a combination that include series of experiment and computational techniques. In the SELEX method, aptamers are selected through iterative rounds in the pool of random oligonucleotides as they interact with the target molecule. Binded molecules are isolated and amplified to obtain the highly specific aptamer toward a particular target [8]. Heterogeneous SELEX involves target immobilization on the surface of solid support with a column or a microarray, and the aptamers bind to this under certain specific conditions [14]. During the washing process, nonspecific binding molecules are washed out and polymerase chain reaction can be used to amplify the remaining bounded molecules. These steps are repeated for several rounds until highly specific aptamers are obtained. Compared to traditional SELEX, heterogeneous SELEX offers several advantages, including increased target specificity and reduced nonspecific binding. However, it can be more technically challenging and time-consuming to perform, especially when working with complex mixtures of target molecules [15, 16]. In the case of homogeneous SELEX, the target and the aptamers are taken in the form of a solution, and there is no involvement of a physical separation step during the selection process [15–17]. This selection is based on a change in different properties that include fluorescence, reflection, and absorption during the interaction of aptamer and sensing target. It allows continuously monitoring of the target and aptamer binding. Homogeneous SELEX is preferred over heterogeneous SELEX method due to its excellent speed, requirement of less sample manipulation, and high specificity to detect target among the complex mixtures. However, the presence of nonspecific interactions limits its specificity and selectivity [14]. The affinity to bind the aptamer pool toward the target molecule is measured using the enzyme-linked oligonucleotide assay [18]. The selected analyte is restrained onto a microtiter plate, and aptamer pool is added. After washing away nonspecific binders, an enzyme-conjugated oligonucleotide is added to the plate, which binds to the aptamers. The bound enzyme is then detected using a chromogenic or fluorescent substrate, allowing quantification of the bound aptamer pool [17]. The affinity and specificity of the complex formed from target and aptamer interaction are measured using the electrophoretic mobility shift assay technique, and unbound aptamers are separated using the gel electrophoresis method. A fluorescent molecule is used to label the target and for incubation in the aptamer pool. After electrophoresis of the mixture, the complex made of aptamer and target is isolated from the unbound aptamer pool. The quantitative measurement of aptamer bonding is done using fluorescence intensity measurements. High-throughput sequencing can be used to identify the sequences and relative abundance of the aptamer pool at different rounds of SELEX [14]. In competitive binding assays there is a competition of target and labeled competitor with analyte mimicking structure. As concentration of the target increases, it displaces a large number of competitor molecules, which reduces signal strength from the labelled competitor. This change is used to measure analyte concentration [19, 20].

5.2.1 Modified Bases

Aptamers are also designed using modified bases e.g. pseudo-uridine, locked nucleic acid, 5-methylcytidine, peptide nucleic acid, inosine and 2′-O-methyl, 2′-fluoro. The locked nucleic acids enhance the binding properties, stability, and specificity [21]. There are various methods for high-quality aptamer synthesis that include particle displays, multi-parametric particle displays, click-chemistry-based particle displays, and non-natural aptamer arrays, as shown in Figure 5.2 [22]. Particle display methods change the solution-phase into particles and fluorescence-activated cell sorting isolation method is used based on its affinity. This requires fewer selection rounds as compared to conventional methods with high-affinity aptamers. In the multi-parametric particle displays method, aptamer particles are isolated using two-color fluorescence-activated cell sorting (FACS) based on affinity and specificity, which produces excellent target binding in the presence of complex matrixes (i.e. serum). Click chemistry-based particle displays that involve principle of biorthogonal chemical reactions without interference with other biological processes using the functional groups of azides or alkynes [23]. These modified functional groups aptamers can detect the required target with high sensitivity specificity and affinity values for challenging or inaccessible targets. The non-natural aptamer arrays method involves the modification in its natural bases called *modified nucleotides* that can detect targets with high-performance parameters and provide them a stability and high affinity. These modified bases can be locked nucleic acid, 5-methylcytidine, peptide nucleic acid, inosine and 2′-O-methyl, 2′-fluoro [24].

5.2.2 Structural Modeling

Aptamers can be designed using computational methods that predict their secondary and tertiary structures. The identification of potential binding sites and aptamer sequence optimization to obtain the highest affinity and specificity can be done through this modeling. Structural modeling of aptamers involves the prediction and visualization of 3D structure of the aptamers. It is an essential step in understanding the molecular interactions of aptamer bio-receptor and sensing analyte and can aid in the optimization of aptamer properties for specific applications [25]. A computer-based modeling method (i.e. homology) is used to investigate the molecular structure on the basis of known structure of a

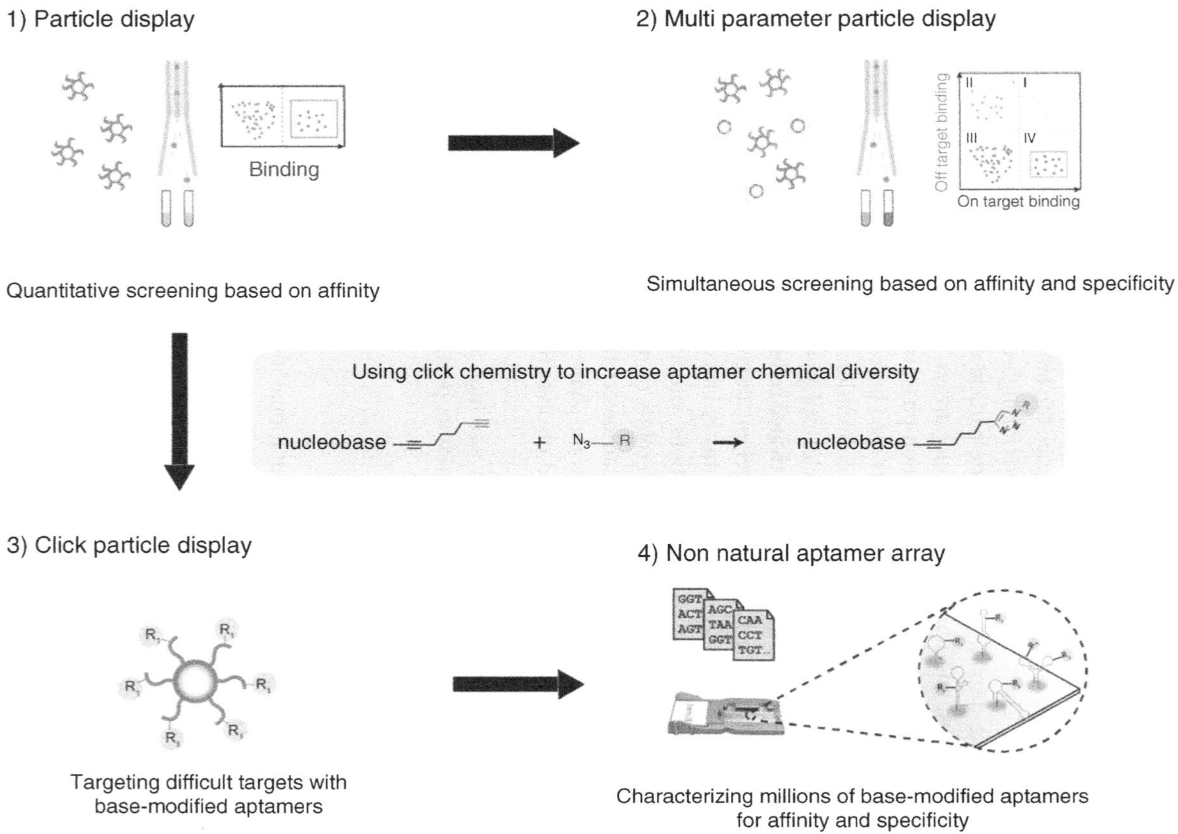

Figure 5.2 Schematic diagram of (1) click particle display that enriches aptamers at a faster rate; (2) multi-parameter particle display method; (3) click particle display; (4) modified nucleotides based non-natural aptamer array. *Source:* [22]/with permission of American Chemical Society.

related molecule. Homology modeling have been explored to find the aptamer structure with the help of known molecule structure (in case of RNA and DNA). The computational method based on molecular docking provides information about the binding affinity with mode and orientation of molecule of small ligand molecules and receptors. There are several software tools to observe the 3D structure of nucleic acids, such as RNA structure [26]. Other algorithms based on thermodynamic and kinetic principles are also reported to study the NA structure. Nuclear magnetic resonance spectroscopy provides the information about the structure of the aptamer by analyzing the chemical shifts of the atoms in the molecule. It provides details about the structure, but it also suffers from several drawbacks that include longer time and complexity in analysis and measurement [27].

5.2.3 Cell-SELEX

The cell-SELEX method involves the use of whole cells or cell surface as the target compared to proteins or small molecules that enable aptamers to recognize the particular cell surface markers [28]. The selection in cell-SELEX is done in two steps: oligonucleotides are used to incubate the target cells screened. In the next step, cells that are not the target are negatively screened. Three advantages are associated with the cell-SELEX system:

1) It can select aptamers to detect a widespread range of cell types and associated surface markers such as cancer cells and microbes.
2) Simultaneous screening of multiple aptamers can target different BREs.
3) It enables direct use of the target aptamer for identification of cells and binding of cells [29].

Cell-SELEX is widely explored to detect cancer on various platforms. Civit et al. reported an aptamer sensor synthesized using cell-SELEX technology to detect breast cancer. Conventional colony, Sanger sequencing methods, and next-generation sequencing methods were applied for the analysis of enriched libraries [30].

5.2.4 Counter-SELEX

The counter-SELEX method, also known as negative selection or subtractive SELEX, is a powerful strategy used for aptamer selection and removal of the nonspecific molecules from the aptamer pool. It is used in cases where the target molecule is complex or contains many epitopes that can lead to the isolation of nonspecific binding sequences through the SELEX process. It is also used in the case of targets available in low abundance that exist in the form of complex matrices that include fluids in the body, cell lysates, and whole blood. This method involves the preparation of a pool of molecules having similar structures, existing in the same biofluids as the target molecule, or sharing similar epitopes. This pool is incubated under specific conditions with the counter-selection pool that strengthens specific target binding and isolates the nonspecific binding with the help of various techniques like centrifugation and magnetic separation. The bound sequences are amplified toward specific aptamers with high affinity. Counter-SELEX makes the selection process easy as it reduces the complexity of the pool by increasing the likelihood of separating aptamers. It is important to mention that the counter-selection pool should be selected carefully to avoid eliminating aptamers with specific binding sites on the target molecule [31]. SELEX processes for individual target selection are expensive, time-consuming, and laborious. Therefore, detection of the different aptamers simultaneously having same structures that can be selected in a single selection can be an alternative solution. Figure 5.3 shows a one-pot SELEX method that was reported to simultaneously detect estradiol, progesterone, and testosterone using counter-SELEX. Steroids estradiol, progesterone, and testosterone were detected due to similarity in structures and their existence in biological samples. A modified steroid molecule attached with magnetic beads toward a specific aptamer among multiple aptamers [32].

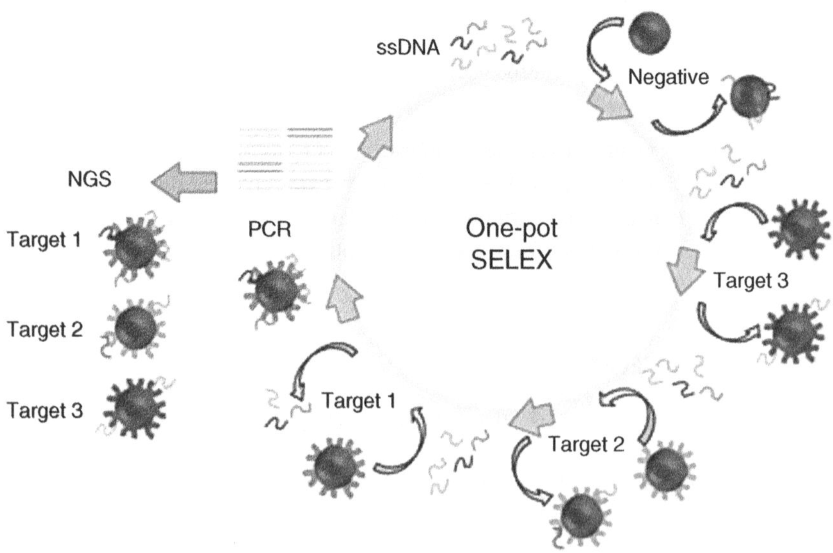

Figure 5.3 Schematic illustration of single-pot SELEX to detect estradiol, progesterone, and testosterone simultaneously. *Source:* [32]/Vasso Skouridou.

5.2.5 High-throughput Sequencing

High-throughput sequencing or massive parallel sequencing or next-generation sequencing is a DNA sequencing method used in case of large DNA and RNA. The process involves the process of library preparation from different sources. These large sample are fragmented into shorter RNA or DNA samples and next step involves the ligation of its ends with unique codes and amplified with PCR and other technologies. This amplified library is loaded onto a next-generation sequencing system such as Ion Torrent that generates millions of short DNA correspond to the individual aptamer sequences. The sequence data is then analyzed using bioinformatics tools to identify the sequences that bind with the highest affinity and specificity to the target molecule.

The selection and design of aptamers depend on the specific needs of the application. The combination of experimental and computational methods allows for the design of aptamers for specific target detection. There are various bead-based, carbon, and other nanomaterial platforms that include magnets, nickel, and agarose to increase the performance of SELEX [33]. Magnetic bead-based platforms use magnetic beads as a solid support that easily separates bound molecules from unbound ones using a magnetic field. The target molecules or SELEX libraries are fixed on magnetic bead surface, and selection process involves incubating the beads with the target molecule or mixture of molecules, applying a magnetic field to separate the bounded particles, washing away unbound particles, and then eluting the bound particles for amplification and further selection rounds [34]. Carbon-based nanomaterial platforms use graphene oxide, carbon nanotube (CNT), or nano-diamonds for support to immobilize the target molecules or SELEX libraries. These materials provide a large surface area that can accommodate a greater number of the target molecules or SELEX libraries. The selection process involves incubating the carbon-based nanomaterials with the target molecule or mixture of molecules, washing away unbound molecules and then eluting the bound molecules for amplification and further selection rounds. Each of these platforms has its advantages, disadvantages, application area, and target molecule. For example, magnetic bead-based platforms are used in case of aptamers against cell surface markers or membrane proteins, whereas carbon-based nanomaterial platforms are utilized to detect the small molecules or toxins [35]. Figure 5.4 shows the magnetic cross-linking precipitation SELEX-based fluorescence biosensor human serum albumin. It does not require capillary electrophoresis, atomic force microscopy, flow cytometry, and microfluidic chips [36].

5.2.6 In Silico SELEX

In silico SELEX is a computational technique that includes docking and molecular dynamics for aptamer design and optimizes the experimental selection and amplification steps. This technique overcomes the difficulties faced by traditional

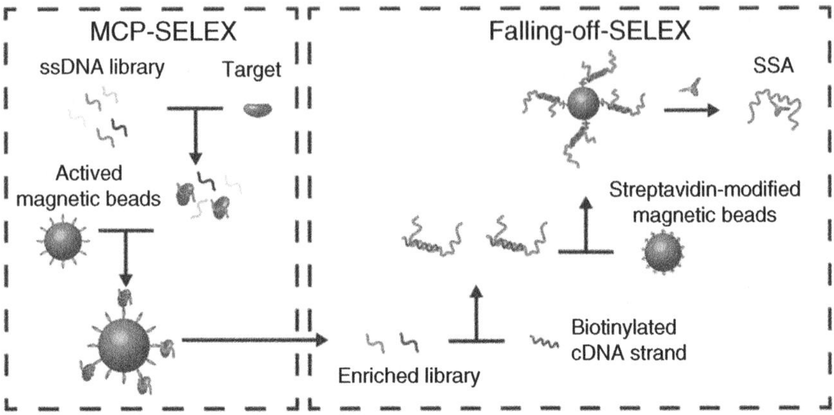

Figure 5.4 Depiction of switching aptamers via SELEX and non-SELEX method through magnetic cross-linking precipitation. *Source:* [36]/with permission of American Chemical Society.

SELEX techniques such as enhanced starting library design, using computational method to calculate affinity and specificity that reduces aptamer number for experimental testing [27]. A virtual library of random DNA/RNA sequences is generated through computer modeling, and a strongly bonded sequence for a specific target is selected. This technique saves time and resources, is less complex, reduces cost, and optimizes various aptamer properties that include selectivity, sensitivity, affinity, and specificity [37]. It is important to mention that in silico predictions may not always accurately reflect the behavior of aptamers *in vivo*, and experimental validation is still necessary to check the efficacy of the selected aptamers. In silico SELEX involves the selection of target, sequence screening using secondary structure, computational docking tools to know the affinities and their ranking based on it [38]. Iterations are repeated to refine the aptamer sequence for a specific target [39–41]. Table 5.1 discusses the different nanomaterials-based platforms to choose aptamer via SELEX method. It is used to design different sensing platforms to detect the various diseases.

5.2.7 Structure-Switching Signaling-Based Aptamers

Structure-switching signaling-based aptamers utilize the conformational change of the aptamer as the binding of sensing analyte and aptamer takes place [63]. In DNAzyme-based aptamers, the aptamer is designed to fold into a specific structure upon binding to the target molecule, which activates a DNAzyme that cleaves a substrate to generate a signal [64]. Various sensing platforms such as fluorescence, colorimetric, and piezoelectric platforms have been reported to detect the

Table 5.1 Various nanomaterial-based platforms for aptamer selection through SELEX.

Material	Analyte/disease	Transduction method	Ref.
Magnetic bead	N-acetylneuraminic acid	Graphene oxide and labeled aptamer based fluorescent biosensor	[35]
	Human serum albumin	Magnetic cross-linking precipitation SELEX-based fluorescence biosensor.	[36]
	Proprotein convertase subtilisin/kexin type 9	RNA aptamer-based fluorescent biosensor to detect the hypercholesterolemia	[42]
	Aleutian mink disease virus	Structural proteins functionalized aptamer-based flow cytometer	[43]
	Autoimmune diseases	Rituximab antibody on protein-A magnetic beads-based aptamer using in silico SELEX	[44]
	Metronidazole	Aptamer- and graphene oxide-based fluorescent biosensor using library-immobilized SELEX	[45]
Agarose bead	Riboflavin and flavin adenine dinucleotide	DNA aptamer-based fluorescence biosensor with streptavidin functional agarose beads	[46]
	Cathinones	Colorimetric biosensor using small aptamers	[47]
	Lucentis	DNA aptamer-based thermo-fluorometric assay	[48]
	3,4-methylenedioxypyrovalerone	Colorimetric biosensor	[49]
	Cannabinoids	trans-Δ9-tetrahydrocannabinol bonded aptamer-based colorimetric assay	[50]
	N-Methyl Mesoporphyrin IX	Chromatography SELEX aptamer-based colorimetric biosensor	[51]
Nickel	N-cadherin	Aptamer-based fluorescent biosensor	[52]

(Continued)

Table 5.1 (Continued)

Material	Analyte/disease	Transduction method	Ref.
Graphene oxide	Okadaic acid	Non-immobilized SELEX and graphene oxide based fluorescence apta-sensor	[53]
	Domoic acid, saxitoxin, and tetrodotoxin	Magnetic reduced graphene oxide and multitarget aptamers-based fluorescent assay	[54]
	miR-215	Graphene oxide–assisted SELEX and Thioflavin T aptamer-based fluorescent sensor	[55]
	Sulfaquinoxaline	Graphene oxide–assisted SELEX fluorescence assay	[56]
AuNPs and agarose beads	Zinc (II)-Protoporphyrin IX	AuNPs-based SELEX fluorescence assay	[57]
	Brassinolide, bisphenol A	AuNPs-based colorimetric assays.	[58]
	Dichlorvos pesticide	AuNPs and aptamer-nanozyme-based colorimetric assays	[59]
Magnetic nanoparticles	Lipopolysaccharides	Capture-SELEX aptamer-based fluorescence sensor	[60]
	RNase B	Glycan- imprinted magnetic nanoparticles-based SELEX	[61]
	Myoglobin and β2-microglobulin	Epitope-imprinted magnetic NPs to detect the protein	[62]

target signal (Table 5.2). Riboswitch-based aptamers cause the conformational change in the RNA structure of the gene expression [81]. Aptamer-mediated proximity ligation assays are labeled with two different oligonucleotides that can hybridize to two complementary oligonucleotides [82].

5.2.8 Folding Aptamer-Based Biosensors

Folding of aptamers refers to the process of the aptamer adopting a specific conformation that allows it to interact with its target. This phenomenon plays an important role, and its three-dimensional structure determines the binding interaction strength and its capability to detect a specific target. Folding structures, including hairpins, stem-loops, pseudoknots (bulge), and G-quadruplexes depend

Table 5.2 Recently reported aptamer-based ECL biosensors on different sensing platforms.

Sensor	Target	LOD	Range	Ref.
Au nanocrystal-based localized surface plasmon resonance (LSPR) apta-sensor	Troponin I	0.1 pg/ml	1–10 nM	[65]
Nitrogen-doped graphene, AuNPs-Apt, and cyclo-metallated iridium (III)-polyvinyl pyridine polymer NPs-based ECL sensor	Troponin I	0.02 pM	0.1 pM–10 nM	[66]
Graphene QDs-based ECL apta-sensor	CEA	3.2 fg/ml	10 fg/ml–200 ng/ml	[67]
Au nanocrystal and multifunctional DNA-based ECL and LSPR combined sensor	Troponin I	1 pg/ml	0.001–100 ng/ml	[68]
Coral-like poly-aniline, AuNPs and peptide-based aptasensor	PSA	0.085 pgml	10^{-4}–100 ng/ml	[69]
Amino functional graphene-Thionin-AuNPs-based ECL aptasensor	CEA	2 pg/ml	0.01–500 ng/ml	[70]
Hybrid chain reaction and Au/Ti_3C_2-MXene-based aptasensor	COVID-19	0.04 fM	0.1–500 fM	[71]
Ag-coated Fe_3O_4-Au NPs-based SERS sensor	CRP	10 fM	0.14–8.7 pM	[72]
AuNPs and anti-methamphetamine aptamer-based ECL sensor	Methamphetamine	5 μM	n.r.	[73]
Polydopamine and hollow metal- frameworks and 6-carboxyfluorescein labeled fluorescent cancer biosensor	CA15–3	2.56×10^{-5} U/ml	10^{-5}–1.28×10^{-2} U/ml	[74]
Fe3O4@Au-teicoplanin NPs-based apata sensor	*S. aureus*	1.09 CFU/ml	7.6×10^1–10^7 CFU/ml	[75]
2D covalent organic framework-based fluorescence biosensor	ATP, Thrombin	100 units/ml	n.r.	[76]

(*Continued*)

Table 5.2 (Continued)

Sensor	Target	LOD	Range	Ref.
Aptamer-modified AuNPs-loaded magnetic reduced graphene oxide-based ECL sensor	Bisphenol A	0.141 pg/ml	0.01–100 ng/ml 2.7%	[77]
SiO_2-Au-ssDNA 2D photonic crystal-based PCF apta-sensor	Kanamycin antibiotic	1.10 pg/ml	5 pg/ml–5 μg/ml	[78]
Chemiluminescence optical fiber apta-sensor	Myco- toxins AFB1, FB1, OTA or ZEN	0.015–0.423 pg/ml	10^5 pg/ml	[79]
Glassy carbon electrode modified chitosan particles electrode and $[Fe(CN)_6]^{3-}$ based apta-sensor	*P. Aeruginosa*	3 CFU/ml	10–10^7 CFU/ml	[80]

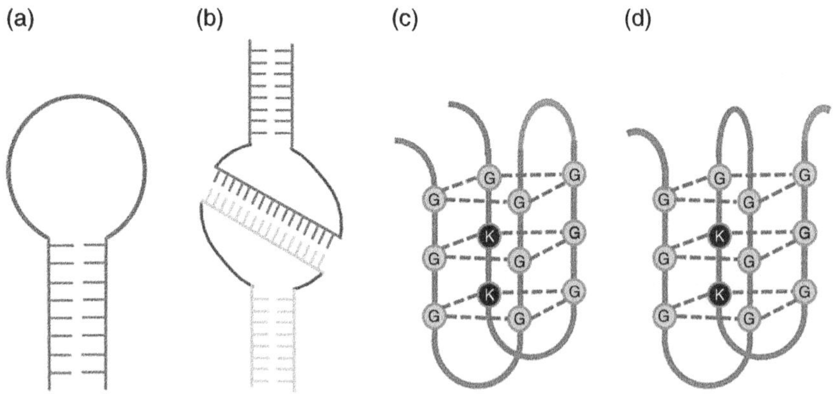

Figure 5.5 Representation of aptamers structures (a) hairpin or stem loop (b) kissing complex (c) quadruplex (d) cross-over. *Source:* [83]/with permission of Springer Nature.

on NA sequence and the nature of the target as depicted in Figure 5.5 [84]. The folding of an aptamer is typically driven by the base-pair interactions between complementary nucleotides within the sequence. The most common folding structures of aptamers are stem-loop structures, where a short region of the sequence folds back on itself to form a stem, which is stabilized by base pairing and a loop, and is often the binding site for the target molecule [85, 86].

Other folding structures of aptamers include G-quadruplex structures that involve a planar arrangement of the guanine bases, and pseudoknot structures, which are formed by the interaction of two or more stem-loop structures [5]. The folding structure of an aptamer can be determined experimentally using techniques such as circular dichroism spectroscopy, nuclear magnetic resonance spectroscopy, and X-ray crystallography [87].

5.2.9 Split Aptamers

Split aptamers are made up of two separate inactive parts that become active as they are brought closer to each other to form a functional aptamer. Most of the apta-sensors are designed using conformational change or structural transformation, but in case of structural transformation aptamer-based biosensors, it is difficult to predict the alterations in structure in advance that can generate false and nonspecific results [88]. Split aptamers overcome the difficulties of binding to two aptamers simultaneously in the presence of steric hindrance because low-molecular-weight molecules have only one epitope or even a part of an epitope (Figure 5.6). In case of split aptamers, there is an absence of secondary structures among the two separated fragments that can eliminate the chances of false-positive as well as nonspecific signals. Various aptamers (more than 100) to detect the small molecules and other targets have been reported to date; among them, only six have been successfully constructed into split aptamers. A very small number of aptamers have been split into fragments to detect the small molecules. Split aptamers include adenosine triphosphate [90], cocaine [91], thrombin [92], 17β-estradiol, D-vasopressin [93], and theophylline [94]. Aptamers have different type of structures such as hairpin-loop, and three-way junction architecture, nonparticipating binding sites of these definite structures can split easily into two parts. Many aptamers have hairpin-like structure and the small target molecules generally binds to nucleobases in the loop region of the hairpin.

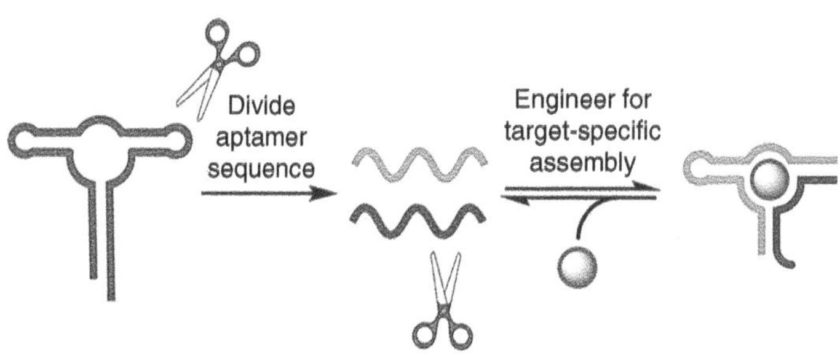

Figure 5.6 Schematic illustration of split aptamers. *Source:* [89]/with permission of American Chemical Society.

An adenosine triphosphate split aptamer with hairpin-like architecture that bind the target in the stem region have been reported [89]. Cocaine split aptamer has a three-way junction architecture and has the advantage of a central binding region, favorable place for small molecules attachment, and it also provide the two loop regions for sequence division without disturbing the target binding region. Thrombin aptamers have a compact 3D structure consisting of two helices and a loop and binds to thrombin through a combination of hydrogen bonding and hydrophobic interactions [95]. A hairpin loop structure consists of an unpaired loop of messenger RNA generated by folding RNA to form base pairs with another section of the same strand, forming a U-shape structure [96]. Split aptamers have potential applications in biosensing, imaging, and drug delivery [93]. In the presence of sensing analyte or target, the split part of an aptamer becomes active and reassembles to procedure a functional aptamer, bringing the two reporter molecules into close proximity and generating a detectable signal. In drug delivery, split aptamers can be used to target specific cells or tissues by conjugating each part to a different component of a drug delivery system, such as a liposome or a nanoparticle [97]. Figure 5.7 shows heterogenous SELEX methods to isolates the aptamers in case of small molecule target such as nucleotides that include target, library, and homogenous SELEX [98].

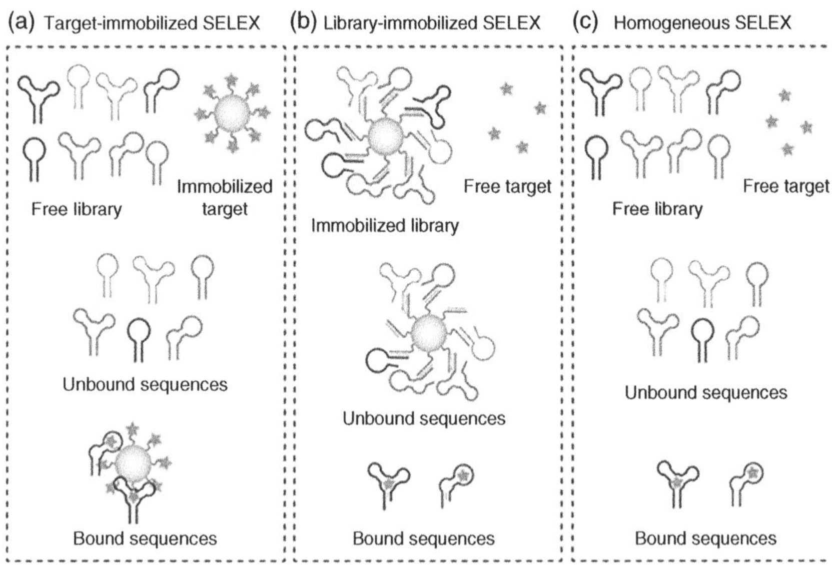

Figure 5.7 Schematic diagram of approaches to isolate the specific and nonspecific targets (a) target-immobilized SELEX, (b) library-immobilized SELEX, and (c) homogeneous SELEX. *Source:* [98]/with permission of John Wiley & Sons.

5.3 Sepsis, Pathogens, and Biomarkers to Detect Disease and Pollutants

An ECL DNA aptamer-based biosensor to detect the *E. coli* immobilizing the DNA aptamers on an Au electrode have been reported. In the presence of *E. coli* bacteria impedance response on the electrode changes was measured using ECL impedance spectroscopy. *E. coli* was detected with limit of detection (LOD), of 50 CFU/ml [99]. Fe_3O_4@SiO_2@Ag magnetic nanoparticles functionalized with aptamers-based SERS biosensor to detect the Staphylococcus aureus (*S. aureus*) and *E. coli* bacteria simultaneously was reported. The aptamers were selected using the SELEX technique, and NPs were tagged with Raman reporters, 4-mercaptobenzoic acid, and 2-mercaptopyridine to detect the target. LOD in case of *S. aureus* and *E. coli* 2.3×10^2 CFU/ml and 1.1×10^2 CFU/ml was achieved [100]. A CRISPR/Cas12a technology and split-aptamer-based biosensor lateral flow strategy was demonstrated to detect the estrogen hormone 17β-estradiol. CRISPR/Cas12a technology activates a nuclease with the help of a target-specific RNA molecule by cleaving a reporter DNA sequence.

The aptamer is split into two parts, and only when it recognizes the target molecule will it reassemble and activate the CRISPR/Cas12a to help cleave the reporter DNA. A gap-enhanced Raman tag, a type of nanoparticle that enhances the Raman signal-based lateral flow strategy, can detect the target with high specificity and sensitivity [101]. A polymer-QD and nanocomposite has been synthesized using fullerene, multiwalled carbon nanotubes (MWCNTs), and polyethylenimine-based ECL apta-sensor for thrombin detection (Figure 5.8). The nanocomposite with a huge number of amine groups has more sites that help in better covalent immobilization of amino-linked aptamers and enhance the performance of the biosensor. Thrombin can be detected with a LOD of 6 fmol/and RSD of 3.6% in the linear range of 50–20 fmol/l [102]. An ECL cancer biosensor to detect the carcinoembryonic antigen (CEA) biomarkers overexpressed in cancer patients using a combination of tetrahedral DNA nanostructures and catalytic hairpin assembly was demonstrated. A catalytic hairpin assembly amplifies the reporter molecule signal with the help of a hairpin-shaped DNA molecule was detected with LOD of 0.04567 pg/ml in the linear range of 1–30 000 pg/ml was achieved with the sensor [104]. Chen et al. describes an aptamer-based biosensor to detect carboxylesterase 2A, an important target enzyme in drug metabolism. The biosensor is based on the modification of green fluorescent protein-like fluorogens (3, 5-difluoro-4-hydroxybenzylidene imidazolinone), which can be engineered to change their fluorescence in response to the target enzyme. Carboxylesterase 2A target can be detected with a detection limit of 8.8 ng/ml [105].

An electrochemical (ECL) biosensor with screen-printed Au electrode and aptamer for diagnosis of periodontal disease biomarker human odontogenic

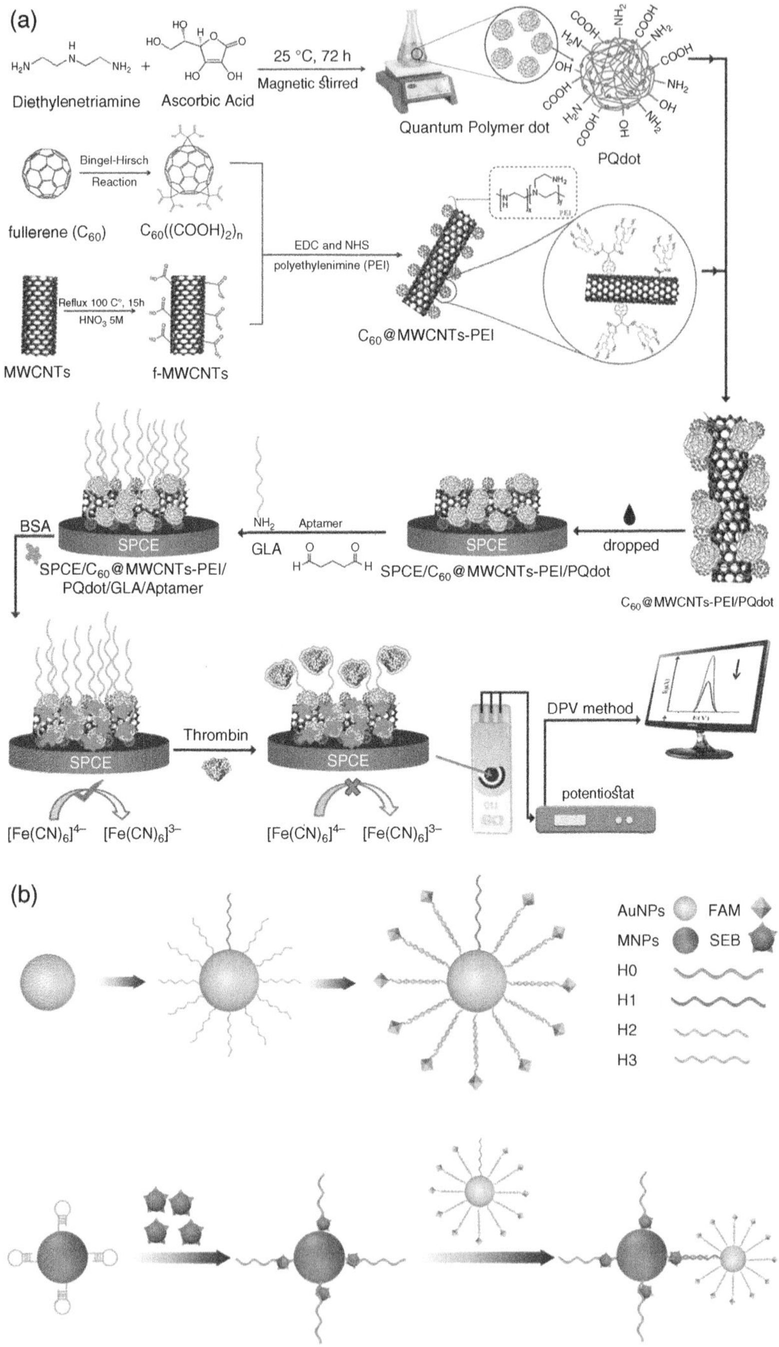

Figure 5.8 Schematic diagram of (a) polymer-QD and nanocomposite-based ECL sensor. *Source:* [102]/with permission of Elsevier. (b) Aptamer-and AuNPs-based fluorescent biosensors to detect *Staphylococcal enterotoxin B*. *Source:* [103]/with permission of Elsevier.

amelo-blast-associated protein is demonstrated in cyclic voltammetry and chronoamperometry mode. The human odontogenic ameloblast-associated protein can be detected with linear range, LOD of 0–15 nM, 0.02 nM and 1 nM in buffer and saliva solution [106]. A split-aptamer sandwich-type fluorescent biosensor was demonstrated to detect the streptomycin antibiotic. The biosensor involves two separate inactive fragments of aptamer immobilized on Au electrode surface. As the target is available, these two inactive fragments become functional and bind with the target molecule. Streptomycin antibiotic was detected with LOD and linear range of 33 nM and 0.06–0.526 μM [107].

A fluorescent biosensor using the split aptamer and N-methyl mesoporphyrin IX fluorophore and G-quadruplex complex-based biosensor to detect cocaine was demonstrated. The split aptamer is attached to a complex molecule that emits light on binding with target cocaine. Cocaine was detected with linear range, relative standard deviations and LOD of 50 pM–25 nM, 2.9–7.5%, 16 pM [108].

Chi and Liu describe the detection of aflatoxin B1 in edible oils using a sandwich biosensor based on a molecularly imprinted polymer and an aptamer-modified CdTe/ZnS QD fluorescent probe. The molecularly imprinted polymer (MIP) was prepared using a template molecule, aflatoxin B1, and a functional monomer, methacrylic acid, to create a specific binding site for aflatoxin B1. The sandwich biosensor was created by immobilizing the MIP onto a glass slide, followed by incubation with a biotinylated aptamer specific to AFB1, and then the aptamer-modified CdTe/ZnS QD fluorescent probe. The sandwich structure allows for the amplification of the fluorescent signal, and aflatoxin B1 was detected with LOD of 4 pg/ml [109].

A peptide-aptamer-based ECL biosensor for the detection of norovirus responsible for gastroenteritis disease. The biosensor is composed of a black phosphorous nanosheet@Ti_3C_2-Mxene nanohybrid modified with the aptamer and a magnetic covalent organic framework modified with the peptide. Norovirus can be detected with the linear range of 0.01–10^5 copies/ml with a LOD of 0.003 copies/ml [110].

A fluorescent biosensor detects *Staphylococcal Enterotoxin B* using aptamer-based recognition and AuNPs as a metal-enhanced fluorescence agent. The biosensor shows an ultrasensitive and fast detection performance with a LOD and concentration range of 1.0 fg/ml and 92–119% in a response time of less than 15 minutes [103]. A peptide-nucleic acid aptamer interferometric biosensor detects vascular endothelial growth factor 165. The biosensor structure consists of a Au and biotin–streptavidin coupling-based 3D aptamer. LOD of 6 pM and a range of 0.01–1 nM was obtained for vascular endothelial growth factor 165 target [111].

A SPR effect-based fiberoptic sandwich assay was reported to detect breast cancer using HER2 protein biomarker. The sensor structure consists of a white light source, unclad fiber, Au metal film thiolated anti-HER2 ssDNA aptamer via SELEX technology and spectrophotometer. Au film of 50 nm thickness deposited on the fiber surface provides a LOD of 0.6 μg/ml in the linear range of 8 fM-8 nm [112]. A cell-SELEX aptamer: tJBA8.1-based biosensor is used to detect the transferrin receptor 1, a cancer biomarker. Aptamer tJBA8.1 is selected among the library of aptamer lakhs using the cell-SELEX method. This method is highly specific, as it targets only cancer cells, depletion rate > 90%, and is scalable at low cost [113].

5.4 Small Biomolecules

Toxins are poisonous substances produced by living organisms that can cause harm to other organisms, including humans, by disrupting cellular function and damaging tissues and organs [114–116]. There are many different types of toxins, including bacterial toxins, fungal toxins, plant toxins, animal toxins, environmental toxins, endogenous toxins, and mycotoxins. Biomolecules are the main components of all living organisms made up of carbohydrates, lipids, proteins, and nucleic acids [40, 117–120]. An ECL paper sensor with aptamer-integrated for multianalyte detection was reported to detect three small molecules in a single sample – acetyl fentanyl, 3,4-methylenedioxypyrovalerone, and adenosine. The sensor structure includes an Ag metal pseudo-reference electrode, Au counter electrode, three other Au working electrodes, and DNA/RNA molecules to detect the target specifically. Acetyl fentanyl, 3,4-methylenedioxypyrovalerone and adenosine were detected with LOD and linear range of the ECL sensor was 0.5, 0.1,1 μM, and 0.5–15, 0.1–10, 1–200 μM [121]. The effect of environmental pollutants such as heavy metals have been widely reported in the literature [122–124]. Table 5.3. discusses various toxins and their examples reported using different sensing platforms.

A coccolith-modified electrodeposited on a screen-printed gold electrode to detect the vaspin biomarker for type 2 diabetes (Figure 5.9). Coccoliths are composed of calcium carbonate and are highly structured micro particles with many nanosized pores derived from *E. huxleyi*. A LOD of 298 pM was achieved to detect the vasodilator [131]. An UiO-66 metallic organic framework and aptamer-based ECL biosensor to detect the cardiac troponin I. The probe is fabricated using a hybrid made of Fe_3O_4, UiO-66 metallic organic framework, and bimetallic Cu and Au nanoparticle and cardiac troponin I was detected with LOD of 16 pg/ml and linear range of 0.05–100 ng/ml [132]. A MIPs, nanoparticles, and aptamer-based ECL biosensor was reported to detect the toxic amyloid-β oligomers found in Alzheimer's disease. Core-shell NPs of Ag and SiO_2 are prepared and aptamer corresponding to target was immobilized on its surface. A molecularly imprinted

Table 5.3 Toxins and their examples reported using different sensing platforms.

Type of toxin	Examples	Ref.
Bacterial toxins	Botulinum toxin, tetanus toxin, cholera toxin, shiga toxin, diphtheria toxin	[125]
Fungal toxins	Aflatoxins, ochratoxins, trichothecenes, ergot alkaloids	[117]
Plant toxins	Ricin, cyanide, solanine, rotenone	[115]
Animal toxins	Snake venom, bee venom, spider venom, pufferfish toxin	[116]
Environmental toxins	Heavy metals (arsenic, lead, mercury), pesticides (dichlorodiphenyltrichloroethane (DDT), glyphosate), PCBs	[117–119]
Endogenous toxins	Urea, bilirubin, homocysteine, lactic acid	[126, 127]
Mycotoxins	Aflatoxins, fumonisins, patulin, zearalenone	[128, 129]
Carbohydrates	Glucose, fructose, sucrose, lactose, starch, cellulose, glycogen	[117]
Lipids	Triglycerides, phospholipids, steroids, waxes, tatty acids	[118, 119]
Proteins	Enzymes, hormones, antibodies, hemoglobin, collagen, actin, myosin	[40, 118, 119, 130]
Nucleic acids	DNA, RNA, adenosine triphosphate	[120]

substrate was fabricated using carbon electrode, that include an AuNPs and reduced graphene oxide layer, and a molecularly imprinted layer. AuNPs and a reduced graphene oxide layer. The oligomer can be detected with a LOD of 1.22 pg/ml and in the concentration range of 5–10 ng/ml [134]. Graphitic carbon nitride nanosheets, aptamer without labeling, and an AuNPs-based fluorescent biosensor to detect digoxin drug used to treat heart failure and found in the human plasma. Nanosheets act as fluorescence material. Digoxin can be detected with a LOD and concentration range of 3.2 ng/l, 10–500 ng/l [133]. A colorimetric biosensor to sense microcystin-LR generated during cyanobacterial metabolism using surface Cu-NPs of polydopamine nanospheres was reported. Fe_3O_4 magnetic nanoparticles are coated with SiO_2 functionalizing using antibodies and then aptamer-functionalized polydopamine nanospheres decorated with Cu NPs were deposited on it. Microcystin-LR catalyzes the reduction of Cu^{2+} ions to Cu (I) on the surface of polydopamine nanospheres that produces the change in color of solution from yellow to orange-red. Microcystin-LR was detected with LOD of 0.25 ng/ml [135]. An up-conversion fluorescent nanoparticle-based immunochromatographic

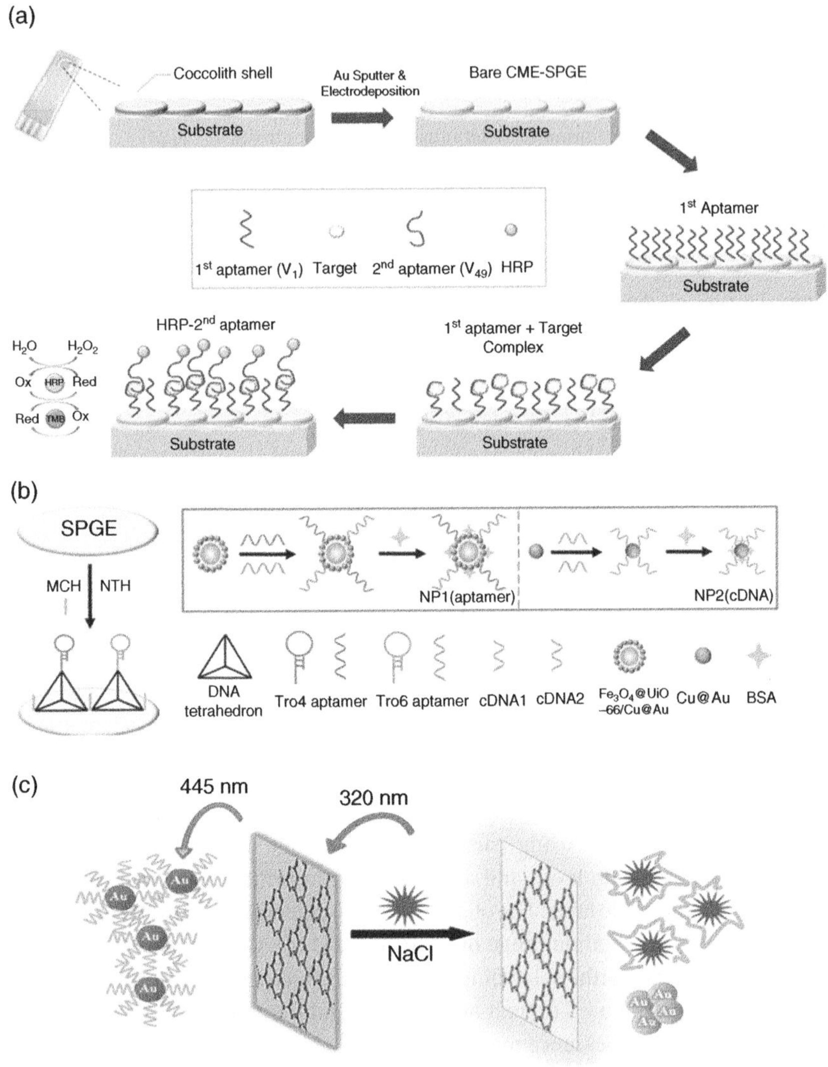

Figure 5.9 Schematic drawing of the (a) coccolith-based aptamer-based ECL biosensor forvaspin detection, a diabetes biomarker. *Source:* [131]/with permission of Elsevier. (b) Fe_3O_4@UiO-66/Cu@Au hybrid nanozyme-based ECL sensor. *Source:* [132]/with permission of Elsevier. (c) aptamer/AuNPs/graphitic carbon nitride nanosheets-based ECL sensor to detect the digoxin. *Source:* [133]/with permission of Elsevier.

colorimetric biosensor dexamethasone sensing can be observed with the bare eye. Antigen was coated on the nitrocellulose membrane for specific target detection. Dexamethasone was detected in a linear range of 0.1–9 ng/ml and LOD of 2 μg/kg [136]. An aptamer and AuNPs based colorimetric sensor to detect the dexamethasone hormone responsible for endocrine-disrupting effect has been demonstrated. As the target is not available, the aptamer is in close contact with AuNPs due to electrostatic bonding and AuNPs remains scattered and yield blue color. In the presence of dexamethasone hormone, aptamer and hormone form a complex and isolate from AuNPs surface results into blue color. The dexamethasone target can be detected in a linear range and LOD of 10–350 nM, 0.5 nM [137]. The performance of two fluorescent aptasensor design that involve turn-on and ratio-metric to detect the adenosine triphosphate was compared and reported. Adenosine triphosphate was detected using a "turn-on" approach without labeling using a guanine-rich aptamer and berberine complex to bind the DNA. In another method, the ratio-metric approach, including Au nanorods, aptamer-red, and carbon QDs, berberine based on the Förster resonance energy transfer (FRET) was used. LOD in case of turn-on and ratio-metric methods are 3.6 and 3.8 μM in the linear range of 0–50 μM.

The results indicate that the ratiometric approach is a more reliable and accurate method for the detection of adenosine triphosphate [138]. The biosensor for the detection of adenosine is based on a split-aptamer-labeled ratiometric fluorescent approach, where the aptamer is split into two fragments (ABA1 and ABA2) and labeled with two blue-emitting carbon dot fluorophores. ABA1 is linked to carbon dots and ABA2 is linked to red-emitting silica-coated CdTe QDs that act as internal references. The two fragments of the aptamer are designed to specifically bind to adenosine, and upon binding, the two fragments are brought together, leading to an increase in FRET between the two fluorophores. The biosensor showed high specificity for adenosine with minimal cross-reactivity with other nucleotides. LOD values of the biosensor was found to be 0.24 μM, which is within the range of adenosine concentrations found in human urine [139]. An amperometric aptamer-based ECL sensor to detect the adenosine triphosphate molecules was demonstrated. A 64-channel array-based Au electrode was used to fabricate the sensor and the aptamer was immobilized on its surface. A sensitivity and LOD of 2.4 nA logC and 0.30×10^{-9} M were reported to measure the adenosine triphosphate [140]. A pH-responsive bioassay using switchable DNA aptamers and metal ion-urease interactions for the colorimetric detect the adenosine triphosphate. A switchable DNA aptamer was used to fabricate biosensors that undergoes a conformational change with target binding adenosine triphosphate. Urease catalyzes urea hydrolysis to yield ammonia, increasing the pH of the solution. A spectrophotometer measures urease activity. Table 5.4 lists various aptamer-based biosensors for detecting toxins.

Table 5.4 Aptamer-based biosensors on different sensing platforms to detect the various toxins.

Aptamer sensor	Target	LOD	Range	Ref.
Anti-STX aptamer with a methylene-based ECL sensor	Saxitoxin	1 nM	1 nM–1 mM	[141]
SiO_2- silicon nitride–SiO_2-based interferometric biosensor	Aflatoxin B1	0.7 pg/ml	10^6–1 μg/ml	[142]
AuNPs and conducting polymer poly-diallyl dimethyl ammonium chloride-based ECL aptasensor	Okadaic acid	41.30 nmol/l	100–1200 nmol/l	[143]
Polymer-based ECL aptasensor	Adenosine	2.3 nM	9.6 nM–600 μM	[144]
Black hole quencher-2-based SERS aptasensor	Adenosine monophosphate	3.4 nM	3.4 nM–200 μM	[145]
Molecular docking simulation-based SPR aptamer	Botulinum neurotoxin	0.2 ng/ml	0.2–1.0 ng/ml	[146]
SELEX-based single-stranded DNA aptamer fluorescent biosensor	Anthrax	n.r.	0.08–10 μM	[147]

The biosensor showed high sensitivity and specificity toward adenosine triphosphate 1.6 nM detection range in the concentration range of 5–500 nM, and an RSD of 2.82% [148]. A semiconductor material 2D-C_3N_4, photo-$BiVO_4$ catalyst and a DNA aptamer photo-ECL biosensor to detect the microcystin-LR toxin generated by cyanobacteria. The 2D-C_3N_4 material was selected due to its greater light absorption capability, good conductivity, and high surface area. On the surface of 2D-C_3N_4 material DNA aptamer was via covalent bonding and then AuNPs was attached. Microcystin-LR toxin target was measured with LOD of 4.2×10^{-8} μg/l [149]. An AuNPs with particle size of 9 nm-based PCF fiber sensor was functionalized with aptamers to detect the aflatoxin B1 toxin responsible for cancer- and liver-related diseases. Linearity, LOD and concentration range of 1 pg/ml −100 ng/ml, 0.28 pg/ml, 0.01 pg/ml–1 μg/ml was achieved [150, 151]. Toxic mercury ion was detected using colorimetric sensor functionalized with poly N-Isopropylacrylamide-acrylic acid, and TiO_2 based one-dimensional photonic crystals was reported. The concentrations of 0–50 nM of mercury ions can be detected [152].

5.5 Summary

Aptamers that include DNA or RNA molecules have been utilized to investigate the various biomarkers for diseases, microorganisms, and small biomolecules. Among all types of biosensor design, ECL aptamer-based sensors are the most commonly studied and commercialized for various applications. Optical sensors are also explored widely for various applications, including environmental monitoring, medical diagnostics, and food safety. They have also shown great potential for detecting a wide range of analytes. Overall, aptamer-based sensors have emerged as a promising alternative to traditional sensors, offering high selectivity, sensitivity, and versatility for a wide range of applications. Aptamers have limitless virtual use, *in vitro* synthesis, and highly specific in nature as they are produced using repeated cycles to eliminate the low-affinity sequences and self-annealing structure that can fold into 3D structures. However, aptamers-based biosensors commercialization suffers from several drawbacks such as high cost, stability issues, and the standardization requirements.

References

1 Zhou, J., Rossi, J., Biology, C., and Rd, E.D. (2018). Aptamers as targeted therapeutics: current potential and challenges. *Nat. Rev. Drug Discov.* 16 (3): 181–202. https://doi.org/10.1038/nrd.2016.199.Aptamers.

2 Chambers, J.P., Arulanandam, B.P., Matta, L.L. et al. (2008). Biosensor recognition elements. *Curr. Issues Mol. Biol.* 10: 1–12.

3 Crivianu-gaita, V. and Thompson, M. (2016). Biosensors and bioelectronics aptamers, antibody scFv, and antibody fab ' fragments : An overview and comparison of three of the most versatile biosensor biorecognition elements. *Biosens. Bioelectron.* 85: 32–45. https://doi.org/10.1016/j.bios.2016.04.091.

4 Berezovski, M., Musheev, M., Drabovich, A., and Krylov, S.N. (2006). Non-SELEX selection of aptamers. *J. Am. Chem. Soc.* 03: 1410–1411.

5 Ning, Y., Hu, J., and Lu, F. (2020). Aptamers used for biosensors and targeted therapy. *Biomed. Pharmacother.* 132: 110902.

6 Zulkeflee Sabri, M., Hamid, A.A.A., Hitam, S.M.S., and Rahim, M.Z.A. (2019). In-silico selection of aptamer: a review on the revolutionary approach to understand the aptamer design and interaction through computational chemistry. *Mater. Today Proc.* 19: 1572–1581. https://doi.org/10.1016/j.matpr.2019.11.185.

7 Parashar, A., Bhushan, V., Mahanandia, N.C., and Kumar, S. (2022). Non-SELEX method for aptamer selection against β-casomorphin-7 peptide. *J. Dairy Sci.* 105 (7): 5545–5560. https://doi.org/10.3168/jds.2021-21569.

8 Kushwaha, A., Takamura, Y., Nishigaki, K., and Biyani, M. (2019). Competitive non-SELEX for the selective and rapid enrichment of DNA aptamers and its use in electrochemical aptasensor. *Sci. Rep.* 9: 1–11. https://doi.org/10.1038/s41598-019-43187-6.

9 Kurdekar, A.D., Chunduri, L.A.A., Manohar, C.S. et al. (2018). Streptavidin-conjugated gold nanoclusters as ultrasensitive fluorescent sensors for early diagnosis of HIV infection. *Sci. Adv.* 4 (11): 1–11. https://doi.org/10.1126/sciadv.aar6280.

10 Mudenkattil, S., Girigoswami, A., Jayaprakash, T., and Girigoswami, K. (2022). Development of nanobiosensors for human immunodeficiency virus detection—a mini review. *Explor. Med.* 3 (5): 479–493. https://doi.org/10.37349/emed.2022.00109.

11 Morales, M.A. and Halpern, J.M. (2018). Guide to selecting a biorecognition element for biosensors. *Bioconjug. Chem.* 29 (10): 3231–3239. https://doi.org/10.1021/acs.bioconjchem.8b00592.

12 Maduraiveeran, G., Sasidharan, M., and Ganesan, V. (2018). Biosensors and bioelectronics electrochemical sensor and biosensor platforms based on advanced nanomaterials for biological and biomedical applications. *Biosens. Bioelectron.* 103: 113–129. https://doi.org/10.1016/j.bios.2017.12.031.

13 Maruccio, G. and Narang, J. (2022). *Electrochemical Sensors from Working Electrodes to Functionalization and Miniaturized Devices*. United Kingdom: Elsevier.

14 Kohlberger, M. and Gadermaier, G. (2022). SELEX: critical factors and optimization strategies for successful aptamer selection. *Biotechnol. Appl. Biochem.* 69 (5): 1771–1792. https://doi.org/10.1002/bab.2244.

15 Blind, M. and Blank, M. (2015). Aptamer selection technology and recent advances. *Mol. Ther. - Nucleic Acids* 4 (1): e223. https://doi.org/10.1038/mtna.2014.74.

16 Yüce, M., Ullah, N., and Budak, H. (2015). Trends in aptamer selection methods and applications. *Analyst* 140 (16): 5379–5399. https://doi.org/10.1039/c5an00954e.

17 Zhuo, Z., Yu, Y., Wang, M. et al. (2017). Recent advances in SELEX technology and aptamer applications in biomedicine. *Int. J. Mol. Sci.* 18 (10): 1–19. https://doi.org/10.3390/ijms18102142.

18 Qu, H., Csordas, A.T., Wang, J. et al. (2016). Rapid and label-free strategy to isolate aptamers for metal ions. *ACS Nano* 10 (8): 7558–7565. https://doi.org/10.1021/acsnano.6b02558.

19 Yoo, H., Jo, H., and Oh, S.S. (2020). Detection and beyond: challenges and advances in aptamer-based biosensors. *Mater. Adv.* 1 (8): 2663–2687. https://doi.org/10.1039/d0ma00639d.

20 Hu, L., Yang, L., Lipchik, A.M. et al. (2013). A quantitative proteomics-based competition binding assay to characterize pITAM-protein interactions. *Anal. Chem.* 85 (10): 5071–5077. https://doi.org/10.1021/ac400359t.

21 Ali, M.H., Elsherbiny, M.E., and Emara, M. (2019). Updates on aptamer research. *Int. J. Mol. Sci.* 20: 2511. https://doi.org/10.3390/ijms20102511.

22 Wu, D., Gordon, C.K.L., Shin, J.H. et al. (2022). Directed evolution of aptamer discovery technologies. *Acc. Chem. Res.* 55 (5): 685–695. https://doi.org/10.1021/acs.accounts.1c00724.

23 Chen, Z., Luo, H., Gubu, A. et al. (2023). Chemically modified aptamers for improving binding affinity to the target proteins via enhanced non-covalent bonding. *Front. Cell Dev. Biol.* 11: 1–12. https://doi.org/10.3389/fcell.2023.1091809.

24 Gordon, C.K.L., Wu, D., Pusuluri, A. et al. (2019). Click-particle display for base-modified aptamer discovery. *ACS Chem. Biol.* 14 (12): 2652–2662. https://doi.org/10.1021/acschembio.9b00587.

25 Xu, X., Dickey, D.D., Chen, S.-J., and Giangrande, P.H. (2018). Structural computational modeling of RNA aptamers Xiaojun. *Physiol. Behav.* 176 (5): 139–148. https://doi.org/10.1016/j.ymeth.2016.03.004.Structural.

26 Bruno, J.G. (2022). Successes and failures of static aptamer-target 3D docking models. *Int. J. Mol. Sci.* 23 (22): https://doi.org/10.3390/ijms232214410.

27 Buglak, A.A., Samokhvalov, A.V., Zherdev, A.V., and Dzantiev, B.B. (2020). Methods and applications of in silico aptamer design and modeling. *Int. J. Mol. Sci.* 21 (22): 1–25. https://doi.org/10.3390/ijms21228420.

28 Song, S., Wang, X., Xu, K. et al. (2019). Selection of highly specific aptamers to Vibrio parahaemolyticus using cell-SELEX powered by functionalized graphene oxide and rolling circle amplification. *Anal. Chim. Acta* 1052: 153–162. https://doi.org/10.1016/j.aca.2018.11.047.

29 Hao, L. and Gu, H. (2018). Introduction of SELEX and important SELEX variants. In: *Aptamers for Analytical Applications* (ed. Y. Dong), 1–25. https://doi.org/10.1002/9783527806799.ch1.

30 Civit, L., Taghdisi, S.M., Jonczyk, A. et al. (2018). Systematic evaluation of cell-SELEX enriched aptamers binding to breast cancer cells. *Biochimie* 145: 53–62. https://doi.org/10.1016/j.biochi.2017.10.007.

31 Feagin, T.A. and Soh, H.T. (2018). Strategies for creating structure-switching aptamers. *ACS Sensors* 3: 1611–1615. https://doi.org/10.1021/acssensors.8b00516.

32 Jauset-Rubio, M. et al. (2019). One-pot SELEX: identification of specific aptamers against diverse steroid targets in one selection. *ACS Omega* 4 (23): 20188–20196. https://doi.org/10.1021/acsomega.9b02412.

33 Baillargeon, K.R., Botero, M.L., Skouridou, V. et al. (2017). Precipitation SELEX: identification of DNA aptamers for calcium phosphate materials synthesis. *Chem. Commun.* 53 (6): 1092–1095. https://doi.org/10.1039/c6cc08687j.

34 Kim, D.M., Go, M.J., Lee, J. et al. (2021). Recent advances in micro/nanomaterial-based aptamer selection strategies. *Molecules* 26 (17): 1–20. https://doi.org/10.3390/molecules26175187.

35 Yue, H., Chen, J., Chen, X. et al. (2021). Systematic screening and optimization of single-stranded DNA aptamer specific for N-acetylneuraminic acid: a comparative study. *Sensors Actuators B Chem.* 344: 130270. https://doi.org/10.1016/j.snb.2021.130270.

36 Qiao, N., Li, J., Wu, X. et al. (2019). Speeding up in vitro discovery of structure-switching aptamers via magnetic cross-linking precipitation. *Anal. Chem.* 91 (21): 13383–13389. https://doi.org/10.1021/acs.analchem.9b00081.

37 Song, S., Wang, L., Li, J. et al. (2008). Aptamer-based biosensors. *TrAC - Trends Anal. Chem.* 27 (2): 108–117. https://doi.org/10.1016/j.trac.2007.12.004.

38 Bayat, P., Nosrati, R., Alibolandi, M. et al. (2018). SELEX methods on the road to protein targeting with nucleic acid aptamers. *Biochimie* 154: 132–155. https://doi.org/10.1016/j.biochi.2018.09.001.

39 Ruscito, A. and DeRosa, M.C. (2016). Small-molecule binding aptamers: selection strategies, characterization, and applications. *Front. Chem.* 4: 1–14. https://doi.org/10.3389/fchem.2016.00014.

40 Kong, H.Y. and Byun, J. (2013). Nucleic acid aptamers: new methods for selection, stabilization, and application in biomedical science. *Biomol. Ther.* 21 (6): 423–434. https://doi.org/10.4062/biomolther.2013.085.

41 Pichon, V., Hennion, M., and Paristech, E. (2012). *Comprehensive Sampling and Sample Preparation: Analytical Techniques for Scientists*, vol. 2, 359–388. Elsevier.

42 Ando, T., Yamamoto, M., Yokoyama, T. et al. (2021). In vitro selection generates RNA aptamer that antagonizes PCSK9–LDLR interaction and recovers cellular LDL uptake. *J. Biosci. Bioeng.* 131 (3): 326–332. https://doi.org/10.1016/j.jbiosc.2020.10.009.

43 Lu, T., Zhang, J., Zhou, Q. et al. (2021). Aptamer-targeting of Aleutian mink disease virus (AMDV) can be an effective strategy to inhibit virus replication. *Sci. Rep.* 11 (1): 1–12. https://doi.org/10.1038/s41598-021-84223-8.

44 Kohlberger, M., Wildner, S., Regl, C. et al. (2020). Rituximab-specific DNA aptamers are able to selectively recognize heat-treated antibodies. *PLoS ONE* 15 (11): 1–19. https://doi.org/10.1371/journal.pone.0241560.

45 Wei, H., Cai, R., Yue, H. et al. (2020). Screening and application of a truncated aptamer for high-sensitive fluorescent detection of metronidazole. *Anal. Chim. Acta* 1128: 203–210. https://doi.org/10.1016/j.aca.2020.07.003.

46 Wang, J., Wang, Q., Luo, Y. et al. (2019). In vitro selection of ssDNA aptamers that can specifically recognize and differentiate riboflavin and its derivative FAD. *Talanta* 204: 424–430. https://doi.org/10.1016/j.talanta.2019.06.039.

47 Yang, W., Yu, H., Alkhamis, O. et al. (2019). In vitro isolation of class-specific oligonucleotide-based small-molecule receptors. *Nucleic Acids Res.* 47 (12): E71. https://doi.org/10.1093/NAR/GKZ224.

48 Bhardwaj, T., Rathore, A.S., and Jha, S.K. (2020). The selection of highly specific and selective aptamers using modified SELEX and their use in process analytical techniques for Lucentis bioproduction. *RSC Adv.* 10 (48): 28906–28917. https://doi.org/10.1039/d0ra03542d.

49 Yu, H., Yang, W., Alkhamis, O. et al. (2018). In vitro isolation of small-molecule-binding aptamers with intrinsic dye-displacement functionality. *Nucleic Acids Res.* 46 (8): E43. https://doi.org/10.1093/NAR/GKY026.

50 Xiao, Y., Yu, H., Luo, Y. et al. (2021). Isolation of natural DNA aptamers for challenging small-molecule targets, cannabinoids. *Anal. Chem.* 93 (6): 3172–3180. https://doi.org/10.1021/acs.analchem.0c04592.

51 Yang, L., Ding, P., Luo, Y. et al. (2019). Exploration of catalytic nucleic acids on porphyrin metalation and peroxidase activity by in vitro selection of aptamers for N-methyl mesoporphyrin IX. *ACS Comb. Sci.* 21 (2): 83–89. https://doi.org/10.1021/acscombsci.8b00129.

52 Yang, L., Gao, T., Li, W. et al. (2020). Ni-nitrilotriacetic acid affinity SELEX method for selection of DNA aptamers specific to the N-cadherin protein. *ACS Comb. Sci.* 22 (12): 867–872. https://doi.org/10.1021/acscombsci.0c00165.

53 Gu, H., Duan, N., Wu, S. et al. (2016). Graphene oxide-assisted non-immobilized SELEX of okdaic acid aptamer and the analytical application of aptasensor. *Sci. Rep.* 6: 1–9. https://doi.org/10.1038/srep21665.

54 Gu, H., Duan, N., Xia, Y. et al. (2018). Magnetic separation-based multiple SELEX for effectively selecting aptamers against saxitoxin, domoic acid, and tetrodotoxin. *J. Agric. Food Chem.* 66 (37): 9801–9809. https://doi.org/10.1021/acs.jafc.8b02771.

55 Islam, M.M., Ghielmetti, V.M., and Allen, P.B. (2021). Graphene oxide assisted light-up aptamer selection against thioflavin T for label-free detection of microRNA. *Sci. Rep.* 11 (1): 1–14. https://doi.org/10.1038/s41598-021-83640-z.

56 Shi, H., Kou, Q., Wu, P. et al. (2021). Selection and application of DNA aptamers against Sulfaquinoxaline assisted by graphene oxide–based SELEX. *Food Anal. Methods* 14 (2): 250–259. https://doi.org/10.1007/s12161-020-01869-2.

57 Li, W., Luo, Y., Gao, T. et al. (2019). In vitro selection of DNA aptamers for a small-molecule porphyrin by gold nanoparticle-based SELEX. *J. Mol. Evol.* 87 (7–8): 231–239. https://doi.org/10.1007/s00239-019-09905-4.

58 Lee, E.S., Kim, E.J., Park, T.K. et al. (2021). Gold nanoparticle-assisted SELEX as a visual monitoring platform for the development of small molecule-binding DNA aptasensors. *Biosens. Bioelectron.* 191: 113468. https://doi.org/10.1016/j.bios.2021.113468.

59 Chatterjee, B., Kalyani, N., Anand, A. et al. (2020). GOLD SELEX: a novel SELEX approach for the development of high-affinity aptamers against small molecules without residual activity. *Microchim. Acta* 187 (11): 618. https://doi.org/10.1007/s00604-020-04577-0.

60 Ye, H., Duan, N., Wu, S. et al. (2017). Orientation selection of broad-spectrum aptamers against lipopolysaccharides based on capture-SELEX by using magnetic nanoparticles. *Microchim. Acta* 184 (11): 4235–4242. https://doi.org/10.1007/s00604-017-2453-3.

61 Ma, Y., Li, X., Li, W., and Liu, Z. (2018). Glycan-imprinted magnetic nanoparticle-based SELEX for efficient screening of glycoprotein-binding aptamers. *ACS Appl. Mater. Interfaces* 10 (47): 40918–40926. https://doi.org/10.1021/acsami.8b14441.

62 Ma, Y., Li, W., Xing, R. et al. (2020). Epitope-imprinted magnetic nanoparticles as a general platform for efficient in vitro evolution of protein-binding aptamers. *ACS Sensors* 5 (8): 2537–2544. https://doi.org/10.1021/acssensors.0c00846.

63 Liu, F., Ding, A., Zheng, J. et al. (2018). A label-free aptasensor for ochratoxin a detection based on the structure switch of aptamer. *Sensors (Switzerland)* 18 (6): https://doi.org/10.3390/s18061769.

64 Deng, B., Lin, Y., Wang, C. et al. (2014). Aptamer binding assays for proteins: the thrombin example-a review. *Anal. Chim. Acta* 837: 1–15. https://doi.org/10.1016/j.aca.2014.04.055.

65 Lee, T., Kim, J., Nam, I. et al. (2019). Fabrication of troponin i biosensor composed of multi-functional dna structure/au nanocrystal using electrochemical and localized surface plasmon resonance dual-detection method. *Nanomaterials* 9 (7): https://doi.org/10.3390/nano9071000.

66 Saremi, M., Amini, A., and Heydari, H. (2019). An aptasensor for troponin I based on the aggregation-induced electrochemiluminescence of nanoparticles prepared from a cyclometallated iridium(III) complex and poly(4-vinylpyridine-co-styrene) deposited on nitrogen-doped graphene. *Microchim. Acta* 186 (4): https://doi.org/10.1007/s00604-019-3352-6.

67 Shekari, Z., Zare, H.R., and Falahati, A. (2019). Electrochemical sandwich aptasensor for the carcinoembryonic antigen using graphene quantum dots, gold nanoparticles and nitrogen doped graphene modified electrode and exploiting the peroxidase-mimicking activity of a G-quadruplex DNAzyme. *Microchim. Acta* 186 (8): https://doi.org/10.1007/s00604-019-3572-9.

68 Chekin, F., Vasilescu, A., Jijie, R. et al. (2018). Sensitive electrochemical detection of cardiac troponin I in serum and saliva by nitrogen-doped porous reduced graphene oxide electrode. *Sensors Actuators B Chem.* 262: 180–187. https://doi.org/10.1016/j.snb.2018.01.215.

69 Li, Z., Yin, J., Gao, C. et al. (2019). The construction of electrochemical aptasensor based on coral-like poly-aniline and au nano-particles for the sensitive detection of prostate specific antigen. *Sensors Actuators B Chem.* 295: 93–100. https://doi.org/10.1016/j.snb.2019.05.070.

70 Wang, Y., Luo, J., Liu, J. et al. (2019). Label-free microfluidic paper-based electrochemical aptasensor for ultrasensitive and simultaneous multiplexed detection of cancer biomarkers. *Biosens. Bioelectron.* 136: 84–90. https://doi.org/10.1016/j.bios.2019.04.032.

71 Mi, X., Li, H., Tan, R. et al. (2021). The TDs/aptamer cTnI biosensors based on HCR and Au/Ti3C2-MXene amplification for screening serious patient in COVID-19 pandemic. *Biosens. Bioelectron.* 192: 113482. https://doi.org/10.1016/j.bios.2021.113482.

72 Hu, Z., Chen, X., Wang, X. et al. (2021). Aptamer-based novel Ag-coated magnetic recognition and SERS nanotags with interior nanogap biosensor for ultrasensitive detection of protein biomarker. *Sensors Actuators B Chem.* 334: 129640. https://doi.org/10.1016/j.snb.2021.129640.

73 Alijanianzadeh, M., Qadami, F., and Molaeirad, A. (2021). Detection of methamphetamine using aptamer-based biosensor chip and cyclic voltammetry technique. *J. Indian Chem. Soc.* 98 (11): 100189. https://doi.org/10.1016/j.jics.2021.100189.

74 Wu, Y., Chen, X., Wang, X. et al. (2021). A fluorescent biosensor based on prismatic hollow metal-polydopamine frameworks and 6-carboxyfluorescein (FAM)-labeled protein aptamer for CA15-3 detection. *Sensors Actuators B Chem.* 329: 129249. https://doi.org/10.1016/j.snb.2020.129249.

75 Qi, X., Ye, Y., Wang, H. et al. (2022). An ultrasensitive and dual-recognition SERS biosensor based on Fe3O4@Au-Teicoplanin and aptamer functionalized Au@Ag nanoparticles for detection of Staphylococcus aureus. *Talanta* 250: 123648. https://doi.org/10.1016/j.talanta.2022.123648.

76 Jouha, J., Li, F., and Xiong, H. (2023). A fluorescence biosensor based on DNA aptamers-COF for highly selective detection of ATP and thrombin. *Spectrochim. Acta Part A Mol. Biomol. Spectrosc.* 295: 122615. https://doi.org/10.1016/j.saa.2023.122615.

77 Hu, L., Cui, J., Wang, Y., and Jia, J. (2023). An ultrasensitive electrochemical biosensor for bisphenol A based on aptamer-modified MrGO@AuNPs and ssDNA-functionalized AuNP@MBs synergistic amplification. *Chemosphere* 311: 137154. https://doi.org/10.1016/j.chemosphere.2022.137154.

78 Li, X., Jia, M., Yu, L. et al. (2023). An ultrasensitive label-free biosensor based on aptamer functionalized two-dimensional photonic crystal for kanamycin detection in milk. *Food Chem.* 402: 134239. https://doi.org/10.1016/j.foodchem.2022.134239.

79 Jia, Y., Zhao, S., Li, D. et al. (2023). Portable chemiluminescence optical fiber aptamer-based biosensors for analysis of multiple mycotoxins. *Food Control* 144: 109361. https://doi.org/10.1016/j.foodcont.2022.109361.

80 Sarabaegi, M. and Roushani, M. (2019). A nano-sized chitosan particle based electrochemical aptasensor for sensitive detection of: P. Aeruginosa. *Anal. Methods* 11 (43): 5591–5597. https://doi.org/10.1039/c9ay01509d.

81 Wang, J., Li, H., Du, C. et al. (2022). Structure-switching aptamer triggering signal amplification strategy for tobramycin detection based on hybridization chain reaction and fluorescence synergism. *Talanta* 243: 123318. https://doi.org/10.1016/j.talanta.2022.123318.

82 Ma, X., Qiao, S., Sun, H. et al. (2019). Development of structure-switching aptamers for kanamycin detection based on fluorescence resonance energy transfer. *Front. Chem.* 7: 1–10. https://doi.org/10.3389/fchem.2019.00029.

83 Allemailem, K.S., Almatroudi, A., Alsahli, M.A. et al. (2020). Recent advances in understanding oligonucleotide aptamers and their applications as therapeutic agents. *3 Biotech* 10 (12): 1–20. https://doi.org/10.1007/s13205-020-02546-1.

84 Sullivan, R., Adams, M.C., Naik, R.R., and Milam, V.T. (2019). Analyzing secondary structure patterns in DNA aptamers identified via compels. *Molecules* 24 (8): 1–18. https://doi.org/10.3390/molecules24081572.

85 Uhuo, O.V., Waryo, T.T., Douman, S.F. et al. (2022). Bioanalytical methods encompassing label-free and labeled tuberculosis aptasensors: a review. *Anal. Chim. Acta* 1234: 340326. https://doi.org/10.1016/j.aca.2022.340326.

86 Golichenari, B., Nosrati, R., Farokhi-Fard, A. et al. (2018). Nano-biosensing approaches on tuberculosis: defy of aptamers. *Biosens. Bioelectron.* 117: 319–331. https://doi.org/10.1016/j.bios.2018.06.025.

87 Thakur, H., Kaur, N., Sabherwal, P. et al. (2017). Aptamer based voltammetric biosensor for the detection of mycobacterium tuberculosis antigen MPT64. *Microchim. Acta* 184 (7): 1915–1922. https://doi.org/10.1007/s00604-017-2174-7.

88 Feng, L., Zhang, Z., Ren, J., and Qu, X. (2014). Functionalized graphene as sensitive electrochemical label in target-dependent linkage of split aptasensor for dual detection. *Biosens. Bioelectron.* 62: 52–58. https://doi.org/10.1016/j.bios.2014.06.008.

89 Kent, A.D., Spiropulos, N.G., and Heemstra, J.M. (2013). General approach for engineering small-molecule-binding DNA split aptamers. *Anal. Chem.* 85 (20): 9916–9923. https://doi.org/10.1021/ac402500n.

90 Park, J.H., Byun, J.Y., Shim, W.B. et al. (2015). High-sensitivity detection of ATP using a localized surface plasmon resonance (LSPR) sensor and split aptamers. *Biosens. Bioelectron.* 73: 26–31. https://doi.org/10.1016/j.bios.2015.05.043.

91 Morris, F.D., Peterson, E.M., Heemstra, J.M., and Harris, J.M. (2018). Single-molecule kinetic investigation of cocaine-dependent Split-aptamer assembly. *Anal. Chem.* 90 (21): 12964–12970. https://doi.org/10.1021/acs.analchem.8b03637.

92 Gray, M.D., Deore, P.S., Chung, A.J. et al. (2020). Lighting up the thrombin-binding aptamer G-quadruplex with an internal cyanine-indole-quinolinium nucleobase surrogate. Direct fluorescent intensity readout for thrombin binding without topology switching. *Bioconjug. Chem.* 31 (11): 2596–2606. https://doi.org/10.1021/acs.bioconjchem.0c00530.

93 Williams, K.P., Liu, X.H., Schumacher, T.N.M. et al. (1997). Bioactive and nuclease-resistant L-DNA ligand of vasopressin. *Proc. Natl. Acad. Sci. USA* 94 (21): 11285–11290. https://doi.org/10.1073/pnas.94.21.11285.

94 Liu, S.G., Zhang, D., He, Y. et al. (2020). A split aptamer sensing platform for highly sensitive detection of theophylline based on dual-color fluorescence colocalization and single molecule photobleaching. *Biosens. Bioelectron.* 166: 1–7. https://doi.org/10.1016/j.bios.2020.112461.

95 Chen, A., Yan, M., and Yang, S. (2016). Split aptamers and their applications in sandwich aptasensors. *TrAC - Trends Anal. Chem.* 80: 581–593. https://doi.org/10.1016/j.trac.2016.04.006.

96 Jeddi, I. and Saiz, L. (2017). Three-dimensional modeling of single stranded DNA hairpins for aptamer-based biosensors. *Sci. Rep.* 7 (1): 1–13. https://doi.org/10.1038/s41598-017-01348-5.

97 Debiais, M., Lelievre, A., Smietana, M., and Müller, S. (2020). Splitting aptamers and nucleic acid enzymes for the development of advanced biosensors. *Nucleic Acids Res.* 48 (7): 3400–3422. https://doi.org/10.1093/nar/gkaa132.

98 Yu, H., Alkhamis, O., Canoura, J. et al. (2021). Advances and challenges in small-molecule DNA aptamer isolation, characterization, and sensor development. *Angew. Chem. Int. Ed.* 60 (31): 16800–16823. https://doi.org/10.1002/anie.202008663.

99 Abdelrasoul, G.N., Anwar, A., MacKay, S. et al. (2020). DNA aptamer-based non-faradaic impedance biosensor for detecting E. Coli. *Anal. Chim. Acta* 1107: 135–144. https://doi.org/10.1016/j.aca.2020.02.004.

100 Mi, F., Guan, M., Wang, Y. et al. (2023). A SERS biosensor based on aptamer-based Fe3O4@SiO2@ag magnetic recognition and embedded SERS probes for ultrasensitive simultaneous detection of Staphylococcus aureus and Escherichia coli. *Microchem. J.* 190: 108605. https://doi.org/10.1016/j.microc.2023.108605.

101 Li, Q., Li, X., Zhou, P. et al. (2022). Split aptamer regulated CRISPR/Cas12a biosensor for 17β-estradiol through a gap-enhanced Raman tags based lateral flow strategy. *Biosens. Bioelectron.* 215: 114548. https://doi.org/10.1016/j.bios.2022.114548.

102 Jamei, H.R., Rezaei, B., and Ensafi, A.A. (2021). Ultra-sensitive and selective electrochemical biosensor with aptamer recognition surface based on polymer quantum dots and C60/MWCNTs- polyethylenimine nanocomposites for analysis of thrombin protein. *Bioelectrochemistry* 138: 107701. https://doi.org/10.1016/j.bioelechem.2020.107701.

103 Chang, X., Cheng, Y., Wang, X. et al. (2023). A novel ultrasensitive and fast aptamer biosensor of SEB based on AuNPs-assisted metal-enhanced fluorescence. *Sci. Total Environ.* 858: 159977. https://doi.org/10.1016/j.scitotenv.2022.159977.

104 Zhang, K. et al. (2021). A novel electrochemical aptamer biosensor based on tetrahedral DNA nanostructures and catalytic hairpin assembly for CEA detection. *J. Electroanal. Chem.* 898: 115635. https://doi.org/10.1016/j.jelechem.2021.115635.

105 Chen, Y., Pei, M., Cheng, Y. et al. (2021). Rational design of a novel aptamer-based biosensor for a target enzyme via modification of GFP-like fluorogens: carboxylesterase 2A as a case study. *Sensors Actuators B Chem.* 330: 129312. https://doi.org/10.1016/j.snb.2020.129312.

106 Joe, C., Lee, B.H., Kim, S.H. et al. (2022). Aptamer duo-based portable electrochemical biosensors for early diagnosis of periodontal disease. *Biosens. Bioelectron.* 199: 113884. https://doi.org/10.1016/j.bios.2021.113884.

107 Zhu, Q., Liu, L., Wang, R., and Zhou, X. (2021). A split aptamer (SPA)-based sandwich-type biosensor for facile and rapid detection of streptomycin. *J. Hazard. Mater.* 403: 123941. https://doi.org/10.1016/j.jhazmat.2020.123941.

108 Esmaelpourfarkhani, M., Mohammad Danesh, N., Ramezani, M. et al. (2023). Split aptamer-based fluorescent biosensor for ultrasensitive detection of cocaine using N-methyl mesoporphyrin IX as fluorophore. *Microchem. J.* 190: 108630. https://doi.org/10.1016/j.microc.2023.108630.

109 Chi, H. and Liu, G. (2023). A fluorometric sandwich biosensor based on molecular imprinted polymer and aptamer modified CdTe/ZnS for detection of aflatoxin B1 in edible oil. *Lwt* 180 (381): 114726. https://doi.org/10.1016/j.lwt.2023.114726.

110 Liu, H., Ma, S., Ning, G. et al. (2023). A 'peptide-target-aptamer' electrochemical biosensor for norovirus detection using a black phosphorous nanosheet@Ti3C2-Mxene nanohybrid and magnetic covalent organic framework. *Talanta* 258: 124433. https://doi.org/10.1016/j.talanta.2023.124433.

111 Gao, S., Li, Q., Zhang, S. et al. (2023). Peptide–nucleic acid aptamer pair biosensor for disease biomarker detection in clinical samples. *Chem. Eng. J.* 458: 141499. https://doi.org/10.1016/j.cej.2023.141499.

112 Loyez, M., Lobry, M., Hassan, E.M. et al. (2021). HER2 breast cancer biomarker detection using a sandwich optical fiber assay. *Talanta* 221: 121452. https://doi.org/10.1016/j.talanta.2020.121452.

113 Cheng, E.L., Cardle, I.I., Kacherovsky, N. et al. (2022). Discovery of a transferrin receptor 1-binding aptamer and its application in cancer cell depletion for adoptive T-cell therapy manufacturing. *J. Am. Chem. Soc.* 144: 13851–13864.

114 Wei, L., Luo, L., Wang, B.-Z. et al. (2023). Trends in Food Science & Technology Biosensors for detection of paralytic shellfish toxins: recognition elements and transduction technologies. *Trends Food Sci. Technol.* 133: 205–218. https://doi.org/10.1016/j.tifs.2023.02.012.

115 Weller, M.G. (2013). Immunoassays and biosensors for the detection of cyanobacterial toxins in water. *Sensors* 13 (11): 15085–15112. https://doi.org/10.3390/s131115085.

116 Gopalakrishnakone, P., Balali-Mood, M., Llewellyn, L., and Singh, B.R. (2015). *Biological Toxins and Bioterrorism*, 1–604. Springer https://doi.org/10.1007/978-94-007-5869-8.

117 Kumar, S. and Singh, R. (2021). Recent optical sensing technologies for the detection of various biomolecules: review. *Opt. Laser Technol.* 134: 106620. https://doi.org/10.1016/j.optlastec.2020.106620.

118 Kumar, R., Pal, S., Prajapati, Y.K. et al. (2022). Sensitivity improvement of a MXene- immobilized SPR sensor with Ga-doped-ZnO for biomolecules detection. *IEEE Sensors J.* 22 (7): 6536–6543. https://doi.org/10.1109/jsen.2022.3154099.

119 Uniyal, S., Choudhary, K., Sachdev, S., and Kumar, S. (2022). Recent advances in K-SPR sensors for the detection of biomolecules and microorganisms: a review. *IEEE Sensors J.* 22 (12): 11415–11426. https://doi.org/10.1109/JSEN.2022.3172115.

120 Li, P., Long, F., Chen, W. et al. (2020). Fundamentals and applications of surface-enhanced Raman spectroscopy–based biosensors. *Curr. Opin. Biomed. Eng.* 13: 51–59. https://doi.org/10.1016/j.cobme.2019.08.008.

121 Liu, Y., Alkhamis, O., Liu, X. et al. (2021). Aptamer-integrated multianalyte-detecting paper electrochemical device. *ACS Appl. Mater. Interfaces* 13 (15): 17330–17339. https://doi.org/10.1021/acsami.1c01822.

122 Cui, X., Zhou, Y., Zheng, Y. et al. (2022). Investigation the effect of antibiotics on the content of N6-methyladenosine in rice seedling tissue and heavy metal on FTO activity based on antibody-free photoelectrochemcial biosensor. *Sensors Actuators B Chem.* 364: 131896. https://doi.org/10.1016/j.snb.2022.131896.

123 Gao, W., Nyein, H.Y.Y., Shahpar, Z. et al. (2016). Wearable microsensor array for multiplexed heavy metal monitoring of body fluids. *ACS Sensors* 1 (7): 866–874. https://doi.org/10.1021/acssensors.6b00287.

124 McConnell, E.M., Nguyen, J., and Li, Y. (2020). Aptamer-based biosensors for environmental monitoring. *Front. Chem.* 8: 1–24. https://doi.org/10.3389/fchem.2020.00434.

125 Varma, A., Mukasyan, A.S., Rogachev, A.S., and Manukyan, K.V. (2016). Solution combustion synthesis of nanoscale materials. *Chem. Rev.* 116 (23): 14493–14586. https://doi.org/10.1021/acs.chemrev.6b00279.

126 Kim, J., Sung, G.Y., and Park, M. (2020). Efficient portable urea biosensor based on urease immobilized membrane for monitoring of physiological fluids. *Biomedicine* 8 (12): 1–11. https://doi.org/10.3390/biomedicines8120596.

127 Daniel, J. (1969). Urea-specific enzyme electrode. *J. Am. Chem. Soc.* 19: 2164–2165.

128 Su, J., Zhu, B., Inoue, A. et al. (2023). The patrol yeast: a new biosensor armed with antibody-receptor chimera detecting a range of toxic substances associated with food poisoning. *Biosens. Bioelectron.* 219: 114793. https://doi.org/10.1016/j.bios.2022.114793.

129 Moon, J., Byun, J., Kim, H. et al. (2018). On-site detection of aflatoxin B1 in grains by a palm-sized surface plasmon resonance sensor. *Sensors (Switzerland)* 18 (2): https://doi.org/10.3390/s18020598.

130 Kumar, V., Raghuwanshi, S.K., and Kumar, S. (2022). Recent advances in carbon nanomaterials based SPR sensor for biomolecules and gas detection-a review. *IEEE Sensors J.* 22 (16): 15661–15672. https://doi.org/10.1109/JSEN.2022.3191042.

131 Kim, S.H., Nam, O., Jin, E.S., and Gu, M.B. (2019). A new coccolith modified electrode-based biosensor using a cognate pair of aptamers with sandwich-type binding. *Biosens. Bioelectron.* 123: 160–166. https://doi.org/10.1016/j.bios.2018.08.021.

132 Sun, D., Luo, Z., Lu, J. et al. (2019). Electrochemical dual-aptamer-based biosensor for nonenzymatic detection of cardiac troponin I by nanohybrid electrocatalysts labeling combined with DNA nanotetrahedron structure. *Biosens. Bioelectron.* 134: 49–56. https://doi.org/10.1016/j.bios.2019.03.049.

133 Shirani, M., Kalantari, H., Khodayar, M.J. et al. (2020). A novel strategy for detection of small molecules based on aptamer/gold nanoparticles/graphitic carbon nitride nanosheets as fluorescent biosensor. *Talanta* 219: 121235. https://doi.org/10.1016/j.talanta.2020.121235.

134 You, M., Yang, S., An, Y. et al. (2020). A novel electrochemical biosensor with molecularly imprinted polymers and aptamer-based sandwich assay for determining amyloid-β oligomer. *J. Electroanal. Chem.* 862: 114017. https://doi.org/10.1016/j.jelechem.2020.114017.

135 Tang, X., Yin, Z., Lei, X. et al. (2019). Colorimetric method for sensitive detection of microcystin-LR using surface copper nanoparticles of polydopamine nanosphere as turn-on probe. *Nanomaterials* 9 (3): 332. https://doi.org/10.3390/nano9030332.

136 Zhang, S., Sun, Y., Sun, Y. et al. (2020). Semiquantitative immunochromatographic colorimetric biosensor for the detection of dexamethasone based on up-conversion fluorescent nanoparticles. *Microchim. Acta* 187 (8): 447. https://doi.org/10.1007/s00604-020-04418-0.

137 Qin, Y., Bubiajiaer, H., Yao, J., and Zhang, M. (2022). Based on unmodified aptamer-gold nanoparticles colorimetric detection of dexamethasone in food. *Biosensors* 12 (4): 1–11. https://doi.org/10.3390/bios12040242.

138 Srinivasan, S., Ranganathan, V., DeRosa, M.C., and Murari, B.M. (2019). Comparison of turn-on and ratiometric fluorescent G-quadruplex aptasensor approaches for the detection of ATP. *Anal. Bioanal. Chem.* 411 (7): 1319–1330. https://doi.org/10.1007/s00216-018-1484-x.

139 You, J., You, Z., Xu, X. et al. (2019). A split aptamer-labeled ratiometric fluorescent biosensor for specific detection of adenosine in human urine. *Microchim. Acta* 186 (1): https://doi.org/10.1007/s00604-018-3162-2.

140 Wu, C., Offenhäusser, A., and Mayer, D. (2020). A highly sensitive Amperometric aptamer biosensor for adenosine triphosphate detection on a 64 channel gold multielectrode array. *Phys. Status Solidi Appl. Mater. Sci.* 217 (13): 1–8. https://doi.org/10.1002/pssa.201900925.

141 Zheng, W., Liu, X., Li, Q. et al. (2022). A simple electrochemical aptasensor for saxitoxin detection. *RSC Adv.* 12 (37): 23801–23807. https://doi.org/10.1039/d2ra03690h.

142 Al-Jawdah, A., Nabok, A., Abu-Ali, H. et al. (2019). Highly sensitive label-free in vitro detection of aflatoxin B1 in an aptamer assay using optical planar waveguide operating as a polarization interferometer. *Anal. Bioanal. Chem.* 411 (29): 7717–7724. https://doi.org/10.1007/s00216-019-02033-4.

143 Yan, X., Qi, X., Zhao, Y. et al. (2022). Development of a label-free colorimetric aptasensor with rationally utilized aptamer for rapid detection of okadaic acid. *J. Ocean Univ. China* 21 (2): 400–408. https://doi.org/10.1007/s11802-022-4849-x.

144 Runsewe, D.O., Haya, G., Betancourt, T., and Irvin, J.A. (2021). Conducting polymer-based electrochemical aptasensor for the detection of adenosine. *ACS Appl. Polym. Mater.* 3 (12): 6674–6683. https://doi.org/10.1021/acsapm.1c01348.

145 Zavyalova, E., Tikhonova, D., Zhdanov, G. et al. (2022). SERS-based biosensor with Raman-active external responsive element for rapid determination of adenosine monophosphate. *Anal. Chim. Acta* 1221: 340140. https://doi.org/10.1016/j.aca.2022.340140.

146 Oh, I.H., Park, D.Y., Cha, J.M. et al. (2020). Docking simulation and Sandwich assay for aptamer-based botulinum neurotoxin type C detection. *Biosensors* 10 (8): 98. https://doi.org/10.3390/bios10080098.

147 Lahousse, M., Park, H.C., Lee, S.C. et al. (2018). Inhibition of anthrax lethal factor by ssDNA aptamers. *Arch. Biochem. Biophys.* 646: 16–23. https://doi.org/10.1016/j.abb.2018.03.028.

148 Zhu, S., Yang, Y., Li, M. et al. (2021). A pH-responsive bioassay for sensitive colorimetric detection of adenosine triphosphate based on switchable DNA aptamer and metal ion–urease interactions. *Anal. Bioanal. Chem.* 413 (6): 1533–1540. https://doi.org/10.1007/s00216-020-03136-z.

149 Li, Y., Bu, Y., Jiang, F. et al. (2020). Fabrication of ultra-sensitive photoelectrochemical aptamer biosensor: based on semiconductor/DNA interfacial multifunctional reconciliation via 2D-C3N4. *Biosens. Bioelectron.* 150: 111903. https://doi.org/10.1016/j.bios.2019.111903.

150 Jia, M., Yu, L., Li, X. et al. (2023). An aptamer-functionalized photonic crystal sensor for ultrasensitive and label-free detection of aflatoxin B1. *Talanta* 260: 124638. https://doi.org/10.1016/j.talanta.2023.124638.

151 Yasli, A. (2021). Cancer detection with surface plasmon resonance-based photonic crystal fiber biosensor. *Plasmonics* 16 (5): 1605–1612. https://doi.org/10.1007/s11468-021-01425-6.

152 Xuan, H., Ren, J., Zhu, Y. et al. (2016). Aptamer-functionalized P(NIPAM-AA) hydrogel fabricated one-dimensional photonic crystals (1DPCs) for colorimetric sensing. *RSC Adv.* 6 (43): 36827–36833. https://doi.org/10.1039/c6ra03831j.

6

Bacteriophage-Based Biosensors

6.1 Introduction

Bacteriophages, also referred to as phages or viruses, are made up of a protein coat surrounded by genetic material, either DNA or RNA, that infect and replicate only within bacteria [1]. In case of phage-based biosensors, the phage and target molecule interact, injecting genetic material inside the bacteria that produces a measurable response [2]. As bacteria enter the cell, its machinery is hijacked and replicates the genetic material to generate new phages.

Bacteriophage replication after the attachment of the selected target occurs in two steps: (i) lytic and (ii) lysogenic cycle. During the lytic cycle, the phage inserts genome material into the cytoplasm of the host cell. It utilizes the ribosomes of the host cell to produce the required proteins. The phage will control the host DNA generation machinery and produce DNA similar to the phage. It produces multiple copies of the phage, kills the host, and explodes or lyses to produce new phages to affect other bacterial cells [3]. Figure 6.1a shows a schematic of stages of the lytic and lysogenic cycles. This process can occur rapidly, leading to the death of the host bacterial population. In lysogenic sequence, the cell is infected by phage and the genome of phage integrates for cell division.

Newly generated cells will consist of prophage DNA during cell division, which does not kill the host cell [6, 7]. Bacteriophage-based biosensors have several advantages over traditional bacterial detection methods, including high specificity due to its strain's specificity, rapidness, and sensitivity, as the signal can be detected within minutes to hours after exposure to the target bacteria [8]. The selection of a suitable host leads to multiplication and cycle completion via lytic or lysis cycle, which is an advantage over the traditional bacteria detection

Biosensors: Nanomaterials, Approaches, and Performance-Enhancement Strategies,
First Edition. Baljinder Kaur, Santosh Kumar, and Brajesh Kumar Kaushik.

Published 2025 by John Wiley & Sons, Inc.
Companion website: www.wiley.com/go/kaur

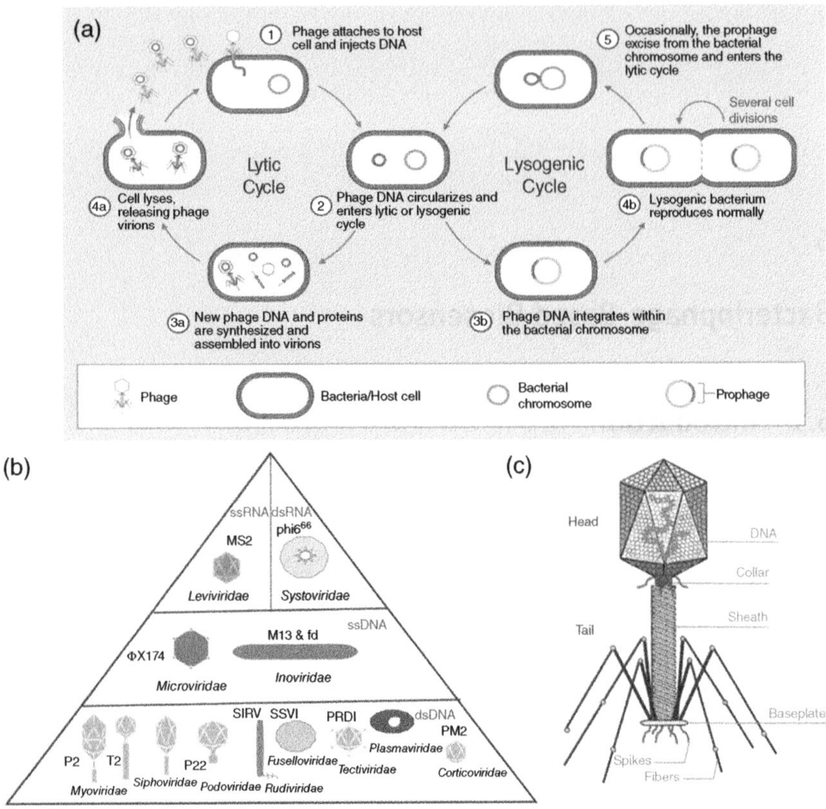

Figure 6.1 Schematic illustration of (a) different stages of the lytic and lysogenic cycle; (b) various shapes. *Source:* [4]/with permission of Elsevier. (c) Structure of a phage. *Source:* [5]/with permission of Elsevier.

methods that can produce false results by detecting dead bacteria [9, 10]. It also offers numerous benefits as it does not require complex pre-sample preparations, can be used in harsh environment, can distinguish dead bacteria from live bacteria, and is cheap and easy to produce at the bulk level [11]. Bacteriophages have been proposed as a potential alternative to biorecognition elements (BREs) to detect various analytes that lead to several diseases due to their high specificity, as shown in Table 6.1 [14]. Phage size varies; among all the phages, T4 is largest – 200 nm in length with diameter in the range of 80–100 nm. Phages with a tail having a genome size bigger than 200 kb are known as "jumbo phages" that harbor large virions [15].

Table 6.1 Common orders and families of bacteriophages, their morphology, examples, and the type of nucleic acid of bacteriophages [12, 13].

S. No.	Order	Family	Morphology	Examples	NA	Replication mode
1	Caudovirales	Myoviridae	Complex (head, long tail)	T4, Mu	DS DNA	Lytic
2	Caudovirales	Siphoviridae	Complex (head, long tail)	Lambda, T5	DS DNA	Lysogenic/Lytic
3	Caudovirales	Podoviridae	Complex (head, long tail)	T7, P22	DS DNA	Lytic
4	Levivirales	Leviviridae	Icosahedral	MS2, Qβ	SS RNA	Lytic
5	Microvirales	Microviridae	Icosahedral	PhiX174	SS DNA	Lytic
6	Inovirales	Inoviridae	Filamentous	M13, fd	SS DNA	Lysogenic
7	Tectivirales	Tectiviridae	Icosahedral	PRD1	DS DNA	Lytic
8	Picornavirales	Cystoviridae	Pleomorphic	Phi6	Segmented DS RNA	Lytic
9	Herpesvirales	Herpesviridae	Complex (Enveloped)	Herpes simplex virus	DS DNA	Lysogenic/Lytic
10	Anellovirales	Anelloviridae	Icosahedral	Torque Teno virus	SS DNA	Lytic
11	Fusellovirales	Fuselloviridae	Lemon-shaped	SIRV2	DS DNA	Lytic
12	Corticoviridae	Corticoviridae	Spherical	PRR1	DS DNA	Lytic
13	Lipothrixviridae	Lipothrixviridae	Filamentous	Acidianus filamentous virus 1	DS DNA	Lysogenic
14	Rudiviridae	Rudiviridae	Rod-shaped	Sulfolobus turreted icosahedral virus	DS DNA	Lytic
15	Phycodnaviridae	Phycodnaviridae	Icosahedral	*Emiliania huxleyi* virus 201	DS DNA	Lytic
16	Geminiviridae	Geminiviridae	Geminate (twin particles)	Tomato yellow leaf curl virus	SS DNA	Not known
17	Baculoviridae	Baculoviridae	Rod-shaped with envelopes	*Autographa californica* nucleopolyhedrovirus	DS DNA	Lytic
18	Adenoviridae	Adenoviridae	Complex icosahedral with fibers	Human adenovirus	DS DNA	Lytic

Bacteriophage types depend on shapes, whether or not they are enveloped, morphology, genetic material, replication mode, host range, and sizes; they are all categorized into one of the two replication methods: lytic and lysogenic, as shown in Table 6.1. Figure 6.1b,c shows the schematic illustration of various shapes of phages and their structure. The number of bacteriophage families may change, as shown in Table 6.1; research is ongoing to discover new phages.

Based on morphology, phages are divided into three main sets: (i) icosahedral (having a 20-sided polygonal shape), (ii) filamentous (having a long, thin, thread-like shape), and (iii) complex (having a nonsymmetrical shape, usually with a head and a tail), and into two groups based on their genetic material: DNA phages and RNA phages [3].

The next subsection discusses the engineered phages used for various applications.

6.1.1 Reporter Bacteriophages

Reporter phages are engineered phages that carries a reporter gene. During the interaction of target and phage it produces a fluorescence or luminescent signal that can be measured using different sensing technologies [1]. The signal can be visual, such as a color change, or measurable, such as fluorescence or luminescence. It can be utilized at different stages and used in case of lysogenic or lytic modes.

Reporter phage-probes are useful tools in bacterial detection and identification in numerous fields [4]. A luminescent nanoluciferase enzyme-based reporter gene has been investigated to detect the *Enterococcus faecalis, Klebsiella,* and *E. coli* among urinary tract infections *E. coli, Enterococcus* spp., and *Klebsiella* spp. Sensitivity of the three bacteria Enterococcus, *E. coli*, faecalis, Klebsiella are 78%, 68%, 87%, specificity of 99% in each case and resolution of 103 CFU/ml have been reported [16]. Another recombinant TUN1 reporter phage and nano-luciferase gene-based biosensor is designed to identify the K64 strains of *Klebsiella pneumoniae.* As a gene-encoded phage interacts with the target pneumoniae bacteria and inserts its gene into bacteria, a luminescent is observed due to a reaction between target and phage and provides LOD of 1 CFU/well [17].

6.1.2 Stained Phages

Phages are stained so they are visible under a microscope. The staining process involves adding a dye to the phage solution and allowing it to bind to the phage particles. Stained phages can be used for visualization and identification of phages in samples [18]. Different staining techniques can be used to highlight different features of the phage, such as the capsid or tail [18]. A nucleic acid–based cyanine dye named as SYBR Green I was used to stain T7 phage. This T7 phage with single-wall carbon nanotubes (CNTs) was used to fabricate an electrochemical (ECL) biosensor that can detect *E. coli*. The strain BL21 *E. coli*. can be detected with 1 CFU/ml and linear range of up to 10^4 CFU/ml [19].

6.1.3 Lytic Phages

Lytic phages are a type of bacteriophage that replicates inside the host bacterium and causes the host cell to lyse, or burst open, releasing new phage particles. T4, T7, and lambda are commonly used lytic bacteriophages. Lytic phages are often used as therapeutic agents to treat bacterial infections [20]. With the help of lytic and temperature phages such as HK620 and ΦV10, reporter phages can be generated [21]. They are also used in research as a tool for genetic engineering and molecular biology. Lytic phages have a short life cycle that can rapidly infect and kill bacterial cells. They have ability to compete against antibiotic-resistant bacteria and are thus a substitute for antibiotics [6].

6.1.4 Capturing Phages

Capturing phages are engineered phages that capture and bind to specific target bacteria or bacterial components. Capturing phages consist of different active groups such as carboxyl group and immobilize on solid matrices. Capturing phages can also be used in environmental remediation to capture and remove specific bacteria from contaminated sites. M13 phage is an example of a capturing phage used to detect the microorganisms. Various colorimetric biosensors that consist of multiple array are constructed using M13 phage to detect the volatile organic compounds, and humidity [22].

6.1.5 Phage Receptor-Binding Proteins

These are the monomeric small-size proteins present on the phages surface that play an important role in binding to specific receptors available on target or bacterial cells [23]. The binding of receptor proteins via specific sequences such as polysaccharide, teichoic acids, and polypeptides exist on the surface of the cell [24]. Phage receptor-binding proteins can be either tail fibers or tail spikes according to morphology [25]. Phage receptor-binding proteins have been extensively studied for their potential use in phage therapy, as they can be engineered to target specific bacterial species or strains [26]. They are also being studied for their potential use in vaccine development, as they can elicit an immune response against specific bacteria [4]. T4, P22, and T7 are the most common examples of receptor-binding proteins phages. Figure 6.2 shows the structure of phage receptor-binding proteins that include wildtype and fusion proteins, their randomization, and the recombination process.

Phage immobilization is an important technique in phage research and applications, as it attaches the phage to substrate surface and allows its interaction with target. There are several methods for immobilizing phages, including poly-L-lysine coating, nitrocellulose membrane immobilization, and adsorption onto a solid support, as shown in Table 6.2 [34, 35]. Poly-L-lysine (PLL) coating provides a positively charged surface for phages to bind to, while nitrocellulose membrane immobilization involves coating a membrane with phages, which are then immobilized on the surface [27]. Adsorption onto a solid support involves binding phages to a solid support, such as glass or magnetic beads, by adsorption [28]. Adsorption has been widely explored in phage-based therapy and diagnostic and treatment applications due to its simplicity and ease of use.

Phage-based probes are an emerging technology with various advantages over traditional methods to detect biospecies. It has been explored in relation to different pathogenic bacteria, viruses, and fungi. High specificity and sensitivity are the prominent advantage of phage-based biosensors because they can detect targets at low levels [29].

Researchers are focusing on improving specificity, sensitivity, stability, and limit of detection (LOD) values of phage-based biosensors. For example, researchers have developed engineered phages that can bind to specific bacterial strains or even specific virulence factors. These engineered phages can be used in phage-based probes to specifically detect the target biospecies [30]. Another advance in phage-based probe technology is the development of rapid detection methods [31, 32].

6.2 Design of Bacteriophage-Based Biosensor

Figure 6.3a depicts a SiO_2@AuNP core-shell NPs based bacteriophage plasmonic sensor using dark-field microscopy and S13′ phage to detect the *S. aureus*. It is based on fact that bound bacteria scatter the light more as compared to unbound and background cells. Dark-field microscopy was used to detect the signal from light scattered from the nanoprobe. The detected LOD values lies in the range of 10^4 CFU/ml in case of *S. aureus* bacteria [36]. Bhardwaj et al. reported a graphene-electrodes immobilized with bacteriophage to detect the *Staphylococcus arlettae* bacteria. After binding of bacteria to phage surface, it changes the electrical resistance due to formation of bacteria layer on the electrodes. This process offers a LOD of 2 CFU and for the concentration range of 10^6 CFU to detect the *Staphylococcus arlettae* bacteria [39]. Octupolar meta-structures with

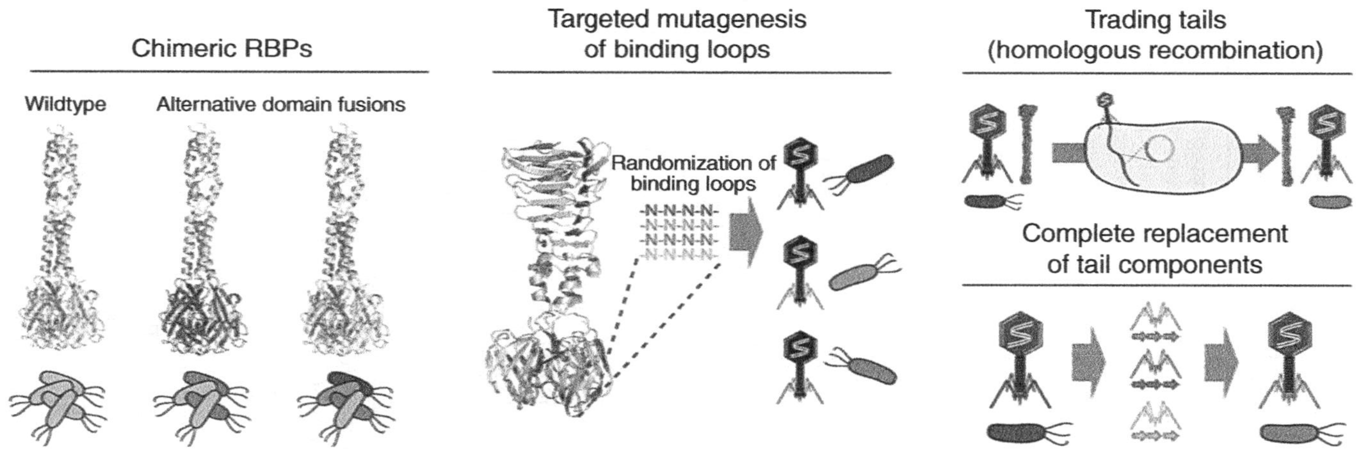

Figure 6.2 Structure of phage receptor-binding proteins. *Source:* Adapted from [4].

Table 6.2 Comparison of immobilization techniques for bacteriophages [27–33].

Immobilization technique	Advantages	Disadvantages
Adsorption to solid surfaces	Simple and quick minimal use of chemicals	Nonspecific binding can lead to reduced activity; phages are arranged; randomly adsorbed phage may detach according to environment condition
Covalent binding	Stable and specific low risk of detachment	Can affect phage structure and activity
Encapsulation	Protects phage from environmental factors	Can reduce phage activity and limit accessibility
Electrostatic binding	Simple and quick	pH and salt concentration have dependent, nonspecific binding
Affinity binding	Highly specific	Can be expensive and time-consuming
Physical entrapment	Gentle and nondestructive	Low loading capacity and limited access to the phage

self-assembled monolayer (SAM) of 4-mercaptobenzoic acid and based plasmonics SERS sensor were reported to detect the Brucella bacteria. The meta-structures are constructed using Au nano-disks in the octupolar shape that enhance the SERS signal by 2100% and offer excellent sensitivity. LOD of 16 fM was reported for the concentration range of 10^4–10^9 CFU/ml [40].

Another SERS sensor combining with polymerase chain reaction (PCR) on Klarite and GaN/Ag-Au-Gamma-phage substrate to detect the *Bacillus anthracis* was investigated. LOD of 10^4 CFU/ml was reported [41]. Figure 6.4b shows that a long-period fiber grating–based immunosensor to detect the T7 bacteriophages. 3-(triethoxysilyl) propyl succinic anhydride was used to functionalize the anti-T7 phage through covalent bonding. The working of this sensor is based on the fact that as a virus binds to phage, it changes the transmission spectrum. The virus can be detected with LOD of 5×10^3 PFU/ml in the RI range of 1.333–1.439 RIU [45]. M-13 bacteriophage has been explored to detect the various analytes such as nitrotoluene, cefadroxil, amoxicillin, and Rifampicin. M13 bacteriophages is of filamentous shape; one end has p6, p3 proteins and the other end has p7 and p9 protein configurations [37]. The structural color of M-13 bacteriophage is determined by the spacing between the p8 proteins on the surface of the phage [46]. An organic–inorganic hybrid nano-flowers made up of glucose oxidase and HRP-$Cu_3(PO_4)_2$-based ECL sensor to detect the *E. coli* during urinary tract infection is shown in Figure 6.3c. Nano-flowers have the capacity to load the large capacity of sample that provide the LOD of 1 CFU/ml and in the concentration range of 10^8 CFU/ml [38]. A surface plasmon resonance (SPR) biosensor that involved

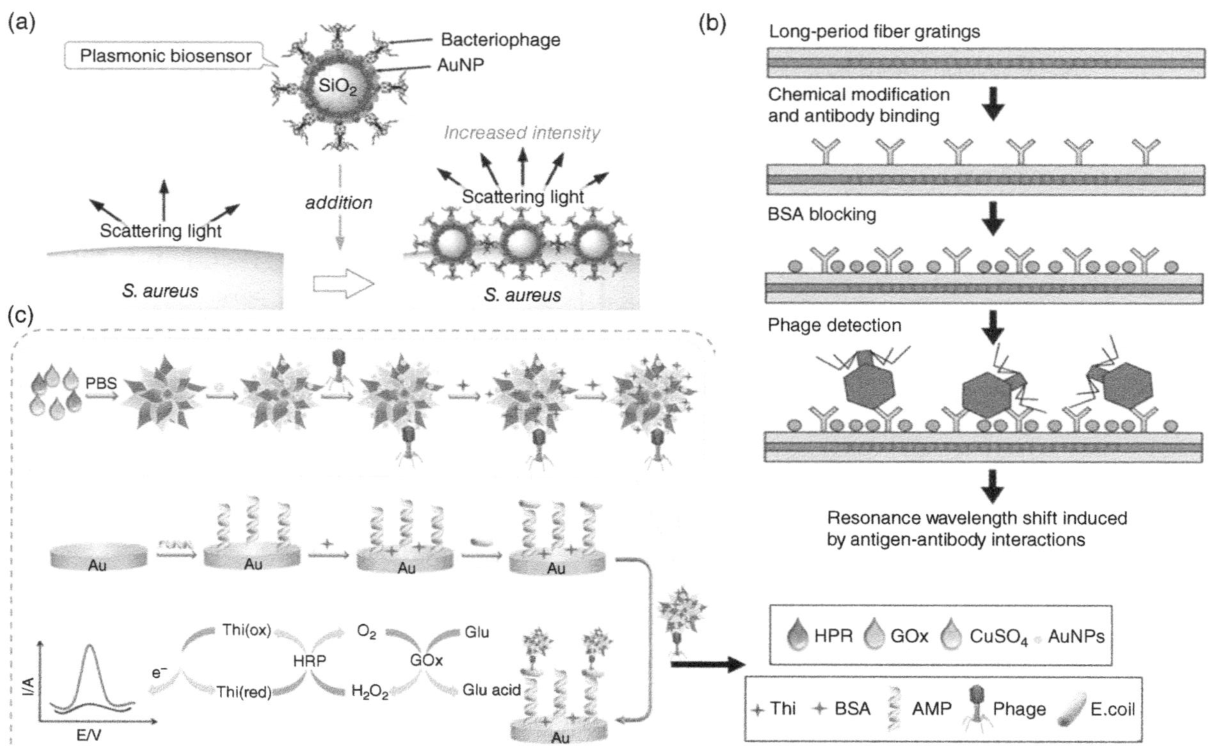

Figure 6.3 Schematic illustration of (a) SiO_2- and AuNP-based core-shell-structure immobilized with S13 phage based sensor to detect the *S. aureus*. *Source:* [36]/with permission of American Chemical Society. (b) Long-period fiber grating–based immunosensor. *Source:* R[37]/with permission of Elsevier. (c) Organic–inorganic hybrid nano-flowers based ECL sensor. *Source:* [38]/with permission of Elsevier.

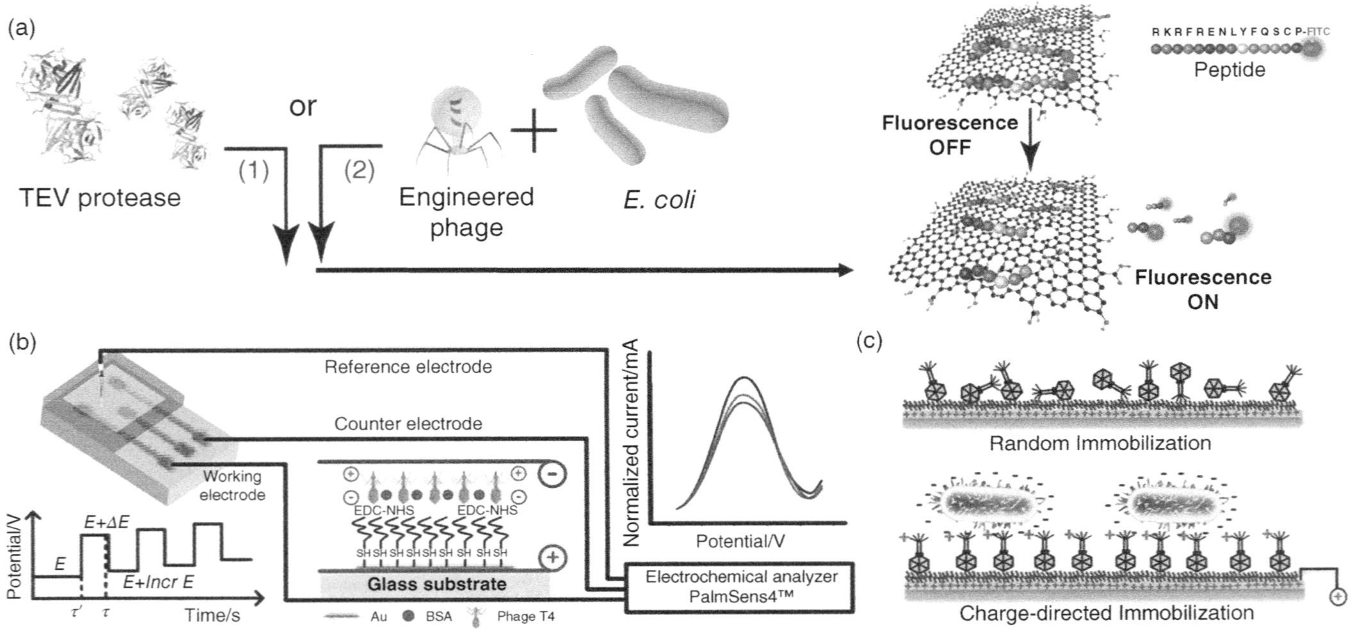

Figure 6.4 Schematic illustration of the (a) fluoro-peptide-graphene oxide nano-sensors. *Source:* [42]/with permission of Springer Nature. (b) T4 bacteriophage-based micro-ECL biosensor. *Source:* [43]/with permission of Elsevier. (c) T2 bacteriophage-CNT functionalized with polyethylenimine based ECL sensor to detect the *E. coli*. *Source:* [44]/with permission of American Chemical Society.

lambda phage has been used to detect the K-12 strain of *E. coli* bacteria. To overcome the host cell lysis issue that lowers the strength of cell signal, a tail fragment of J protein of lambda phage with a (His)6-tag was used *E. coli* K-12 can be detected in the concentration range of 10^4–10^9 CFU/ml and LOD of 2×10^4 CFU/ml [47].

A colorimetric sensor has been developed to create programmable micro-color patterns using the self-assembly of M13 bacteriophage. The method is based on the fact that the color of M13 bacteriophage can be tuned by changing the temperature at which the self-assembly occurs. M13 bacteriophage can self-assemble into long, helical filaments. The color of the filaments depends on the temperature at which the self-assembly occurs. At low temperatures, the filaments are blue, while at high temperatures, the filaments are red [48]. *Salmonella enterica* serovar typhimurium has been detected using Det7 phage tail protein through SPR biosensor. Sensors are constructed by immobilizing the Au metal with Det7T proteins via amine-coupling that can detect the *Salmonella enterica* in the concentration range of 10^4–10^7 CFU/ml and LOD of 10^4 CFU/ml [49]. Bacteriophage-based nano-biosensors have been explored to detect the pathogenic bacteria's in food samples. An AuNPs- multi-walled CNT-tungsten oxide nanostructures-based ECL nano-biosensor to detect the *E. coli O157:H7* in food samples. 4-aminothiophenol was used as a linker molecule to create SAM. *E. coli* can be detected with LOD of 3.0 CFU/ml in the concentration range of 10^1–10^7 CFU/ml [50]. A colorimetric approach based on chimeric phages, engineered bacteriophages that specifically bind to target bacteria, coupled with AuNPs, is demonstrated. Chimeric M13 phage was immobilized on AuNPs through a covalent bonding. This sensor was designed to detect the different stains of *E. coli* and two strains of the plant pathogen *Xanthomonas campestris*. It can detect ~100 cells with high sensitivity [51]. A lyophilized engineered T7 phage-based colorimetric biosensor for detecting *E. coli* bacteria through overexpressed β-galactosidase in food samples was developed. The concentration of 100 CFU/mL can be measured [52]. A fluoro-peptide-graphene oxide nano-sensor with engineered phages to infect bacterial cells and express a protease enzyme that cleaves a peptide substrate, leading to a detectable change in *E. coli* was reported as shown in Figure 6.4a. Tobacco etches virus concentrations of 51 ng/μl with a LOD of 10^4 CFU/ml were reported [42]. The detection of *Salmonella typhimurium* was reported using E2 phage on the surface of a quartz crystal. This sensor can detect *Salmonella typhimurium* through changes in mass and viscosity on binding of bacteria and phages. The biosensor provides a LOD of 10^5 CFU/ml of the bacteria in the romaine lettuce samples [53].

A biosensor based on CTXφ phage coated with pIII protein fixed on an Au can detect *Vibrio cholerae* in the lytic cycle through changes in RI using SPR sensor structure. CTXφ bacteriophage is a thin-diameter and wormlike structure that can detect the cholera virus. *Cholerae* was detected in the concentrations of 10^3–10^9 CFU/ml and LOD of 2×10^4 CFU/ml [54]. A gold-coated sensor chip allows for the detection of the biomarkers through changes in color caused by the gap plasmonic effect. The M13 bacteriophage was chosen as a recognition element because the structural protein capsid can be readily modified to target the desired analyte [55]. Xu et al. describe the development of a biosensor for the diagnosis of lung cancer using gap plasmonic color films. The biosensor shown in Figure 6.4b is based on the immobilization of lung cancer biomarkers on a T4 bacteriophage-based micro-ECL biosensor using an Au chip to detect the *E. coli* B bacteria with detection limit of 14 CFU/ml in the concentration range of 10^1–10^8 CFU/ml [43]. A capacitive biosensor constructed using M13 bacteriophage immobilized on Au metal cross-linked with glutaraldehyde to detect gram-negative Salmonella. Sensor provides relative standard deviation (RSD), linear range, and LOD of 1.1%, 10^2–10^7 CFU/mL, 200 CFU/ml. A vB_YepM_ZN18 phage-based ECL biosensor fabricated using poly-(indole-5-carboxylic acid), reduced graphene oxide, and AuNPs to detect *Yersinia pseudotuberculosis*. It can detect the bacteria with linear range, correlation coefficient, and LOD of 5.30×10^2–1.05×10^7 CFU/ml 0.992 and 3 CFU/ml [56].

Figure 6.4c shows a T2 bacteriophage, CNT functionalized with polyethylenimine-based ECL sensor for detection of *E. coli, K* strain. It provides the LOD of 1000 CFU/ml in *E. coli* concentrations of 10^3–10^6 CFU/ml [44]. AuNPs-modified 3D-printed graphene electrodes-based ECL biosensor was reported to detect the severe acute respiratory syndrome (SARS)-CoV-2 cDNA virus. The biosensor has a LOD of 1.9 fM. The biosensor's performance was also evaluated using clinical samples, and it showed comparable results to the RT-qPCR method, which is considered the gold standard for COVID-19 diagnosis. The use of 3D-printed graphene electrodes and AuNPs modifications improved the ECL performance of the biosensor, enabling the SARS-CoV-2 cDNA detection. The current methods for detecting sepsis are not always accurate, so there is a need for new diagnostic tools. The authors developed a M13 bacteriophage and mesoporous substrate-based SERS sensor to detect the soluble triggering receptor expressed on myeloid cells-1, C-reactive protein and procalcitonin. This substrate allows for the detection of multiple biomarkers simultaneously, making it a useful tool in sepsis diagnosis. The sensor provides LOD values of 27, 103, and 78 pM for C-reactive protein, procalcitonin, and soluble triggering receptors expressed on myeloid cells-1 [57]. The authors used genetically engineered phages to improve the binding of biosensors to specific molecules. They screened a large library of phages to identify those with high affinity and selectivity for the target molecule. They then used the selected phages to improve the performance of the biosensor. The authors found that this method improved the binding affinity and selectivity of the biosensor, making it a more accurate and reliable tool for detecting specific molecules. They also established a LOD of 8 ng/cm^2 for the biosensor [58].

Table 6.3 discusses various other bacteriophage-based biosensors to detect the diseases. Rippa et al. made a 2D SERS substrate based on phages. It is made of plasmonic nano-cavities arranged in a photonic quasicrystal pattern with 12-fold (dodecagonal) rotational symmetry. A SERS biosensor that involves Tbilisi, Podoviridae family of phages as bioreceptors was investigated to detect the Tbilisi virus. Phage immobilization amplifies the SERS signal 62 times and provides the LOD of 1.7 fM [68]. Methicillin-resistant *S. aureus* was detected using ECL biosensors that utilize SATA-8505 bacteriophages and CNT-based biosensors. SATA-8505 phage was immobilized using 1-dodecanethiol on the electrode surface by forming a SAM. The results showed that the biosensor is capable of detecting Methicillin-resistant *S. aureus* with LOD values of 1.23×10^2 and 1.29×10^2 CFU/ml in aqueous solution and blood plasma having concentration range of 10–10^8 CFU/ml [66]. *Listeria monocytogenes* causes various disease arising in different food samples. The biosensor was designed using Au electrode-CNT modified with polyethylenimine-P100 phage. The results showed that the biosensor was capable of detecting *L. monocytogenes* concentrations as low as 8.4 CFU/ml, in the concentration range of 10–10^4 CFU/ml [64]. A CRISPR technology-based fluorescent bacteriophage biosensor was designed to detect the *E. coli* EV36-RFP strain using phage K1F. The bacteriophages used in the study were engineered to express a cell-penetrating peptide on their capsid surfaces. The ability of the engineered bacteriophages to penetrate human cells was demonstrated using fluorescent microscopy and flow cytometry techniques. The engineered bacteriophages can detect the bacteria in the range of 10^6–10^3 CFU/ml [69].

Figure 6.5a T7 presents bacteriophages-based ECL sensor to detect *E. coli*. Three electrodes – working, counter, and a reference electrode – were used to construct the biosensor. The working electrode is made of a gold surface functionalized with SAMs of mercapto hexanol. The gold surface is then modified with a layer of carboxylate-terminated polyethylene glycol (PEG) to minimize nonspecific binding of the engineered phages. The engineered phages are then immobilized onto the PEG layer through covalent bonding with the carboxylic acid groups. The biosensor operates based on the principle of ECL impedance spectroscopy. The engineered phages on the surface of working electrode bind the *E. coli* in the aqueous sample, causing a change in the properties of the electrode surface. This change was detected by measuring the changes in impedance of the electrode-electrolyte interface at different frequencies [70]. Chen et al. reported a genetically engineered bacteriophage-based fluorometric sensor for *E. coli* bacteria detection. The sensor is constructed by modifying a lytic bacteriophage called T7, which is specific to *E. coli*, as shown in Figure 6.5b. Figure 6.5c also shows an another ECL sensor constructed using T2 bacteriophage and CNT functionalized with polyethylenimine to detect the *E. coli*.

Table 6.3 Recently reported bacteriophage-based ECL, optical, and piezoelectric, SERS, colorimetric, and fluorescence biosensors for various diseases.

Sensor structure with transduction method	Analyte	LOD	Linear range	Phages	Refs.
ECL sensor made up of T7 bacteriophage genetically engineered using phoA gene and CNT	*E. coli*	1 CFU/ml	$1–10^4$ CFU/ml	T7	[19]
MS2 phage amplification-based sandwich-type immunoassay	*E. coli*	10^2 CFU	$10^6–10^9$ PFU/ml	MS2	[59]
Fluorescence microscopy	*E. coli*	10 CFU/ml	$10^2–10^4$ CFU/ml	T7	[60]
Optical absorbance	*S. enterica* serovar *Typhimurium*	10^3 CFU/ml	10^7, 10^6 and 10^5 CFU/ml	Phage 10	[61]
Fluorophores labeled phage-based fluorescence biosensor	*Tuberculosis*	0.6 million CFU/ml	7–227 nM	D29	[62]
Fluorescent phage-based biosensor	*Salmonella*	10 cells/ml	$10^2–10^4$ cells/ml	Det7T	[63]
Phage-based ECL biosensor	*L. monocytogenes*	8.4 CFU/ml	$10–10^5$ CFU/ml	P100	[64]
Engineered T7lacZ phage-based colorimetric biosensor	*E. coli*	10 CFU/ml	$10^1–10^7$ CFU/ml	T7	[65]
CNT-based ECL phagosensor	*S. aureus*	10^3 CFU/ml	$10^3–10^5$ CFU/ml	SATA-8505	[66]
M13/carbon nano fiber/Cysteine-based ECL sensor	Cysteine	20 μM	20 μM–1 mM	M13	[67]

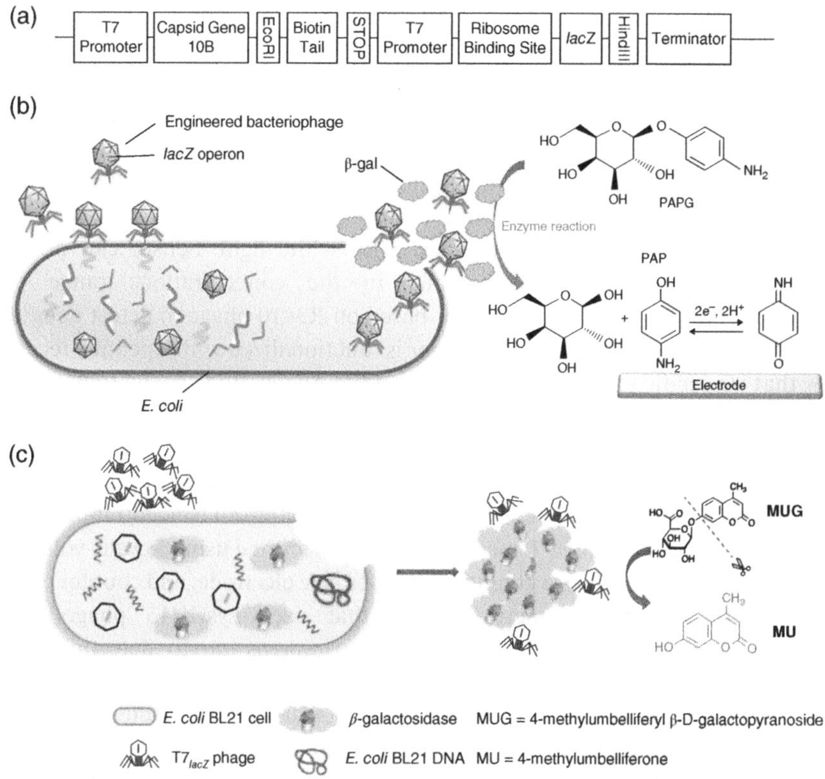

Figure 6.5 Design of (a) engineered bacteriophage Genome to detect *E. coli* and overexpresses of β-galactosidase through lacZ gene. (b) ECL biosensor using T7 bacteriophage. *Source:* [70]/with permission of American Chemical Society. (c) T7 phage-based fluorescent biosensor to detect the *E. coli*. *Source:* Adapted from [71].

The researchers inserted a gene encoding a green fluorescent protein into the genome of T7, so that when the phage infects *E. coli* cells, the protein is expressed and fluoresces green. Ground beef samples are first incubated with the modified T7 phage. In the presence of *E. coli*, the phage infects the bacteria and the green fluorescent protein is expressed, causing the sample to fluoresce green. The fluorescence can then be measured using a fluorometer as shown in Figure 6.5a. The sensor can detect *E. coli* with a LOD of 100 CFU/ml and a range of 10^2–10^5 CFU/ml [71]. A sensor for detecting *Shigella flexneri* pathogens using the tail spike protein of the bacteriophage Sf6 was reported. The tail spike protein binds specifically to the lipopolysaccharides on *Shigella flexneri* cells surface. The bacteria were bound on the surface, then separated from the rest of the sample using a magnet, and the number of bound bacteria was quantified using a spectrophotometer. This sensor provides LOD of 10^3 *Shigella flexneri* cells in a sample, with a linear range of detection up to 10^6 cells [72].

A colorimetric biosensor made of M13 bacteriophage with p8 protein was demonstrated with a smartphone and cloud server to detect toxic chemicals. These chemicals are xylene, hexane, benzene, toluene, and aniline. The sensor was made up of a thin film of dried bacteriophages that produces a colorful interference pattern when illuminated with white light. Sensor can detect xylene concentration of 5 ppm and in the concentrations range of 5–11 500 ppm [73]. An ECL biosensor based on R3#10 phage to detect dengue with the help NS1 biomarker. The sensor is functionalized with a peptide receptor that is specific to the NS1 biomarker on the Au electrode as the transducer to convert the binding event between the NS1 biomarker and the peptide receptor into an ECL signal Figure 6.6a. A buffer solution is added to stabilize the environment and optimize the pH and ionic strength conditions between the peptide and biomarker that can detect the 0.025–3.5 μg/ml concentrations and LOD of 0.025 μg/ml. The ECL measurement is performed using a cyclic voltammetry setup, that includes a potentiostat, reference electrode, and counter electrode [74]. An interferometric sensor that uses LysGH15 phage and streptavidin-coated biosensor chip for *Staphylococcus aureus* detection was reported. The detection principle, based on bio-layer interferometry technology, measures the change in optical interference caused by the bacteria binding on substrate surface. The binding of bacteria to the LysGH15-functionalized chip causes a shift in the interference pattern, detected in real time by a bio-layer interferometry instrument. *S. aureus* was detected with LOD and concentration range of 13 CFU/ml, 10^7–0^8 CFU/ml [20].

An immunosensor that consists of glassy carbon electrode and M13 bacteriophage to detect the total prostate-specific antigen. The phage library was then screened using PSA as the target molecule, and the landscape phage probe that exhibited the highest binding affinity and selectivity for PSA biomarker was selected for use in the immunosensor as shown in Figure 6.6b. The M13 phage probe has a high binding affinity and is sensitive for total PSA, with a dissociation constant, range, and LOD values of 3.44 nM, 0.01–100 ng/ml, and 3 pg/ml [75]. Figure 6.7a shows an M13 phage-based ECL sensor design to detect the neutrophil gelatinase-associated lipocalin, an acute kidney injury indicator, using peptide-displayed. The transducer in this study is a gold electrode that is used to convert the binding event between the lipocalin and the affinity peptide into a measurable ECL signal. An ECL workstation that is used to measure the current changes resulting from the binding event between the affinity peptide and analyte. Lipocalin was detected for concentrations of 25 ng/ml–100 μg/ml and LOD of 1.74 ng/ml [76]. Ovomucoid was detected using a M13 phage-based ECL

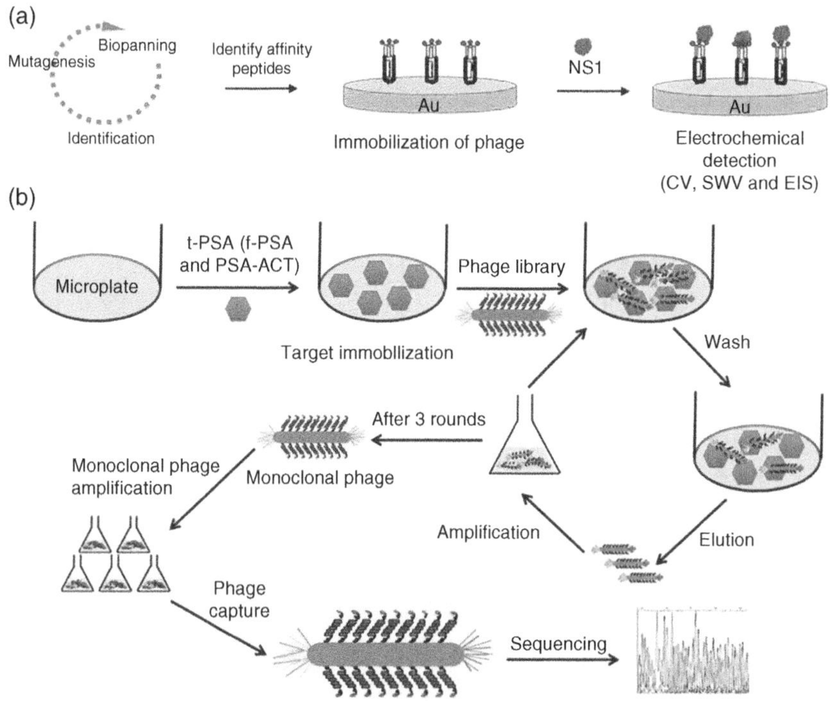

Figure 6.6 Schematic depiction of (a) R3#10 phage bacteriophage-based ECL biosensor to detect the dengue virus. *Source:* [74]/with permission of Elsevier. (b) Total prostate-specific antigen (PSA) detection using M13 bacteriophage-based ECL immunosensor. *Source:* [75]/with permission of Elsevier.

biosensor on a screen-printed carbon electrode; ovomucoid is a major allergen in egg white. ECL sensor design can detect allergens for concentration range of 1.55–12.38 μg/ml and LOD of 0.12 μg/ml [78]. M13 phages and AuNPs based ECL sensor to detect the mercury ions. The M13 phages used in this study were genetically engineered to display cysteine-rich peptides that can bind to Hg^{2+} ions with high affinity and selectivity. AuNPs were synthesized through the reduction of Au ions using sodium borohydride. This process allowed for the immobilization of the phages onto an Au electrode, resulting in a stable and sensitive biosensor platform. Mercury ion concentration in μM range, and LOD of 10^{-8} M can be detected [79]. The QuantiPhage test is used to detect the coliphages called viruses that infect *E. coli* bacteria using the colorimetric method. This QuantiPhage assay consists of a cellulose pad as a solid support that allows the retention of coliphages and passes other particles due to its filtration property and plaque formation on which a sample containing coliphages is applied. The cellulose pad is incubated in

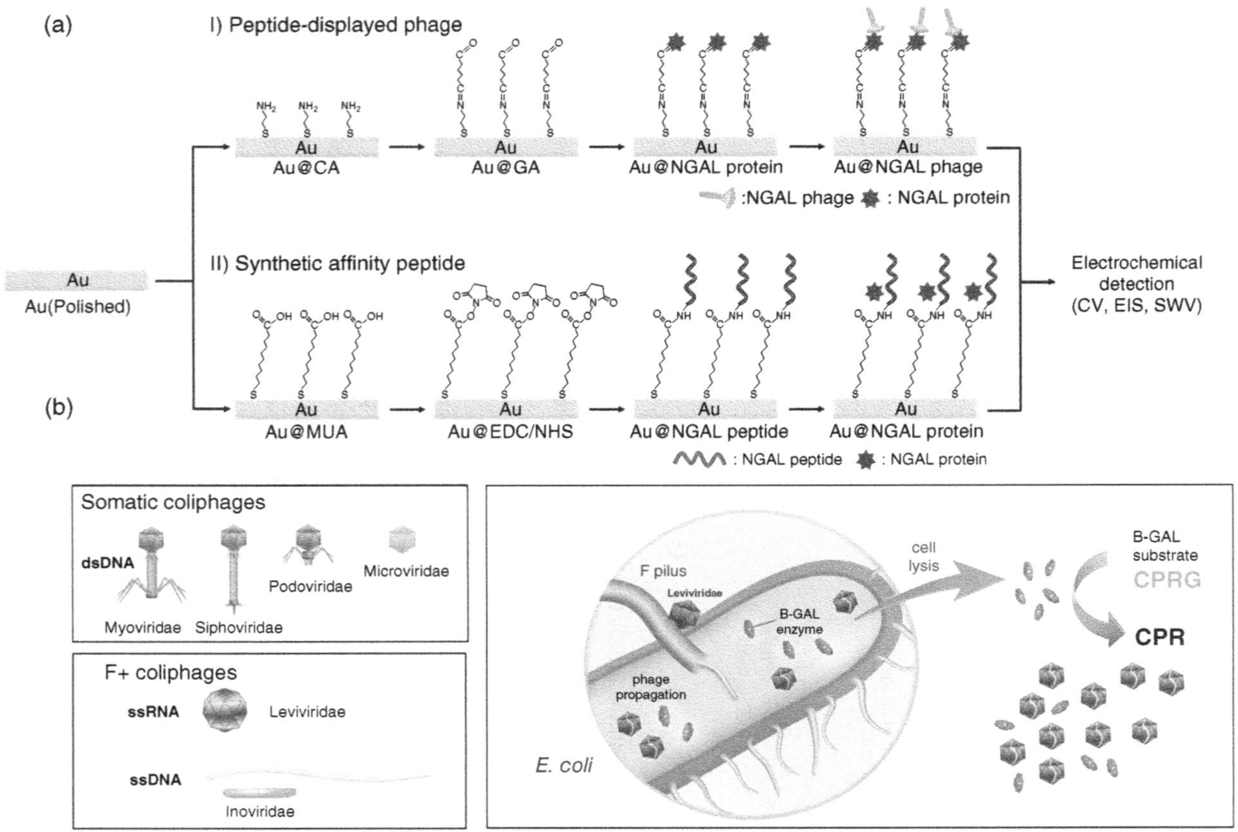

Figure 6.7 A schematic illustration of the (a) M13 phage-based ECL sensor to detect the lipocalin. *Source:* [76]/with permission of Elsevier. (b) QuantiPhage assay-based colorimetric sensor for *E. coli* detection. *Source:* [77]/with permission of Elsevier.

the presence of coliphage specific indicator bacteria strains. Somatic and F+ coliphages are a group of coliphages that infect and replicate within *E. coli* bacteria. After the incubation, 2,3,5-triphenyl tetrazolium chloride is added for colorimetric detection of *E. coli*, which produces changes after the reaction of indicator bacteria present inside the plaques with detected bacteria, as indicated in Figure 6.7b. The indicator bacteria play the role of targets to detect the coliphages; in the presence of coliphages, plaque formation takes place. The plaques can be easily seen on the surface of the cellulose pad. QuantiPhage assays are simple, have high speed, and allow rapid detection that does not require complex equipment or specialists and has a LOD of 1 CFU/ml [77].

6.3 Future Prospects

The efficiency of immobilized phages depends on the type of immobilization method used for bio-receptor molecule functionalization. The commonly used methods that include physical adsorption, covalent bonding, and entrapment are also used to immobilize phages on different support materials. The selection of the immobilization method plays a crucial role in the stability of the bacteriophages and its capacity to recognize and bind to the target bacteria. Another factor is that the properties of the support material affect the efficiency of immobilized phages significantly. The support material should be biocompatible and should not interfere between phage and target bacteria binding. Properties of the support materials that include shape and charge distribution can also affect the immobilization efficiency and stability of the phages. There are several disadvantages related to whole phages, such as the large size of the whole phage and the fact that the basal lytic activity has the capability to kill the bacteria before detection. Phage proteins do not have these drawbacks and thus represent an alternative to whole phages for detecting various types of targets. Phages have limited host ranges and exhibit specificity, which allows them to infect and recognize certain bacterial strains. It limits their use for certain target bacteria and therefore requires the use of multiple phages for different strains of bacteria. Phages degrade with the passage of time and become unstable due to their sensitivity to temperature, pH, and other environmental conditions. The bulk production of phages with high quality is a challenging task, as bacteria may develop resistance to the bacteriophages via genetic mutations that reduce their efficiency in detecting the resistant strains. Monitoring the phages is another challenge because they are alive, and that requires regulation. It's important to note that despite these drawbacks, phages still offer unique advantages in terms of specificity, sensitivity, and their ability to target specific bacteria.

6.4 Summary

This chapter presents a comprehensive overview of phage-based biosensors, focusing on their principles and applications. Different types of ECL, optical, and piezoelectric biosensors designs have been discussed in detail for various biomedical applications. Types of phages, structures, and families have also been discussed in detail. Phages have advantages that include availability in abundance (i.e. 10^{32} bacteriophage in the water, soil, dung, and thermal vents), lyse ability, ability to kill the host, capacity to multiply during infection, and genetic modification. Furthermore, we have discussed techniques for immobilizing phages on suitable substrates, which is a critical step in the designs of bacteriophage biosensors. Lytic and lysogenic processes in phage detection were discussed in detail.

References

1 Schofield, D., Sharp, N.J., and Westwater, C. (2012). Phage-based platforms for the clinical detection of human bacterial pathogens. *Bacteriophage* 2 (2): 105–121. https://doi.org/10.4161/bact.19274.

2 Anany, H., Brovko, L., El Dougdoug, N.K. et al. (2018). Print to detect: a rapid and ultrasensitive phage-based dipstick assay for foodborne pathogens. *Anal. Bioanal. Chem.* 410 (4): 1217–1230. https://doi.org/10.1007/s00216-017-0597-y.

3 Campbell, A. (2003). The future of bacteriophage biology. *Nat. Rev.* 4 (June): 471–477.

4 Hussain, W., Ullah, M.W., Farooq, U. et al. (2021). Bacteriophage-based advanced bacterial detection: concept, mechanisms, and applications. *Biosens. Bioelectron.* 177: https://doi.org/10.1016/j.bios.2021.112973.

5 Ye, M., Sun, M., Huang, D. et al. (2019). A review of bacteriophage therapy for pathogenic bacteria inactivation in the soil environment. *Environ. Int.* 129: 488–496. https://doi.org/10.1016/j.envint.2019.05.062.

6 Giri, N. (2021). Bacteriophage structure, classification, assembly and phage therapy. *Biosci. Biotechnol. Res. Asia* 18 (2): 239–250. https://doi.org/10.13005/bbra/2911.

7 Singh, S., Dhanjal, D.S., Thotapalli, S. et al. (2020). An insight in bacteriophage based biosensors with focus on their detection methods and recent advancements. *Environ. Technol. Innovation* 20: 101081. https://doi.org/10.1016/j.eti.2020.101081.

8 Abd-Allah, I.M., El-Housseiny, G.S., Yahia, I.S. et al. (2021). Rekindling of a masterful precedent; bacteriophage: reappraisal and future pursuits. *Front. Cell. Infect. Microbiol.* 11: 1–22. https://doi.org/10.3389/fcimb.2021.635597.

9 Paczesny, J., Richter, Ł., and Hołyst, R. (2020). Recent progress in the detection of bacteria using bacteriophages: a review. *Viruses* 12 (8): https://doi.org/10.3390/v12080845.

10 Paczesny, J. and Bielec, K. (2020). Application of bacteriophages in nanotechnology. *Nanomaterials* 10 (10): 1–25. https://doi.org/10.3390/nano10101944.

11 Burlage, R.S. and Tillmann, J. (2017). Biosensors of bacterial cells. *J. Microbiol. Methods* 138: 2–11. https://doi.org/10.1016/j.mimet.2016.12.023.

12 Sutcliffe, S.G., Reyes, A., and Maurice, C.F. (2023). Bacteriophages playing nice: lysogenic bacteriophage replication stable in the human gut microbiota. *iScience* 26 (2): 106007. https://doi.org/10.1016/j.isci.2023.106007.

13 Drew, R.E., Clarke, P.H., and Brammar, W.J. (1980). The construction in vitro of derivatives of bacteriophage lambda carrying the amidase genes of Pseudomonas aeruginosa. *Mol. Gen. Genet.* 177 (2): 311–320. https://doi.org/10.1007/BF00267444.

14 Chibani, C.M., Farr, A., Klama, S. et al. (2019). Classifying the unclassified: a phage classification method. *Viruses* 11 (2): https://doi.org/10.3390/v11020195.

15 Yuan, Y. and Gao, M. (2017). Jumbo bacteriophages: an overview. *Front. Microbiol.* 8: 403. https://doi.org/10.3389/fmicb.2017.00403.

16 Meile, S., Du, J., Staubli, S. et al. (2022). Engineered reporter phages for rapid detection of Escherichia coli, Klebsiella spp., and Enterococcus spp. in urine. *Nat. Commun* 14: 4336. https://doi.org/10.1038/s41467-023-39863-x.

17 Braun, P., Raab, R., Bugert, J.J., and Braun, S. (2023). Recombinant reporter phage rTUN1::nLuc enables rapid detection and real-time antibiotic susceptibility testing of Klebsiella pneumoniae K64 strains. *ACS Sens.* 8 (2): 630–639. https://doi.org/10.1021/acssensors.2c01822.

18 Singh, J., Kumar, M., Sharma, A. et al. (2016). We are IntechOpen, the world's leading publisher of open access books built by scientists, for scientists TOP 1%. *Intech* 11 (tourism): 13. [Online]. https://www.intechopen.com/books/advanced-biometric-technologies/liveness-detection-in-biometrics.

19 El-Moghazy, A.Y., Wisuthiphaet, N., Yang, X. et al. (2022). Electrochemical biosensor based on genetically engineered bacteriophage T7 for rapid detection of Escherichia coli on fresh produce. *Food Control* 135: 108811. https://doi.org/10.1016/j.foodcont.2022.108811.

20 Liu, X., Huang, C., Qiu, C. et al. (2022). Rapid and sensitive detection of Staphylococcus aureus using biolayer interferometry technology combined with phage lysin LysGH15. *Biosens. Bioelectron.* 198: 113799. https://doi.org/10.1016/j.bios.2021.113799.

21 Al-Hindi, R.R., Teklemariam, A.D., Alharbi, M.G. et al. (2022). Bacteriophage-based biosensors: a platform for detection of foodborne bacterial pathogens from food and environment. *Biosensors* 12 (10): 1–22. https://doi.org/10.3390/bios12100905.

22 Kim, S.J., Lee, Y., Choi, E.J. et al. (2023). The development progress of multi-array colourimetric sensors based on the M13 bacteriophage. *Nano Convergence* 10 (1): 1–14. https://doi.org/10.1186/s40580-022-00351-5.

23 Jiang, J., Yang, Q., Wajid Ullah, M., and Wang, S. (2010). Principle and development of phage-based biosensors. *Intech* 57–67. [Online]. https://doi.org/10.5772/intechopen.86419.

24 Costa, S.P., Cunha, A.P., Freitas, P.P., and Carvalho, C.M. (2022). A phage receptor-binding protein as a promising tool for the detection of Escherichia coli in human specimens. *Front. Microbiol.* 13: 1–14. https://doi.org/10.3389/fmicb.2022.871855.

25 Farooq, U., Ullah, M.W., Yang, Q. et al. (2020). High-density phage particles immobilization in surface-modified bacterial cellulose for ultra-sensitive and selective electrochemical detection of Staphylococcus aureus. *Biosens. Bioelectron.* 157: 112163. https://doi.org/10.1016/j.bios.2020.112163.

26 Dunne, M., Prokhorov, N.S., Loessner, M.J., and Leiman, P.G. (2021). Reprogramming bacteriophage host range: design principles and strategies for engineering receptor binding proteins. *Curr. Opin. Biotechnol.* 68: 272–281. https://doi.org/10.1016/j.copbio.2021.02.006.

27 Rosner, D. and Clark, J. (2021). Formulations for bacteriophage therapy and the potential uses of immobilization. *Pharmaceuticals* 14 (4): 359. https://doi.org/10.3390/ph14040359.

28 Wang, C., Sauvageau, D., and Elias, A. (2016). Immobilization of active bacteriophages on polyhydroxyalkanoate surfaces. *ACS Appl. Mater. Interfaces* 8 (2): 1128–1138. https://doi.org/10.1021/acsami.5b08664.

29 Durr, H.A. and Leipzig, N.D. (2023). Advancements in bacteriophage therapies and delivery for bacterial infection. *Mater. Adv.* 4 (5): 1249–1257. https://doi.org/10.1039/d2ma00980c.

30 Paramasivam, K., Shen, Y., Yuan, J. et al. (2022). Advances in the development of phage-based probes for detection of bio-species. *Biosensors* 12 (1): https://doi.org/10.3390/bios12010030.

31 Turner, D., Shkoporov, A.N., Lood, C. et al. (2023). Abolishment of morphology-based taxa and change to binomial species names: 2022 taxonomy update of the ICTV bacterial viruses subcommittee. *Arch. Virol* 168 (2): 1–9. https://doi.org/10.1007/s00705-022-05694-2.

32 Zhu, Y., Shang, J., Peng, C., and Sun, Y. (2022). Phage family classification under Caudoviricetes: a review of current tools using the latest ICTV classification framework. *Front. Microbiol.* 13: https://doi.org/10.3389/fmicb.2022.1032186.

33 El-Shibiny, A. and El-Sahhar, S. (2017). Bacteriophages: the possible solution to treat infections caused by pathogenic bacteria. *Can. J. Microbiol.* 63 (11): 865–879. https://doi.org/10.1139/cjm-2017-0030.

34 O'Connell, L., Marcoux, P.R., and Roupioz, Y. (2021). Strategies for surface immobilization of whole bacteriophages: a review. *ACS Biomater. Sci. Eng.* 7 (6): 1987–2014. https://doi.org/10.1021/acsbiomaterials.1c00013.

35 Henschke, L., Frese, M., Hellmuth, S. et al. (2019). Identification of bioactive small molecule inhibitors of Separase. *ACS Chem. Biol.* 14 (10): 2155–2159. https://doi.org/10.1021/acschembio.9b00661.

36 Imai, M.M., Mine, K., Tomonari, H. et al. (2019). Dark-field microscopic detection of bacteria using bacteriophage-immobilized SiO_2@AuNP core–shell nanoparticles. *Anal. Chem.* 91: 12352–12357.

37 Moon, J.S., Choi, E.J., Jeong, N.N. et al. (2019). Research progress of M13 bacteriophage-based biosensors. *Nanomaterials* 9: 1448. https://doi.org/10.3390/nano9101448.

38 Li, Y., Xie, G., Qiu, J. et al. (2018). A new biosensor based on the recognition of phages and the signal amplification of organic-inorganic hybrid nanoflowers for discriminating and quantitating live pathogenic bacteria in urine. *Sens. Actuators, B* 258: 803–812. https://doi.org/10.1016/j.snb.2017.11.155.

39 Bhardwaj, N., Bhardwaj, S.K., Mehta, J. et al. (2016). Bacteriophage immobilized graphene electrodes for impedimetric sensing of bacteria (Staphylococcus arlettae). *Anal. Biochem.* 505: 18–25. https://doi.org/10.1016/j.ab.2016.04.008.

40 Rippa, M., Castagna, R., Pannico, M. et al. (2017). Octupolar metastructures for a highly sensitive, rapid, and reproducible phage-based detection of bacterial pathogens by surface-enhanced Raman scattering. *ACS Sens.* 2 (7): 947–954. https://doi.org/10.1021/acssensors.7b00195.

41 Lai, A., Almaviva, S., Spizzichino, V. et al. (2017). Bacillus spp. cells captured selectively by phages and identified by surface enhanced Raman spectroscopy technique. *Proceedings* 1: 519. https://doi.org/10.3390/proceedings1040519.

42 Chen, J. and Nugen, S.R. (2019). Detection of protease and engineered phage-infected bacteria using peptide-graphene oxide nanosensors. *Anal. Bioanal. Chem.* 411: 2487–2492. https://doi.org/10.1007/s00216-019-01766-6.

43 Xu, J., Zhao, C., Chau, Y., and Lee, Y.K. (2020). The synergy of chemical immobilization and electrical orientation of T4 bacteriophage on a micro electrochemical sensor for low-level viable bacteria detection via differential pulse voltammetry. *Biosens. Bioelectron.* 151: 111914. https://doi.org/10.1016/j.bios.2019.111914.

44 Zhou, Y., Marar, A., Kner, P., and Ramasamy, R.P. (2017). Charge-directed immobilization of bacteriophage on nanostructured electrode for whole-cell electrochemical biosensors. *Anal. Chem.* 89 (11): 5734–5741. https://doi.org/10.1021/acs.analchem.6b03751.

45 Janczuk-Richter, M., Dominik, M., Roźniecka, E. et al. (2017). Long-period fiber grating sensor for detection of viruses. *Sens. Actuators, B* 250: 32–38. https://doi.org/10.1016/j.snb.2017.04.148.

46 Moon, J.S., Park, M., Kim, W.G. et al. (2017). M-13 bacteriophage based structural color sensor for detecting antibiotics. *Sens. Actuators, B* 240: 757–762. https://doi.org/10.1016/j.snb.2016.09.050.

47 Shin, H.J. and Lim, W.K. (2018). Rapid label-free detection of E. coli using a novel SPR biosensor containing a fragment of tail protein from phage lambda. *Prep. Biochem. Biotechnol.* 48 (6): 498–505. https://doi.org/10.1080/10826068.2018.1466154.

48 Nguyen, T.M., DoáKim, Y., JungáChoi, E. et al. (2021). Programmable self-assembly of M13 bacteriophage for micro-color pattern with a tunable colorization. *RSC Adv.* 11 (51): 32305–32311. https://doi.org/10.1039/d1ra04302a.

49 Hyeon, S.H., Lim, W.K., and Shin, H.J. (2021). Novel surface plasmon resonance biosensor that uses full-length Det7 phage tail protein for rapid and selective detection of Salmonella enterica serovar Typhimurium. *Biotechnol. Appl. Biochem.* 68 (1): 5–12. https://doi.org/10.1002/bab.1883.

50 Abdelhamied, N., Abdelrahman, F., El-Shibiny, A., and Hassan, R.Y.A. (2023). Bacteriophage-based nano-biosensors for the fast impedimetric determination of pathogens in food samples. *Sci. Rep.* 13 (1): 1–11. https://doi.org/10.1038/s41598-023-30520-3.

51 Peng, H. and Chen, I.A. (2019). Rapid colorimetric detection of bacterial species through the capture of gold nanoparticles by chimeric phages. *ACS Nano* 13 (2): 1244–1252. https://doi.org/10.1021/acsnano.8b06395.

52 Chen, J., Picard, R.A., Wang, D., and Nugen, S.R. (2017). Lyophilized engineered phages for Escherichia coli detection in food matrices. *ACS Sens.* 2 (11): 1573–1577. https://doi.org/10.1021/acssensors.7b00561.

53 Mack, J.D., Yehualaeshet, T., Park, M.K. et al. (2017). Phage-based biosensor and optimization of surface blocking agents to detect salmonella typhimurium on Romaine lettuce. *J. Food Saf.* 37 (2): https://doi.org/10.1111/jfs.12299.

54 Shin, H.J., Hyeon, S.H., Cho, J.H., and Lim, W.K. (2021). Minor coat protein pIII domain (N1N2) of bacteriophage CTXϕ confers a novel surface plasmon resonance biosensor for rapid detection of vibrio cholerae. *Microbiol. Biotechnol. Lett.* 49 (4): 510–518. https://doi.org/10.48022/mbl.2109.09013.

55 Nguyen, T.M. et al. (2023). Multiarray biosensor for diagnosing lung cancer based on gap plasmonic color films. *ACS Sens.* 8 (1): 167–175. https://doi.org/10.1021/acssensors.2c02001.

56 Yang, Q., Deng, S., Xu, J. et al. (2021). Poly(indole-5-carboxylic acid)/reduced graphene oxide/gold nanoparticles/phage-based electrochemical biosensor for highly specific detection of Yersinia pseudotuberculosis. *Microchim. Acta* 188 (4): 107. https://doi.org/10.1007/s00604-020-04676-y.

57 Nguyen, A.H., Shin, Y., and Sim, S.J. (2016). Development of SERS substrate using phage-based magnetic template for triplex assay in sepsis diagnosis. *Biosens. Bioelectron.* 85: 522–528. https://doi.org/10.1016/j.bios.2016.05.043.

58 Lee, J.M., Choi, E.J., Park, J. et al. (2019). Improvement of high affinity and selectivity on biosensors using genetically engineered phage by binding isotherm screening. *Viruses* 11 (3): 1–11. https://doi.org/10.3390/v11030248.

59 Mido, T., Schaffer, E.M., Dorsey, R.W. et al. (2018). Sensitive detection of live Escherichia coli by bacteriophage amplification-coupled immunoassay on the Luminex® MAGPIX instrument. *J. Microbiol. Methods* 152: 143–147. https://doi.org/10.1016/j.mimet.2018.07.022.

60 Yang, X., Wisuthiphaet, N., Young, G.M., and Nitin, N. (2020). Rapid detection of Escherichia coli using bacteriophage-induced lysis and image analysis. *PLoS One* 15: 1–19. https://doi.org/10.1371/journal.pone.0233853.

61 Tamariz, J., Guevara, V., and Guerra, H. (2018). Rapid detection of salmonellosis due to Salmonella enterica serovar typhimurium in peruvian commercially bred cavies, using indigenous wild bacteriophages. *Germs* 8 (4): 178–185. https://doi.org/10.18683/germs.2018.1144.

62 Franch, O., Han, X., Marcussen, L.B. et al. (2019). A new DNA sensor system for specific and quantitative detection of mycobacteria. *Nanoscale* 11 (2): 587–597. https://doi.org/10.1039/c8nr07850e.

63 Vinay, M., Franche, N., Grégori, G. et al. (2015). Phage-based fluorescent biosensor prototypes to specifically detect enteric bacteria such as E. coli and Salmonella enterica Typhimurium. *PLoS One* 10 (7): 1–17. https://doi.org/10.1371/journal.pone.0131466.

64 Zolti, O., Suganthan, B., Maynard, R. et al. (2022). Electrochemical biosensor for rapid detection of listeria monocytogenes. *J. Electrochem. Soc.* 169 (6): 067510. https://doi.org/10.1149/1945-7111/ac7a63.

65 Chen, J., Alcaine, S.D., Jackson, A.A. et al. (2017). Development of engineered bacteriophages for Escherichia coli detection and high-throughput antibiotic resistance determination. *ACS Sens.* 2 (4): 484–489. https://doi.org/10.1021/acssensors.7b00021.

66 Patel, D., Zhou, Y., and Ramasamy, R.P. (2021). A bacteriophage-based electrochemical biosensor for detection of methicillin-resistant Staphylococcus aureus. *J. Electrochem. Soc.* 168 (5): 057523. https://doi.org/10.1149/1945-7111/abef85.

67 Szot-Karpińska, K., Leśniewski, A., Jönsson-Niedziółka, M. et al. (2019). Electrodes modified with bacteriophages and carbon nanofibres for cysteine detection. *Sens. Actuators, B* 287: 78–85. https://doi.org/10.1016/j.snb.2019.01.148.

68 Rippa, M., Castagna, R., Zhou, J. et al. (2018). Dodecagonal plasmonic quasicrystals for phage-based biosensing. *Nanotechnology* 29 (40): https://doi.org/10.1088/1361-6528/aad2f5.

69 Møller-Olsen, C., Ho, S.F.S., Shukla, R.D. et al. (2018). Engineered K1F bacteriophages kill intracellular Escherichia coli K1 in human epithelial cells. *Sci. Rep.* 8 (1): 1–18. https://doi.org/10.1038/s41598-018-35859-6.

70 Wang, D., Chen, J., and Nugen, S.R. (2017). Electrochemical detection of Escherichia coli from aqueous samples using engineered phages. *Anal. Chem.* 89 (3): 1650–1657. https://doi.org/10.1021/acs.analchem.6b03752.

71 Chen, A., Wang, D., Nugen, S.R., and Chen, J. (2021). An engineered reporter phage for the fluorometric detection of Escherichia coli in ground beef. *Microorganisms* 9 (2): 1–13. https://doi.org/10.3390/microorganisms9020436.

72 Kunstmann, S., Scheidt, T., Buchwald, S. et al. (2018). Bacteriophage Sf6 tailspike protein for detection of Shigella flexneri pathogens. *Viruses* 10 (8): 431. https://doi.org/10.3390/v10080431.

73 Lee, J.H., Fan, B., Samdin, T.D. et al. (2017). Phage-based structural color sensors and their pattern recognition sensing system. *ACS Nano* 11 (4): 3632–3641. https://doi.org/10.1021/acsnano.6b07942.

74 Lim, J.M., Kim, J.H., Ryu, M.Y. et al. (2018). An electrochemical peptide sensor for detection of dengue fever biomarker NS1. *Anal. Chim. Acta* 1026: 109–116. https://doi.org/10.1016/j.aca.2018.04.005.

75 Han, L., Xia, H., Yin, L. et al. (2018). Selected landscape phage probe as selective recognition interface for sensitive total prostate-specific antigen immunosensor. *Biosens. Bioelectron.* 106: 1–6. https://doi.org/10.1016/j.bios.2018.01.046.

76 Cho, C.H., Kim, J.H., Song, D.K. et al. (2019). An affinity peptide-incorporated electrochemical biosensor for the detection of neutrophil gelatinase-associated lipocalin. *Biosens. Bioelectron.* 142 (May): 111482. https://doi.org/10.1016/j.bios.2019.111482.

77 Rames, E. and Macdonald, J. (2019). The QuantiPhage assay: a novel method for the rapid colorimetric detection of coliphages using cellulose pad materials. *Water Res.* 149: 98–110. https://doi.org/10.1016/j.watres.2018.10.089.

78 Shin, J.H., Park, T.J., Hyun, M.S., and Park, J.P. (2022). A phage virus-based electrochemical biosensor for highly sensitive detection of ovomucoid. *Food Chem.* 378 (September 2021): 132061. https://doi.org/10.1016/j.foodchem.2022.132061.

79 Wang, X., Yang, T., Zhang, X. et al. (2017). In situ growth of gold nanoparticles on Hg^{2+}-binding M13 phages for mercury sensing. *Nanoscale* 9 (43): 16728–16734. https://doi.org/10.1039/c7nr06292c.

7

Peptide-Based Biosensors

7.1 Introduction

Peptides are made up of amino acids chains of small length connected via peptide bonds and are smaller than proteins, which typically consist of 2–100 amino acids. Peptides that are 2–10 amino acids long are called dipeptides, tripeptides, tetrapeptides, and so on. Peptides that are 11–50 amino acids long are called oligopeptides. Peptides that are 51 or more amino acids long are called polypeptides. Peptide bonds are partial double bonds in nature, which makes them strong and shows stability under strong heating and dense concentration of salts [1]. Peptide bonds break easily in the presence of strong acids, bases kept for a long time, and some enzymes at an elevated temperature. Both partial positive and negative charge groups are present inside the peptides. The size of a peptide can affect its properties and function. For example, smaller peptides are typically more soluble in water, while larger peptides are typically more soluble in organic solvents. Smaller peptides are also typically more easily absorbed by the body, while larger peptides are typically more difficult to absorb [2]. Smaller peptides are typically more effective at binding to receptors, while larger peptides are typically more effective at catalyzing chemical reactions [3]. Therefore, peptide solubility depends on its size and can be used to design biosensors in different analytes or other applications [4].

Peptides can be used as receptors to bind specific analytes, such as proteins, DNA, or ions, that can target the particular analyte for various applications. They can also be combined with enzyme substrates to measure the activity of enzymes. These molecules are also utilized in signal transducers, as they produce a measurable signal as target bind with peptide. This is done by changing the

Biosensors: Nanomaterials, Approaches, and Performance-Enhancement Strategies,
First Edition. Baljinder Kaur, Santosh Kumar, and Brajesh Kumar Kaushik.

Published 2025 by John Wiley & Sons, Inc.
Companion website: www.wiley.com/go/kaur

electrical properties of the peptide or by generating a chemical signal. The other advantage in using peptides in biosensors is that their small size allows them to easily diffuse across cell membranes. This makes them ideal for use in biosensors that are designed to detect analytes inside cells. The interaction of peptides with target analyte in case of biosensors is similar to antigen–antibody interactions that generate measurable output signal [5].

The structure of peptides is simple compared to antibodies and enzymes; they can be easily engineered via chemical methods. Peptides provide more control on optical properties – for example: hydrophobicity and interface charge distribution can be altered by number and type of residue peptides in a reaction [6]. It can make assembly with other nanomaterial to provide a large surface area that enhances the biosensor performance [6]. Peptides have been explored to bind to specific analytes with high affinity for single-analyte detection [7]. Peptides have the ability to detect analytes at very low concentrations. Peptides has significant role during the biochemical reactions such as cell adhesion, control of blood pressure, and anti-inflammatory responses [3]. Peptides act as signaling molecules in the endocrine system and neurotransmitters or neuromodulators in the nervous system. Examples of peptide hormones include insulin, glucagon, oxytocin, and growth hormones, which regulate processes such as metabolism, growth, and reproduction. Neuropeptides participate in the regulation of pain, mood, appetite, and other neurological functions [8]. Examples include substance P, endorphins, and enkephalins. Antimicrobial peptides are naturally occurring molecules capacity to kill or prevent the growth of different microorganisms [9, 10]. Peptides also play the roles of enzymes, enzyme inhibitors, and cell signaling, which ease biochemical reactions in the body. Peptides play the role of cell-signaling molecules between cells, mediating communication, and regulating cellular processes [11].

7.2 Synthesis Methods

Solution-phase synthesis or liquid phase is the oldest method to synthesize the peptides. In this method, amino acids are dissolved in a solvent, coupled together using a chemical reaction as shown in Figure 7.1. It is an older, simpler method that can synthesize peptides of any length, but it suffers from the drawback of low yields [13]. Various steps involve protection of the N-terminus, coupling, deprotection, repeated cycles, and final deprotection. A protecting group is used to stop unwanted reactions at the N-terminus group. As it is activated after interaction with the protecting group, this is further coupled with peptide chains using a coupling reagent such as dicyclohexylcarbodiimide that generates a peptide bond between growing chain amino acids and the carboxyl group of the activated amino acid. These steps are repeated to obtain the desired sequence. After this step,

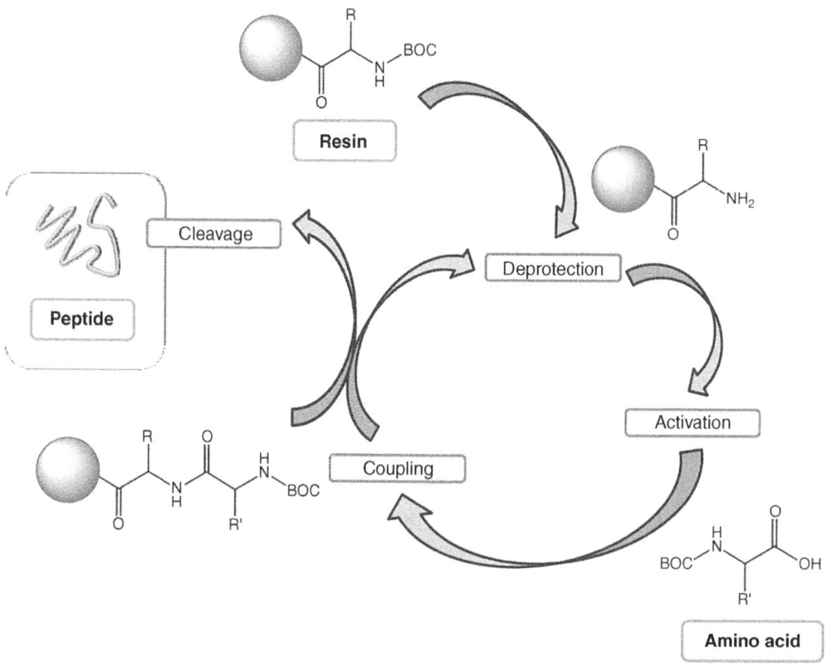

Figure 7.1 Schematic illustration of various steps involved in commonly used solid-phase synthesis. *Source:* [12]/MDPI/CC BY 4.0.

protecting groups on any remaining side chains and the N-terminus are removed to obtain the final peptide product [14]. Another method to synthesize the peptides is solid-phase synthesis method and is commonly used for peptides. In this case, solid support is used to attach amino acids such as a resin bead, and they are coupled together one at a time using a chemical reaction. The amino acids are deprotected, which means that the protecting groups are removed. It can be used to synthesize peptides of any length but suffers from complexity and requires specialized equipment [12].

7.2.1 Design of ECL Biosensors

A novel ECL biosensor was developed to detect the matrix metalloproteinase-14, a biomarker for cancer types (colorectal, breast) and heart diseases. The biosensor was based on a sandwich assay that uses two different inhibitory peptides to capture and detect biomarker through MDA-MB-231 cancer cells. The inhibitory peptide, AP1, was covalently bounded on the carbon electrode surface and explored as a capture probe. The second inhibitory peptide, AP2, is labeled with a ruthenium complex to use as a signal probe. In the presence of biomarkers, it binds to AP1, which further binds to AP2 – which forms the sandwich and brings the ruthenium complex into close proximity to the electrode surface. The ruthenium complex is then electrochemically oxidized, which generates a chemiluminescent signal and enhances the sensor's performance. This biosensor design was able to detect matrix metalloproteinase-14 with a limit of detection (LOD) of 0.05 ng/ml and high specificity and sensitivity [15].

Figure 7.2 illustrates an AuNPs and conducting polymer poly (3,4-ethylenedioxythiophene) (PEDOT) modified electrode-based ECL biosensor that was reported to detect the human epidermal growth factor receptor 2 (HER2) in the concentration range of 1 pg/ml μg/mL in complex biological media. The biosensor was based on a sandwich assay that uses a designed-recognizing peptide and polyethylene glycol to reduce nonspecific bindings and antifouling materials. In the presence of HER2, the binding of peptide and analyte target generates a measurable signal and leads to LOD of 0.44 pg/ml [16].

An AuNPs ECL biosensor was designed using carbon electrode to detect the caspase-9 that removes the cells during apoptotic death process. ZnO/CuO nanocrystal was deposited on borosilicate glass and anti-caspase-9 antibodies to construct biosensor. It can achieve LOD of 0.07 U/ml and a linear range of 0.1–1 U/ml [17]. A peptide-based ECL biosensor to detect the breast cancer using a poly 3-(3-aminophenyl) propionic acid matrix was designed. The sensor consisted of a glassy carbon electrode (GCE) modified with a peptide-PPA conjugate. The peptide-PPA conjugate was used to bind to breast cancer cells. The sensor had a LOD of 100 cells/ml and a linear range of 0.1–1000 cells/ml.

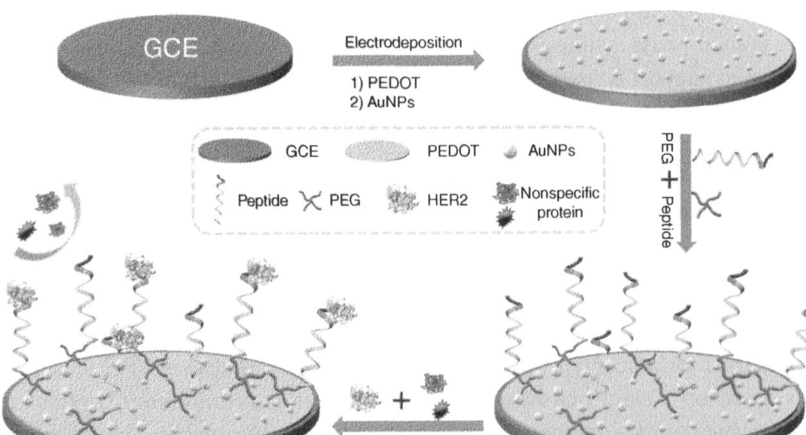

Figure 7.2 Schematic of HER2 detection using PEDOT and AuNPs ECL biosensor. *Source:* [16]/with permission of Elsevier.

Silva-Junio et al. developed an ECL biosensor based on the temporin-PTA peptide for the detection of microorganisms. The sensor consisted of a GCE modified with a temporin-PTA peptide. The temporin-PTA peptide was used to bind to microorganisms. The sensor had a LOD of 10 CFU/ml and a linear range of 0.1–1000 CFU/ml [17–19]. Table 7.1 highlights the others recently reported peptide-based ECL biosensors.

Li et al. [33] describe a novel ECL biosensor based on an analyte-restrained peptide nucleic acid displacement reaction constructed on different AuNPs-deposited carbon electrodes. The sensor is constructed on different AuNPs-deposited carbon electrodes using an analyte-restrained peptide nucleic acid displacement reaction. The sensor structure involves the immobilization of NF-κB binding peptide and peptide nucleic acid (PNA) on the gold nanoparticle-deposited carbon electrodes. The PNA serves as a displacement probe; in the absence of NF-κB, it hybridizes with the immobilized peptide, blocking the electrode surface. However, in the presence of NF-κB, the analyte displaces the PNA, resulting in a change in the ECL signal. The biosensor demonstrated a LOD of 2.7 pg/ml for NF-κB and a linear range of 0.02–0.1 ng/ml [33]. Liu et al. made an ultrasensitive ECL biosensor that can find tumor exosomes by recognizing peptides and amplifying the signal from a luminol-AuNPs@g-C3N4 nanoprobe. The sensor structure involves the use of peptide recognition and signal amplification using luminol-AuNPs@g-C_3N_4 nanoprobe, shown in Figure 7.3a. The peptide recognition element specifically binds to tumor exosomes, enabling their selective detection. The luminol-AuNPs@g-C3N4 nanoprobe is employed to amplify the electrochemiluminescence signal, enhancing the sensitivity of the biosensor. The sensor demonstrated a LOD of 39 exosomes/μL and a linear range from 1×10^2 to 10^6 exosomes/μL [34]. Zheng et al. describe a peptide-antibody sandwich ECL biosensor for prostate-specific antigen (PSA) detection, utilizing the signal amplification of a MnO_2-functionalized covalent organic framework (COF). The sensor structure involves the utilization of a signal amplification strategy using MnO_2-functionalized COF. The COF serves as a support matrix for the immobilization of antibodies, and the affinity peptide specifically binds to PSA, forming a sandwich complex. The presence of PSA triggers the release of MnO_2, leading to enhanced ECL signals. The biosensor demonstrated a LOD of 16.7 fg mL^{-1} for PSA and a linear range from 0.00005–10 ng mL^{-1} [38].

Sfragano et al. summarized the role of peptides in the design of ECL biosensors for clinical diagnostics. The authors provide an overview of peptide-based recognition elements and their applications in biosensing. It highlights the advantages of using peptides, such as their high selectivity and affinity toward target analytes, as well as their versatility in accommodating different sensing platforms [6].

An AuNPs@ZIF-8/Ti_3C_2 MXene immobilized T1R1-VFT peptide-based biosensor has been developed by Liu et al. to detect umami. The sensor structure involves

Table 7.1 Recently reported peptide-based ECL biosensors.

Sensor structure	Analyte	LOD	Linear range	Ref.
AuNPs modified glassy carbon electrode	Human norovirus	10^2 fg/ml	0.1–10^3 ng/ml	[20]
AuNPs functionalized with a peptide-streptavidin conjugate	Neutrophil gelatinase-associated lipocalin			[21]
AuNPs functionalized with a peptide nucleic acid probe	Hepatitis C virus RNA			[22]
GO modified GCE functionalized with a peptide	Glucose	100 pM	0.1–10 mM	[23]
GO-Au/methylene blue-sodium alginate hydrogel nanocomposites substrate-based ECL sensor	Matrix metalloproteinase-7	3.1 fg/ml	10 fg/ml –10 ng/ml	[24]
AuNPs /CNT ECL sensor	Matrix metalloproteinase-7	6 pg/ml	1×10^{-2} to 1×10^{3} ng/ml	[25]
Carbon microspheres modified GCE with a peptide-Au-ZIF-8 conjugate	Protein kinase A	100 ng/ml	0.1–1000 ng/ml	[26]
Ferrocene group deposited on Au electrode	Matrix metalloproteinase-14	0.1 ng/l	0.2–0.9 ng /l	[27]
TiO_2/g-C3N4 modified GCE functionalized with a peptide-PNA probe	Multiple microRNAs from cancer cells	100 pM	0.1–1000 nM	[28]
GCE modified with a nisin-chitosan composite film	Salmonella spp.	10 CFU/ml	0.1–100 CFU/ml	[29]
Paper-based ECL PNA biosensor	MicroRNA-492	100 pM	0.1–1000 nM	[27]

Recombinant engineered fructosyl peptide oxidase modified GCE	Glycated hemoglobin	100 ng/dL	0.1–1000 mg/dL	[30]
GCE functionalized with a peptide-AuNPs conjugate	Matrix metalloproteinase-14	100 ng/ml	0.1–1000 ng/ml	[31]
QD-modified GCE functionalized with a bi-functional peptide	Cancer cells overexpressing MMP-14	1000 cells/ml	0.1–10 000 cells/ml	[32]
GCE functionalized with a peptide-G-quadruplex conjugate	Glutathione	100 nM	0.1–1000 nM	[33]
Y-shaped peptide modified GCE	IgG in human serum	100 ng/ml	0.1–1000 ng/ml	[34]
AuNPs modified GCE functionalized with a peptide nucleic acid (PNA) probe	Nuclear factor kappa B	100 pM	0.1–1000 nM	[6]
Luminol-AuNPs@g-C3N4 nanoprobe modified GCE	Tumor exosomes	100 exosomes/ml	0.1–1000 exosomes/ml	[35]

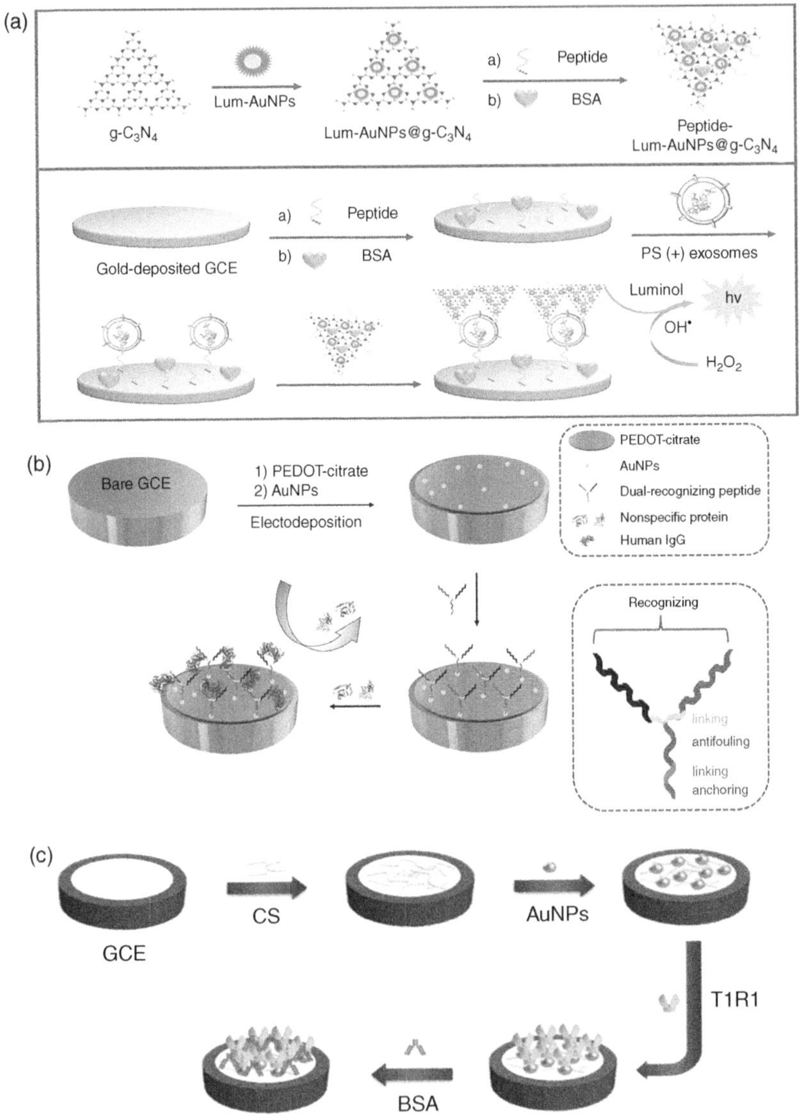

Figure 7.3 Schematic of ECL biosensor (a) (b) synthesis of peptide-Lum-AuNPs@g-C_3N_4 nanoprobe, structure of ECL biosensor. *Source:* [34]/with permission of Elsevier. (c) multifunctional peptide with two branches recognizing two different sites of the target IgG. *Source:* [36]/with permission of Elsevier. T1R1 receptor immobilized on the AuNPs/reduced graphene oxide/chitosan-based ECL sensor. *Source:* [37]/with permission of Elsevier.

the immobilization of T1R1-VFT (taste receptor) on AuNPs@ZIF-8/Ti_3C_2 MXene nanocomposites. The nanocomposite serves as a robust and stable platform for the immobilization of T1R1-VFT, enabling the specific recognition of umami taste substances. The biosensor demonstrated a LOD of 0.06 μM for umami taste substances and a linear range from 10^{-11} to 10^{-3} M. This research highlights the potential of AuNPs@ZIF-8/Ti_3C_2 MXene-based sensor platforms and the specific immobilization of taste receptors for the development of sensitive ECL biosensors for umami taste detection in food samples [39].

Li et al. designed a multifunctional peptide with two recognizing branches for highly sensitive and low-fouling ECL protein assays in human serum. Figure 7.3b shows the sensor structure that involves the synthesis of designed peptides that possess two distinct branches, each specifically recognizing a target protein. The immobilization of these peptides on the electrode surface enables the selective capture and detection of the target protein in human serum. The designed peptides exhibit high sensitivity and low fouling characteristics, ensuring accurate and reliable protein detection. The assay demonstrated a LOD of 0.031 pg/ml for the target protein and a linear range from 0.1 pg/ml to 0.1 mg/ml [36].

Da Silva-Junio et al. [19] develop an ECL biosensor based on the temporin-PTA peptide for the detection of microorganisms. The sensor structure involves the immobilization of temporin-PTA, a peptide with antimicrobial properties, onto the electrode surface. This enables the specific recognition and capture of microorganisms, facilitating their detection. The biosensor demonstrated a LOD of 10 CFU/ml for the target microorganism and a linear range from 10 to 10^6 CFU/ml. This research highlights the potential of using temporin-PTA peptide-based ECL biosensors for the sensitive and selective detection of microorganisms [19]. Fedacı et al. describe a citropin-A modified impedimetric biosensor for the detection of LNCaP prostate cancer cells as shown in Figure 7.3c. The sensor structure involves the modification of the biosensor's surface with citropin-A, a specific bio-recognition receptor for LNCaP cells. The immobilization of citropin-A enables the selective capture and detection of LNCaP cells, facilitating their identification and quantification. The biosensor demonstrated a LOD of 10 cells/ml for LNCaP cells and a linear range from 10 to 10^6 cells/ml [40].

Chen et al. present a non-faradaic impedimetric biosensor for monitoring caspase-9 in mammalian cell culture. The sensor consists of a gold electrode modified with a self-assembled monolayer (SAM) of thiolated DNA. The DNA is designed to bind specifically to caspase-9. As caspase-9 binds to the DNA, it changes the impedance of the electrode. This change in impedance can be used to quantify the amount of caspase-9 in the sample. The sensor has a LOD of 10 pM and a linear range of 10 pM–100 nM. The sensor was used to successfully monitor caspase-9 activity in mammalian cell culture [17].

Soto and Orozco [41] propose a peptide-based ECL biosensor for the simple detection of SARS-CoV-2. The sensor structure involves the utilization of a specific peptide that exhibits high affinity and selectivity toward the SARS-CoV-2 virus. This peptide is immobilized on the electrode surface, enabling the capture and recognition of the virus. The biosensor utilizes an ECL readout method for detection, providing a rapid and sensitive response. The biosensor demonstrated a LOD of 2.1 pg/ml for SARS-CoV-2 and a linear range from 10 pg/ml to 1 μg/ml [41]. Wang et al. [42] develop a peptide aptamer-based ECL amperometric sensor for sensitive L-glutamate detection. The sensor structure involves the utilization of a specific peptide aptamer that possesses high affinity and selectivity for L-glutamate. This peptide aptamer is immobilized on the sensor surface, allowing for the capture and recognition of L-glutamate molecules. The sensor utilizes an amperometric detection method, which measures the current generated by the ECL reaction between L-glutamate and the sensor. The biosensor exhibited a LOD of 0.1 nM for L-glutamate and a linear range from 0.1 nM to 1 μM [42].

Zhang et al. made a biosensor that can detect metal matrix protease-7 that is both antifouling and sensitive. It is based on a multifunctional peptide and urease@zeolite imidazole frameworks (urease@ZIFs). The sensor structure incorporated the multifunctional peptide and urease@ZIFs. The specific peptide sequence and the analyte, metal matrix protease-7, were mentioned. The LOD of 24.34 fg/ml and linear range values 0.1 pg/ml–100 ng/ml were obtained [43]. Wang et al. developed a sensitive and stable ECL impedimetric biosensor based on the T1R1 receptor for the detection of umami substances. The sensor structure included the T1R1 receptor immobilized on the AuNPs/reduced graphene oxide/chitosan electro-deposited onto a glassy carbon electrode surface. The investigated analyte of interest was umami substance, i.e. concentrations of the detected targets, monosodium glutamate and inosine-5′-monophosphate, within their respective linear ranges of 10^{-14} to 10^{-9} M and 10^{-16} to 10^{-13} M and LOD of 10^{-15} M and 10^{-16} M were obtained with the proposed sensor. Liang et al. developed a chimeric peptide-DNA probe-based ECL biosensor for severe acute respiratory syndrome coronavirus-2 (SARS-CoV-2) detection based on its papain-like cysteine protease and protease inhibitor screening. The sensor structure involved the detection of protease activity using a designed peptide substrate. These nanoprobes are composed of a chimeric peptide sequence that is specific to SARS-CoV-2 PLpro and a DNA sequence that is immobilized on the electrode surface. The DNA2 strand of DNA is complementary to the DNA sequence on the pDNA nanoprobe. The sensor detects the ECL signal generated when the released DNA fragment hybridizes with the DNA2 strand. The analyte SARS-CoV-2 papain-like cysteine protease can be detected with a LOD of 27.18 fM and linear range values 1 pg/ml–10 μg/ml [44]. Filippova et al. developed an ECL biosensor for trypsin activity assays based on the cleavage of an immobilized tyrosine-containing peptide. The sensor structure included the immobilization of the peptide substrate on the screen-printed electrodes modified with AuNPs.

Tyrosine-containing peptides are specific peptides containing tyrosine residues used as the substrate for trypsin. Trypsin enzyme, a protease enzyme, is the target analyte that specifically recognizes and cleaves peptide bonds adjacent to lysine or arginine residues. The LOD of trypsin was calculated from this dependence as 22 nM in the concentration range of 2.68 pM–2.9 nM [45]. A clustered regularly interspaced Short Palindromic repeats (CRISPR)/Cas13a-based ECL biosensor has been developed for the detection of metalloproteinase-2 (MMP-2), a critical biomarker for early cancer detection. The biosensor is based on the use of a PNA/crRNA duplex that can be specifically cleaved by MMP-2. As MMP-2 is present, it cleaves the PNA/crRNA duplex, releasing the crRNA. The released crRNA then binds to CRISPR/Cas13a, which activates the enzyme and cleaves the DNA sequence. The ECL sensor detects the ECL signal generated by the DNA cleavage. The ECL signal is proportional to the concentration of MMP-2 in the sample. The biosensor has a detection limit of 15.56 fM and a linear detection range from 10 pM to 100 nM [46]. An α/β-peptides recognition element with an ECL sensor based on anti-enzymolysis and antifouling capabilities was designed to detect the IgG. The designed α/β-peptides have the ability to resist enzymatic degradation. This ensures that the peptides remain stable and functional in the presence of enzymes that could potentially degrade them. The α/β-peptides also possess antifouling properties, which minimize nonspecific binding and fouling of the sensor surface. The α/β-peptides are first immobilized on the electrode surface. When the target biomarker is present, it binds to the α/β-peptides. The binding of the target biomarker to the α/β-peptides changes the ECL properties of the electrode, which can be detected by the biosensor. The biosensor has a detection limit of 33.7 pg/ml and a linear detection range of 100 pg/ml to 10 μg/ml [47].

7.2.2 Design of Plasmonics Biosensors

The focus on biosensor-surface plasmon resonance (SPR) is a strategy to establish a new generation of RNA-specific small molecules to analyze the interactions of different RNA sequences with proteins and small molecules [48]. Platelet-derived growth factor (PDGF)-BB is a growth factor that plays a role in cell proliferation, migration, and differentiation. It is overexpressed in a number of cancer cells, and its levels are correlated with tumor progression. Therefore, there is a need for sensitive and specific methods for detecting PDGF-BB. Qian made a fiberoptic SPR biosensor for detecting PDGF-BB in serum, as shown in Figure 7.4. It is based on a self-assembled aptamer-antifouling peptide monolayer, which is coated on the

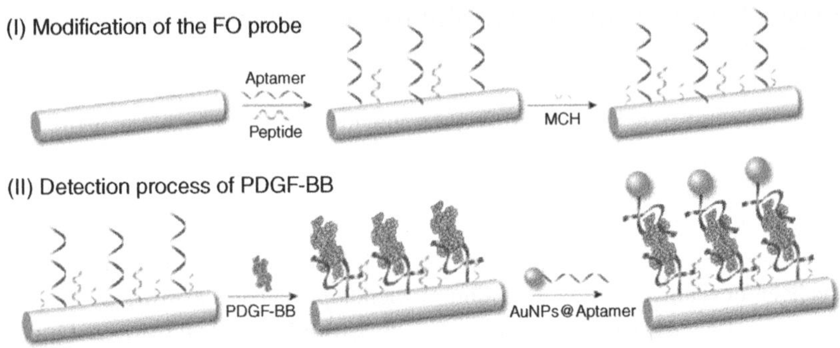

Figure 7.4 Schematic illustration of (A) platelet-derived growth factor -BB FO-SPR biosensor. *Source:* [49]/with permission of Elsevier.

fiberoptic surface to support the plasmon excitation. An antifouling peptide monolayer is introduced onto the metal surface before the aptamer immobilization to enhance the sensor's performance. The biosensor system includes a sample delivery system where serum samples containing PDGF-BB are introduced and flowed over the fiberoptic sensor surface. Changes in the SPR signal resulting from the binding interactions between the aptamer and PDGF-BB are monitored and analyzed to quantify the concentration of PDGF-BB in the serum. The biosensor was able to detect PDGF-BB in serum with a detection limit of 0.35 pM and a broad detection range of 1–1000 pM of PDGF-BB [49].

Zhu developed an ultra-sensitive detection method for caspase-3, a biomarker in various biological processes. This SPR sensor uses Cucurbit [7] urils (induced bimetallic nanoparticle network) in conjunction with bimetallic NPs to enhance the detection sensitivity and selectivity of caspase-3. Cucurbit [7] urils (Cucurbit [7] urils): Cucurbit [7] urils is a macrocyclic compound known for its ability to host guest molecules within its cavity. In this study, cucurbit [7] urils are used as a key component to induce the formation of a bimetallic nanoparticle network. Three-dimensional (3D) bimetallic nanonetworks were formed through Cucurbit [7] urils integrated self-assembly of AuNPs and AgNPs using the one-pot synthesis method. An LOD of 5.39 pg mL1 and a linear range of 10 pg/ml–100 ng/ml were reported [50]. An Au film-based SPR sensor was developed to detect the O-linked N-acetylglucosamine (O-GlcNAc). A single peptide sequence containing three recognition sites for the detection of the O-GlcNAc transferase enzyme was involved in the post-translational modification of proteins with O-linked β-N-acetylglucosamine, which plays a crucial role in various biological processes.

The biosensor consists of three recognition sites involved in detecting the target, specifically (i) protease K cleavage site, (ii) O-GlcNAcylated site by enzyme transferase, and (iii) six histidine residues that are used as a signal-report probe to recognize Ni^{2+}. As the immobilized peptide is cleaved by protease K, the His-tag residue part will be released and bind to Ni^{2+}, which will cause a change in the SPR signal. The developed biosensor was used to detect O-GlcNAc with a detection limit of 0.01 nM and a linear range of 2×10^{-13} to 5×10^{-8} M, which is much lower than the existing methods [35]. Tables 7.2 and 7.3 discuss the sensor structure, LOD, and linear range of peptide-based plasmonic and ECL biosensors to detect the various analytes.

Figure 7.5a discusses the various steps used to pre and post-immobilization used for peptide on the Au film. Figure 7.5b shows a chitosan and GO-based SPR biosensors that consist of layer-by-layer assembly to detect the Aβ antigen, β-amyloid in cases of Alzheimer's disease. Assembly was designed using chitosan and polystyrene sulphonate on the surface of AgNPs, and then antibodies of Aβ were fixed on layer-by-layer assembly (AgNPs-CS-PSS-CS@anti-Aβ). Chitosan is a natural biopolymer that stabilizes and provides a biocompatible matrix for the biosensor and GO enhance the sensitivity due to its high surface area and excellent electrical properties. Specific antibodies or probes are immobilized onto the biosensor surface, which selectively bind to β-amyloid. This sensor provides the

Table 7.2 Recently reported peptide-based plasmonic biosensors.

Sensor structure	Transducer type	LOD	Linear range	Disease	Ref.
Rhodamine B-labeled peptides	Fluorescence	1 μM	0.1–10 μM	Heparin	[51]
Interface peptide nano-network	SPR	100 nM	0.1–10 μM	Alzheimer's	[53]
Antifouling peptide	ECL	10 μM	0.1–100 μM	S. pneumonia	[54]
SPR sensor	SPR	10 nM	0.1–10 μM	Artificial nose	[55]
Peptide and hairpin DNA	SPR	1 μM	0.1–10 μM	Volatile organic compound	[56]
Ultrasmall noble metal nanoparticles	SPR	10 μM	0.1–100 μM	Bovine serum albumin	[57]
One peptide sequence with three recognition sites	ECL	100 nM	0.1–10 μM	O-GlcNAc transferase	[35]

Table 7.3 Recently reported peptide-based plasmonic and ECL biosensors.

Sensor structure	LOD	Linear range	Disease	Ref.
Photofuel cell-based self-powered ECL biosensor	0.02 pg/ml	0.1–500 pg/ml	HER2	[58]
Peptide-templated copper nano-clusters-based surface acoustic wave sensor	0.02 U/ml	0–50 U/ mL	Protein kinase A	[59]
Au-PDMS with interdigitated electrode array and flow-cell-based sensor SPR sensor	n.r.	10^6–10^8 CFU/ml	*Staphylococcus aureus*	[60]
AuNPs-Bi_2Se_3 peptide electrode-based ECL sensor	1.07×10^{-11} mg/ml	3.6×10^{-10}–10^{-5} mg/ml	Programmed cell death-1, Anti-hemagglutinin tag antibody	[61]
Cytop-Au-peptide-long-range SPR aptasensor	n.r.	0.78–100 μM	vancomycin	[62]
Signal peptide-based luminescent biosensor	n.r.	1–10 μg/ml	SARS-CoV-2	[63]

linearity range of 2 fg/ml–400 ng/ml and LOD of 1.21 fg/ml [52]. Qi developed an SPR biosensor for the accurate and sensitive quantitation of small molecules (i.e. chloramphenicol) in blood samples. Chloramphenicol is a therapeutic drug used in the management and treatment of superficial eye infections such as bacterial conjunctivitis and otitis externa. The sensor was fabricated on an Au-coated SPR chip that was functionalized with antibodies specific to the target molecule. The magnitude of the shift was proportional to the concentration of the target molecule. The SPR biosensor was used to detect the small molecule CAP in rat blood samples. The sensor was able to detect chloramphenicol at concentrations as low as 0.099 ng/ml and in a linear range of 0.1–50 ng/ml [64]. A surface plasmon-enhanced spin selectivity sensor for the ultrafast purification of chiral peptides is fabricated on an Au surface functionalized with chiral molecules. Figure 7.5c shows that an AuNPs-decorated ZnO nanorod electrodes were used to modulate the polarization of spintronic in order to enhance the charge mobility of excitons for hydrogen generation. As polarized light passes through the metal surface,

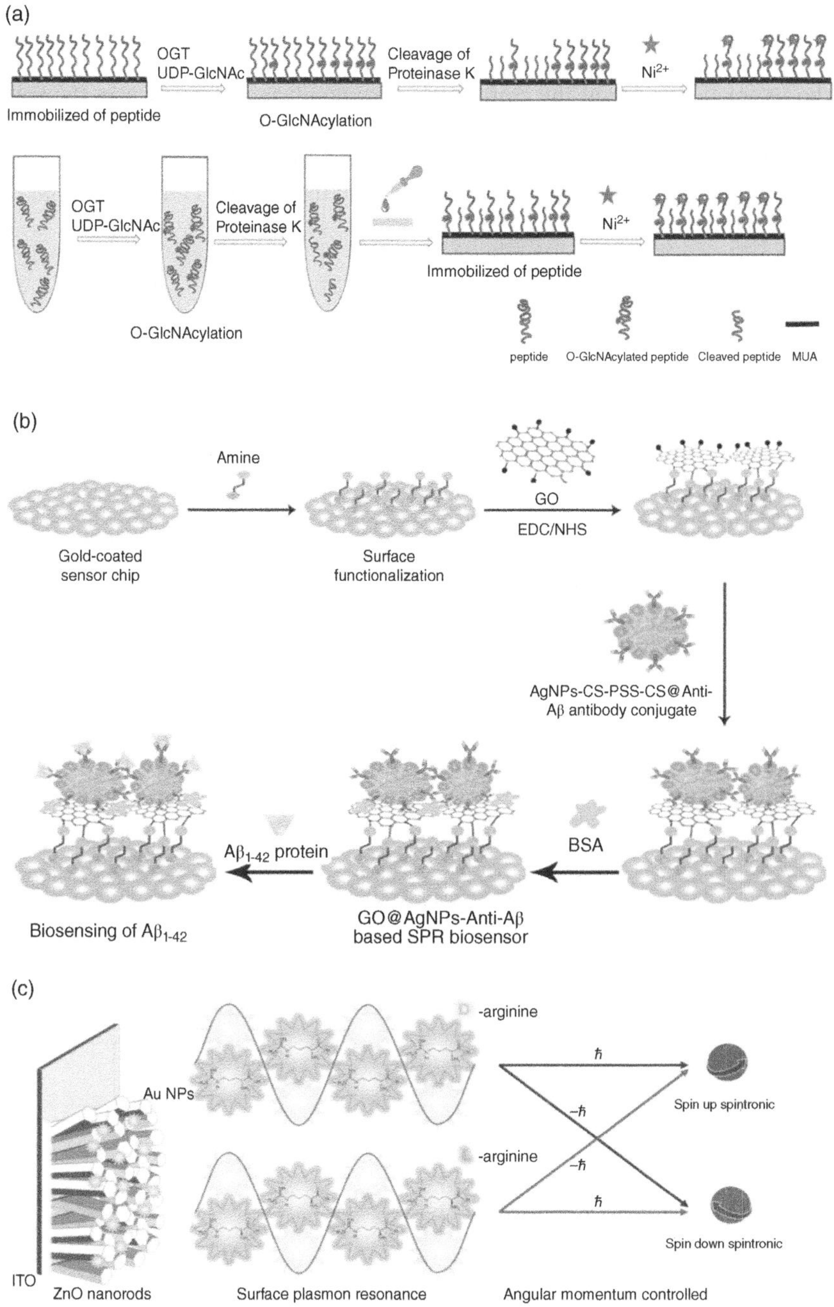

Figure 7.5 Schematic of (a) pre-immobilized and post-immobilized method used for peptide immobilization on the Au film. *Source:* [30]/with permissison of Elsevier. (b) AgNPs-CS-PSS-CS@anti-Aβ based sensor. *Source:* [52]/with permission of Elsevier. (c) Mechanism of surface plasmon resonance enhancement photons to spintronic conversion devices by SPR effects from Au NPs decorated ZnO nanorod electrode. *Source:* [54]/with permission of Elsevier.

the interaction between the chiral molecules produces a difference in the spin relaxation rate of the chiral molecules that is used to separate the chiral molecules. Two chiral peptides, leucine enkephalin and methionine enkephalin, are used for the purification process. A linear range of 0–300 ppm and a LOD of 200 ppm of chiral peptide can be detected [65].

7.2.3 Design of Colorimetric Biosensors

Figure 7.6 shows a turn-on unlabeled colorimetric biosensor based on aptamer-AuNPs conjugates was developed for the detection of amyloid-β oligomers, core biomarkers for early diagnosis of Alzheimer's disease. The aptamer polythymine-polyadenine was designed to specifically bind to Aβ oligomers, and the AuNPs were conjugated to the aptamer via a linker. As the aptamer-AuNPs conjugates were exposed to Aβ oligomers, the AuNPs were aggregated, which resulted in a color change. The biosensor was able to detect Aβ oligomers in the range of 10–100 nM with a detection limit of 3.03 nM. The biosensor was also able to distinguish between Aβ oligomers and Aβ monomers. The results of this study demonstrate

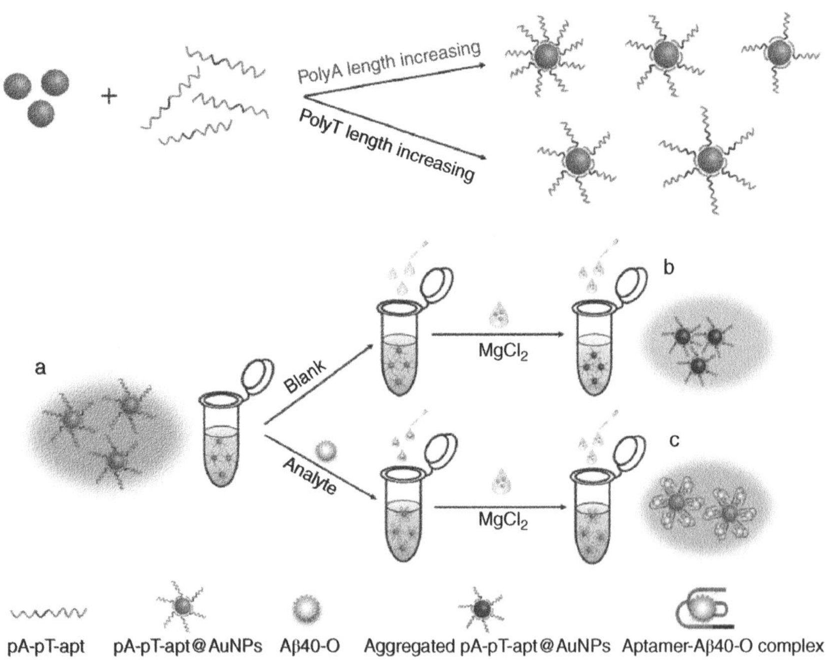

Figure 7.6 Schematic of aptamer-AuNPs-peptide-based colorimetric biosensors for amyloid-β oligomer detection. *Source:* [66]/with permission of Elsevier.

Table 7.4 Recently reported peptide-based plasmonic biosensors.

Sensor structure	Transducer type	LOD	Linear range	Disease	Ref.
Photo-fuel cell-based self-powered biosensor	ECL	0.02 pg/ml	0.1–500 pg/ml	HER2	[58]
Peptide-templated copper nanoclusters-based sensor	Surface acoustic wave	0.02 U/ml	0–50 U/ml	Protein kinase A	[59]
Au-PDMS with interdigitated electrode array and flow-cell-based sensor	SPR	10 nM	100–1000 nM	*S. aureus*	[60]
Topological insulator Bi_2Se_3	SPR	1 nM	10–100 nM		[61]
Long-range surface plasmon aptasensor	SPR	1 nM	10–100 nM	vancomycin	[62]
SpACE-CCM	SPR	100 pM	1–100 nM	SARS-CoV-2	[63]

the potential of the aptamer-AuNPs conjugates for the development of a simple, sensitive, and specific biosensor for the detection of Aβ oligomers [66]. Some of recently reported plasmonic and colorimetric biosensor designs have been presented in Tables 7.4 and 7.5.

7.2.4 Design of Fluorescence Biosensors

Horseradish peroxidase (HRP) metalloenzyme is widely explored for various applications, but it also suffers from several drawbacks involving high cost, low stability, and degradation in some food matrices with time. Therefore, different low-cost inorganic nanomaterials with peroxidase-like activity have been explored in the last few years, such as manganese dioxide nanosheets (MnO_2NSs), iron-based nanomaterials, graphene, carbon nanotubes, and CuNPs. Liu et al. explored an MnO_2NSs-based colorimetric sensor by immobilizing specific nonapeptides to detect *Vibrio parahaemolyticus* in water and seafood samples. In this case, a MnO_2NSs@peptide complex is created by fusing the 9-mer phage display peptides to MnO_2NSs using the physical adsorption method. A sandwich immunoassay is fabricated by incubating the bacteria for 2 hours to ensure binding to the peptide-grafted surface. Then a sandwich complex is formed from MnO_2NSs and peptide fusion. Finally, chromogenic tert-butyl carbamate was added for 30 minutes, which changes the color depending on the bacterial concentration,

Table 7.5 Recently reported peptide-based colorimetric biosensors.

Sensor structure	Transducer type	Analyte	Linear range	LOD	Ref.
Alginate microcapsules incorporated onto cotton fabric	Colorimetric	Urea	0.1–10 μg/ml	0.05 μg/ml	[67]
Nano-cellulose	Colorimetric	Human neutrophil elastase	0.01–10 μg/ml	0.01 μg/ml	[68]
Peptide nucleic acid	Colorimetric	Influenza A virus	0.05–10 μg/ml	0.05 μg/ml	[69]
Nanomaterial-mediated paper-based biosensors	Colorimetric	Pathogen detection	0.01–1 μg/ml	0.01 μg/ml	[70]
Not specified	Colorimetric	Virus detection	0.01–1 μg/ml	0.01 μg/ml	[71]
Hemin-carbon nanotube nanocomposites	Colorimetric	Single-nucleotide polymorphisms	0.01–1 μg/ml	0.01 μg/ml	[72]
Blended chitosan-poly(vinyl alcohol) nanofibers	Colorimetric	Glucose detection	0.01–1 μg/ml	0.01 μg/ml	[73]
Not specified	Colorimetric	Copper (II) binding	Not specified	0.01 μg/ml	[74]
Peptide-modified gold nanoparticles	Colorimetric	Allergenic fungal spore	Not specified	0.1 μg/ml	[75]
Dual-modified gold nanoparticles	Colorimetric	Mercury ion	Not specified	0.01 μg/ml	[76]
Not specified	Colorimetric	Shiga toxins	Not specified	0.1 μg/ml	[77]
hACE2-based affinity peptide pair	Colorimetric	SARS-CoV-2	Not specified	0.1 μg/ml	[78]
Two-dimensional (2D) nanomaterial and Au nanoparticles	Colorimetric	Heavy metal ions	Not specified	0.1 μg/ml	[79]

and forms absorbance measurements at 652 nm. A linear range of 20–10^4 CFU/ml and LOD of 15 CFU mL^{-1} were reported [80].

Li et al. developed an innovative approach for the bio-functionalization of MoS_2 nanosheets with peptides as intracellular fluorescent biosensors for the detection of caspase-3 activity, an important indicator of cellular apoptosis. It can detect caspase-3 activity in living cells. The MoS_2 NSs were first functionalized with polydopamine to improve their biocompatibility. The PDA-modified MoS_2 NSs were then further functionalized with peptides that specifically bind to caspase-3. The resulting MoS_2@PDA-PEG-Peptide biosensor. The large surface area and unique electronic properties of MoS_2 nanosheets contribute to improved sensitivity, stability, and enhanced fluorescence upon interaction with caspase-3. The LOD of the target was 0.33 ng/ml [81].

Bacterial endotoxin, known as lipopolysaccharide, is a Gram-negative bacteria that causes fever, chills, and shock. The detection of lipopolysaccharide in the bloodstream is important to the diagnosis and treatment of sepsis. A fluorescent biosensor that can detect lipopolysaccharide in living cells based on aggregation-induced emission was reported that involves an increase in fluorescence of a fluorophore on its aggregation. A lipopolysaccharide-specific peptide binds to it form aggregation-induced emission fluorophore, 1-(4-carboxylbenzene)-1,2,2-triphenyl. The LOD of the biosensor was 6.97 nM, which is comparable to the ELISA method [82].

Protein tyrosine phosphatase 1B (PTP1B) is an enzyme that dephosphorylates proteins, affects cell signaling in various types of diabetes mellitus, is responsible for insulin resistance, and is overexpressed in different types of cancer. A fluorescence biosensor based on a titanium dioxide-decorated single-walled carbon nano-horn nanocomposite for the detection of PTP1B was reported. The nanocomposite was functionalized with a peptide that specifically binds to PTP1B. In the presence of PTP1B, the peptide binds to the composite and causes its fluorescence to be quenched, which is proportional to the concentration of PTP1B. PTP1B can be detected in the range of 0.1–100 nM with a LOD of 0.01 ng/ml [83].

Transforming growth factor-β (TGF-β) regulates multiple fundamental physiological processes and is closely related to severe diseases such as cancer, fibrosis, immune disorders, and cardiovascular diseases. A green fluorescent protein (GFP) reporter gene-based fluorescence sensor was reported to detect TGF-β. The biosensor cells are engineered to express a fusion protein of GFP and a TGF-β binding domain. When active TGF-β is present, the binding domain binds to TGF-β and activates the GFP reporter gene. This results in an increase in the fluorescence of the biosensor cells. The biosensor was able to detect active TGF-β in the range of 0.024–6.25 ng/ml and a LOD of 2.300–18.75 pg/ml [84].

Figure 7.7a depicts a sensitive "turn-on" fluorescent biosensor for the detection of biomarkers based on three-dimensional DNA walkers. The biosensor consists

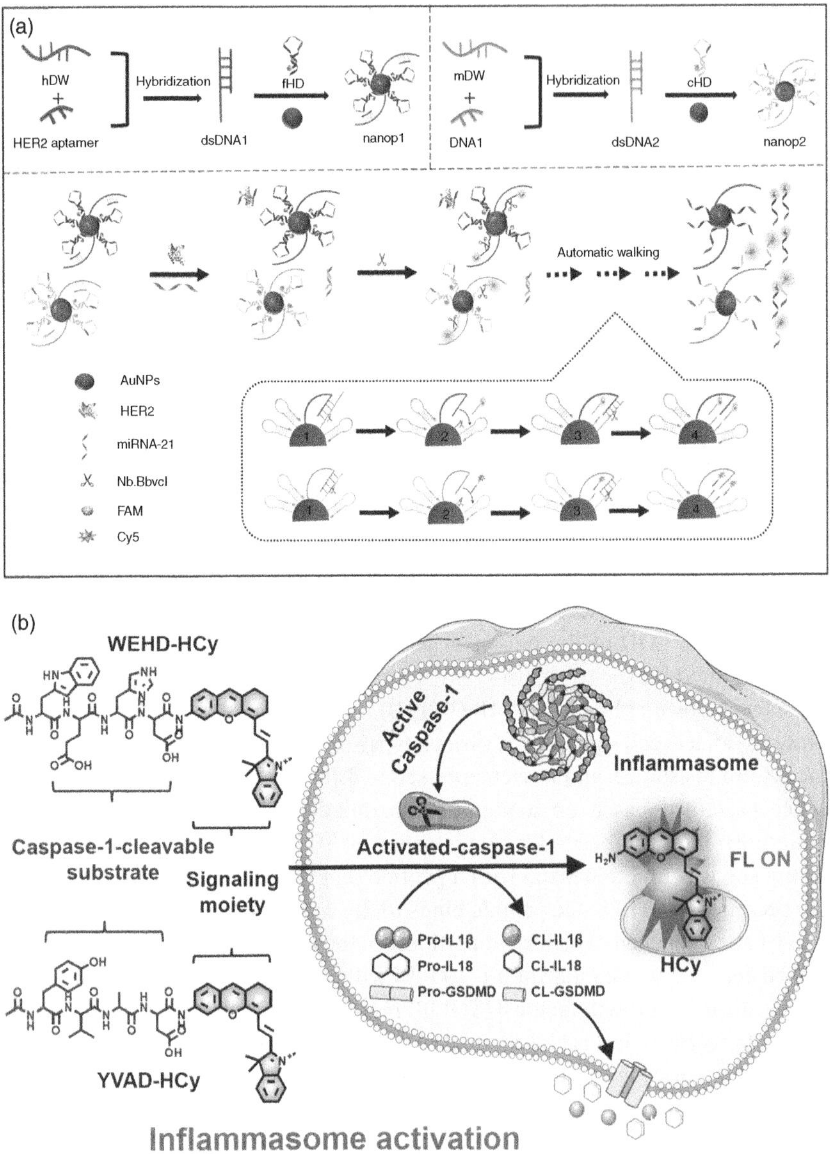

Figure 7.7 Schematic illustration of the (a) fluorescent biosensor for HER2 and miRNA-21 detection. *Source:* [85]/with permission of Elsevier. (b) Chemical structures of WEHD-HCy and YVAD-HCy and schematic illustration of mitochondria-targeted WEHD-HCy and YVAD-HCy responses to inflammasome activation. *Source:* [86]/with permission of Elsevier.

of a three-dimensional DNA walker immobilized on a surface. The DNA walker is designed to bind to a specific biomarker. When the biomarker is present, the DNA walker is activated and its fluorescence is enhanced. The biosensor was evaluated using a series of experiments. The biosensor was able to detect a variety of biomarkers, including cancer biomarkers, in the range of 0.1–100 nM. The LOD of the biosensor was 0.1 nM [85]. Caspase-1 is an enzyme that plays a critical role in the activation of the inflammasome, a protein complex that is involved in the immune response. The activation of the inflammasome leads to the release of inflammatory cytokines, which can cause inflammation and tissue damage. Caspase-1-responsive fluorescence biosensors are a new type of biosensor that can be used to monitor the activation of the inflammasome. These biosensors are based on the use of a fluorescent probe that is quenched by caspase-1. As caspase-1 is activated, it cleaves the fluorescent probe, which results in an increase in fluorescence. The range of caspase-1-responsive fluorescence biosensors is typically 0.1–100 nM. The LOD of these biosensors is typically in the range of 0.1–1 nM. Figure 7.7b shows the structure of caspase-1-responsive fluorescence biosensors that typically consists of a fluorescent probe attached to a caspase-1 binding domain [86].

A fluorometric biosensor of α-amylase, an enzyme involved in starch digestion, has been developed using an artificial allosteric biosensor immobilized on a nanostructured interface. This biosensor offers a sensitive and selective method for detecting α-amylase activity in biological samples. The biosensor design involves the immobilization of an allosteric sensor on a nanostructured interface, which enhances the sensitivity and stability of the system. The allosteric sensor undergoes a conformational change in the presence of α-amylase, leading to a fluorescent signal that can be measured and quantified. The biosensor was able to detect α-amylase in the range of 0.1–100 nM with a LOD of 0.1 nM [87]. Peptide-based fluorescence biosensors with seven lysine residues linked to a cysteine through a three-glycine residue linker with attached fluorescent probes (fluorescein-5-maleimide and tetramethylrhodamine-5-maleimide) were reported to detect the negatively charged nanoparticles (ZnO, Fe_3O_4, CeO, and SWCNT). These biosensors utilize the unique binding properties of peptides to selectively recognize and bind to target nanoparticles, leading to the generation of fluorescence signals. Peptide-based biosensors offer several advantages, including their ability to be easily modified with fluorophores or signaling molecules, enabling sensitive and selective detection [88]. Pan et al. explored a fluorescent biosensor based on a Cd^{2+}-fueled wheel DNAzyme walker for the detection of cadmium (Cd^{2+}) in water samples. The DNAzyme walker is a DNA molecule that can catalyze the cleavage of a specific DNA strand. As Cd^{+2} ions are present, it binds to the DNAzyme walker and activates it. The activated DNAzyme walker then cleaves the specific DNA strand, which releases a fluorescent dye. The amount of fluorescence is proportional to the concentration of Cd^{2+} ions in the sample. The biosensor was tested with a series of Cd^{2+} solutions with known concentrations. The detection limit of the biosensor was found to be 0.2 pM. The linear range of the biosensor was 0.2 pM–100 nM [89].

A fluorometric biosensing technique based on an artificial allosteric biosensor immobilized on a nanostructured interface detects the α-amylase, an enzyme responsible for starch hydrolysis. In the presence of α-amylase, it causes a change in the conformation of the biosensor, which in turn causes a change in the fluorescence of the biosensor. The fluorescent dye is attached to the artificial allosteric biosensor, and when the biosensor binds to α-amylase, it causes a change in the fluorescence of the dye. This change in fluorescence can be used to quantify the concentration of α-amylase in the sample. It involves the immobilization of the chimeric enzymes on the SiO_2-NPs. LOD of 2 pM, and the linear range of the biosensor was from 2 pM–100 nM [87].

7.2.5 Design of Interferometric Biosensors

Shumeiko developed a single-wall carbon nanotube (SWCNT) paper-based near-infrared optical biosensor for the quantitative detection of protease activity. The SWCNTs are modified with a peptide that is specific to the protease of interest. As the protease binds to the SWCNTs, it causes a change in the near-infrared absorption of the SWCNTs. This change in absorption can be used to quantify the concentration of protease activity in the sample. The biosensor was tested with a series of protease solutions with known concentrations. The detection limit of the biosensor was found to be 10 nM and the linear range of the biosensor was from 10 nM to 100 μM [90]. A self-reference interference sensor based on coherence multiplexing based on a Mach-Zehnder interferometer (MZI) with two sensing arms and one reference arm was reported. The proposed sensor has two reaction chambers and sensing chips of different thicknesses, which define two interferometric paths with different optical path differences. This allows the proposed sensor to achieve self-reference based on coherent multiplexing. The sensing arms are used to detect the target analyte, while the reference arm is used to track environmental disturbances. Coherence multiplexing is a technique that uses multiple wavelengths of light to measure the same analyte. This technique allows the sensor to cancel out the effects of environmental disturbances such as temperature and vibration. The detection limit of the sensor was found to be 10 pM and the linear range of the sensor was from 10 pM to 100 nM [91]. Zaraee developed a label-free interferometric reflectance imaging (IRI) based sensor that uses LEDs, and photodetectors with interferometric reflectance imaging technology to detect whole *E. coli* bacterial cells. It captures the interference patterns generated by the interaction of light with the bacterial cells immobilized on

Table 7.6 Summary of recently reported peptide-based interferometric biosensors.

Sensor structure	LOD	Linear range	Analyte	Ref.
LED-based interferometric reflectance imaging sensor	10 pM	100 nM	Amyloid-β aggregation	[94]
Chitosan-nickel-film-based interferometric optical fiber sensor	0.8368 ng/ml	0–78 ng/ml	Histidine-tagged proteins	[95]
Paper-based near-infrared optical biosensor	12.5 ng/ml	1–20 μg/ml	Protease activity	[90]
Common-path interferometric label-free protein sensing with resonant dielectric nanostructures	1.8×10^{-6} RIU	1 pg/ml	Proteins	[96]
Peptide-based using porous silicon biosensor	n.r.	n.r.	Chikungunya virus	[97]
Optical interferometric based biosensor	n.r.	n.r.	SARS-CoV-2 immunoglobulins	[98]
Peptide–nucleic acid aptamer pair biosensor	6 pM	0.01–1 nM	$VEGF_{165}$ for disease biomarkers	[99]

a surface. The sensitivity of the IRI sensor was demonstrated by detecting as few as 100 *E. coli* cells in a sample with a LOD of 2.2 CFU/ml [92]. Kaur et al. investigated biolayer interferometry-SELEX to select specific aptamers for the detection of Shiga toxin, a bacterial toxin associated with foodborne illnesses. The biosensor is designed by immobilizing the aptamers onto a chitosan-WSe_2 hybrid material. Chitosan, a biocompatible and adhesive polymer, served as a support matrix for the aptamers, while WSe_2 acted as a transducer, converting the binding events into measurable signals. When Shiga toxin binds to the apta-sensors, it causes a change in the refractive index of the apta-sensors. This change in refractive index is detected by the biolayer interferometry platform. This label-free detection approach enabled real-time monitoring of the toxin concentration. The biosensor provides a LOD of 44.5 pg/ml and a linear range of 44.5 pg/ml–413 pg/ml [93]. Detailed structures with performance parameters of peptide-based interferometric biosensors have been summarized in Table 7.6.

7.2.6 Design of SER-Based Biosensors

A surface-enhanced Raman scattering (SERS) bioassay for the simultaneous detection of two important bacterial pathogens, *Acinetobacter baumannii* and Klebsiella pneumonia, is demonstrated. It consists of a dual-target detection system by combining a vancomycin-modified polyethyleneimine-interlayered nanocomposite with aptamer-functionalized SERS tags. Vancomycin, a glycopeptide antibiotic, was functionalized to detect the *A. baumannii*, while the aptamer targeted K. pneumonia. The polyethyleneimine-interlayered nanocomposite served as a substrate for the immobilization of the vancomycin and aptamer-functionalized SERS tags. The nanocomposite enhanced the Raman signals, enabling sensitive detection of the captured bacteria. The SERS tags, functionalized with specific aptamers, provided high specificity for the targeted bacterial strains. The bioassay exhibited excellent sensitivity, with an LOD of 10 cells/ml in the range of 10^5 cells/ml for both *A. baumannii* and *Klebsiella pneumoniae* [100]. The paper introduces a novel quantitative assay for the detection of ultratrace levels of copper ions (Cu^{2+}) using a peptide-mediated COF nanocatalytic amplification (SERS) approach. The researchers developed a unique peptide-based COF nanocatalyst that selectively binds to Cu^{2+} ions. This COF nanocatalyst acts as a scaffold to amplify SERS signals, significantly enhancing the sensitivity of the detection method. The specific peptide sequence ensures high selectivity for Cu^{2+} ions, enabling accurate quantification. The assay involves capturing Cu^{2+} ions with the peptide-mediated COF nanocatalyst, resulting in the formation of a stable complex. This interaction triggers a catalytic reaction on the COF surface, leading to the generation of amplified SERS signals. The intensity of the SERS signals is directly proportional to the concentration of Cu^{2+} ions present in the sample. The assay demonstrates exceptional sensitivity, capable of detecting Cu^{2+} ions at ultra-trace levels. It offers a wide linear range, allowing for precise quantification over a broad concentration range. The peptide-mediated COF nanocatalytic amplification approach provides improved signal amplification, enhances detection sensitivity, and enables accurate quantification of Cu^{2+} ions even at low concentrations [101]. It exhibited a LOD of 0.0045 nM and linear range of 0.005–0.115 nM [101]. A magnetic (M) SERS biosensor based on Ag nanorods deposited on neodymium magnetic substrates at a low temperature of 120 K was reported to detect hemozoin, a biomarker associated with malaria infection, using an external magnetic field. Hemozoin is a metabolic by-product of malaria parasites that exhibits paramagnetic properties. The presence of high-spin trivalent iron in the hemozoin structure led to the magnetic field-induced agglomeration of these molecules in the vicinity of the electromagnetic "hotspots" available on the SERS substrates. It has been shown that the magnetic field can be used to induce the agglomeration of hemozoin molecules, which further enhances the SERS signal. Figure 7.8a shows the pyridine-AgNRs-based M-SERS sensor with modulated intensity. The LOD for hemozoin for M-SERS was obtained as low as 10^{-11} M (<10 parasites/μL), which is significantly lower than the detection limits of other methods for malaria diagnosis [102]. Zhong developed a ratiometric peptide SERS nanoprobe for in situ imaging of protease activity in single living cancer cells as shown in

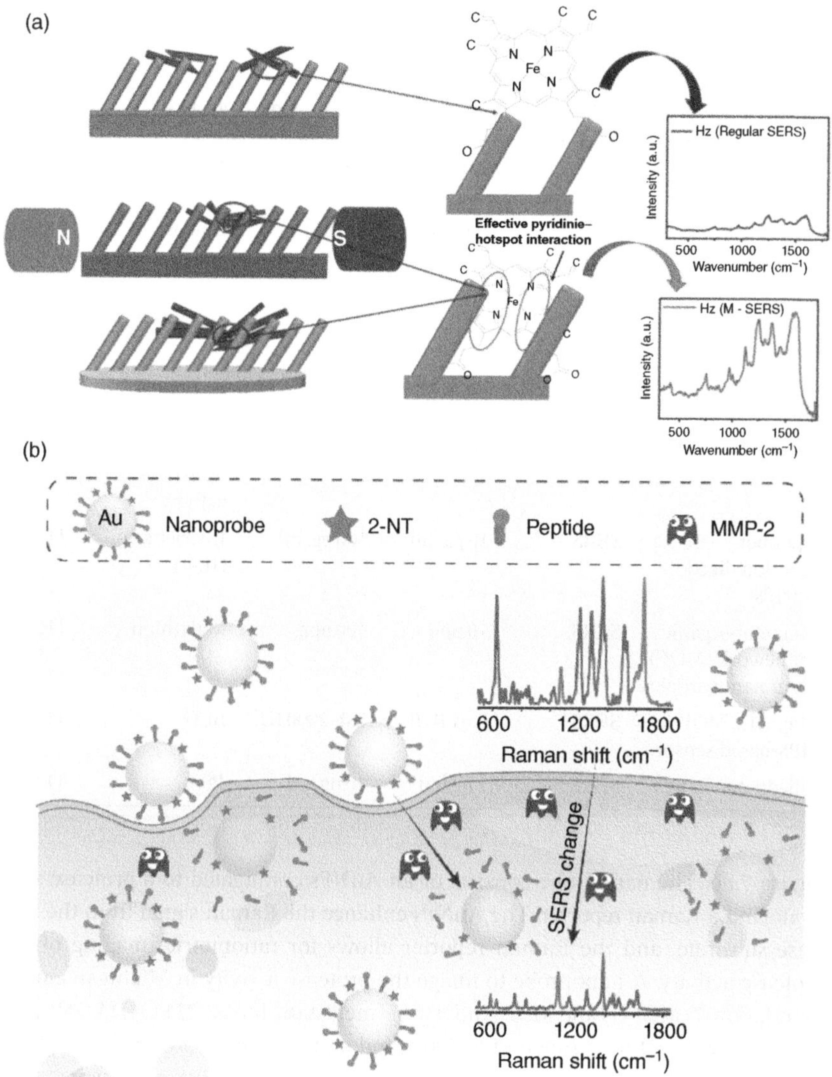

Figure 7.8 Schematic diagram of (a) pyridine-AgNRs-based M-SERS sensor. *Source:* [102]/with permission of Elsevier. (b) SERS nanoprobe to detect the protease activity in MCF-7 and MDA-MB-231. *Source:* [103]/with permission of Elsevier.

Table 7.7 Recently reported peptide-based SERS biosensors.

Sensor structure	Transduction method	LOD	Linear range	Analyte	Ref.
AuNPs	SERS	10 pg/ml	100 pg/ml	Tumor necrosis factor alpha	[104]
Core-shell Au @silver hollow nanocubes	SERS	100 pM	100 nM	Glucose	[105]
Paper-based biosensor	ECL	100 pM	100 nM	miRNA-492	[28]
M13 phage-based nanoprobe	SERS	10 CFU/ml	100 CFU/ml	*S. Aureus*	[106]
AuNPs	SERS	10 nM	100 nM	O-GlcNAc transferase activity	[107]
Aptamer-functionalized AuNPs	SERS	10 pg/ml	100 pg/ml	Interleukin-6 (IL-6)	[108]
Tb metal-organic framework (MOF) @Au nanoparticles	SERS	10 ppb	100 ppb	Malathion	[109]
Magnetic MOF NPS-based sensor	SERS	0,61 IU/l	2.0–2000 IU/l	hCG	[110]
Silicon nanowires	SERS	1 ng/ml	10 ng/ml	PSA	[111]

Figure 7.8b. The nanoprobe consists of an AuNPs conjugated to a protease substrate and a Raman reporter. The AuNPs enhance the Raman signal from the protease substrate, and the Raman reporter allows for ratiometric imaging of the protease activity. A nanoprobe to image the protease activity in Michigan cancer foundation-7 (MCF-7) and M.D. Anderson – metastatic breast-231 (MDA-MB-231) was used, with a linear range of 8–400 ng/ml and LOD of 1×10^3 cells/ml [103]. Table 7.7 summarizes the recently reported peptide-based SERS biosensors.

7.3 Summary

Peptide-based biosensors are a potential candidate to detect a wide range of analytes, including biomolecules, diseases, toxins, and pathogens. Peptide-based biosensors offer a number of advantages that include high sensitivity, low cost, and easy fabrication. Peptides can be designed to have high affinity and specificity for target analytes, which can lead to high sensitivity in the detection of these analytes. Peptides are relatively inexpensive to produce and can be easily fabricated using a variety of methods, which can make peptide-based biosensors more affordable than traditional biosensors. Peptides also suffer from several drawbacks, as they are relatively unstable and can be easily degraded by heat, pH, and other environmental factors. This can lead to poor performance of the biosensor, as the peptide may not be able to bind to the target analyte or may not be able to generate a measurable signal. They are not as specific as other bio-recognition element (BREs), such as antibodies and aptamers. This could lead to false positives and false negatives that reduce the accuracy of the biosensor. The other drawback is the lower sensitivity of the currently used transducers, which is not enough to detect low concentrations of analytes. Despite these challenges, peptide-based biosensors have the potential to revolutionize the field of biosensing.

References

1 Masuda, Y. (2021). Bioactive 3D structures of naturally occurring peptides and their application in drug design. *Biosci. Biotechnol. Biochem.* 85 (1): 24–32. https://doi.org/10.1093/bbb/zbaa008.

2 Akbarian, M., Khani, A., Eghbalpour, S., and Uversky, V.N. (2022). Bioactive peptides: synthesis, sources, applications, and proposed mechanisms of action. *Int. J. Mol. Sci.* 23 (3): https://doi.org/10.3390/ijms23031445.

3 Wang, L., Wang, N., Zhang, W. et al. (2022). Therapeutic peptides: current applications and future directions. *Signal Transduct. Target. Ther.* 7 (1): 48. https://doi.org/10.1038/s41392-022-00904-4.

4 Shechter, G. and Schwartz, A. (2018). Peptide solubility limits: backbone and side-chain interactions. *Physiol. Behav.* 176 (1): 139–148. https://doi.org/10.1021/acs.jpcb.7b10734.Peptide.

5 Wang, M., Li, L., Zhang, L. et al. (2022). Peptide-derived biosensors and their applications in tumor immunology-related detection. *Anal. Chem.* 94 (1): 431–441. https://doi.org/10.1021/acs.analchem.1c04461.

6 Sfragano, P.S., Moro, G., Polo, F., and Palchetti, I. (2021). The role of peptides in the design of electrochemical biosensors for clinical diagnostics. *Biosensors* 11 (8): 1–20. https://doi.org/10.3390/bios11080246.

7 Sun, X., Fan, J., Fu, C. et al. (2017). $WS_2$2 and $MoS_2$2 biosensing platforms using peptides as probe biomolecules. *Sci. Rep.* 7 (1): 1–8. https://doi.org/10.1038/s41598-017-10221-4.

8 Zhang, Q.Y., Yan, Z.B., Meng, Y.M. et al. (2021). Antimicrobial peptides: mechanism of action, activity and clinical potential. *Mil. Med. Res.* 8 (1): 1–25. https://doi.org/10.1186/s40779-021-00343-2.

9 Whitesides, G.M. (2001). Moving from structure to function. *Abstr. Pap. Am. Chem. Soc.* 221: U318–U318.

10 Huan, Y., Kong, Q., Mou, H., and Yi, H. (2020). Antimicrobial peptides: classification, design, application and research progress in multiple fields. *Front. Microbiol.* 11: 1–21. https://doi.org/10.3389/fmicb.2020.582779.

11 Langer, J., Jimenez de Aberasturi, D., Aizpurua, J. et al. (2020). Present and future of surface-enhanced Raman scattering. *ACS Nano* 14 (1): 28–117. https://doi.org/10.1021/acsnano.9b04224.

12 Duro-Castano, A., Conejos-Sánchez, I., and Vicent, M.J. (2014). Peptide-based polymer therapeutics. *Polymers (Basel).* 6 (2): 515–551. https://doi.org/10.3390/polym6020515.

13 Chandrudu, S., Simerska, P., and Toth, I. (2013). Chemical methods for peptide and protein production. *Molecules* 18 (4): 4373–4388. https://doi.org/10.3390/molecules18044373.

14 Sotirios Koutsopoulos (2018). *Peptide Applications in Biomedicine, Biotechnology and Bioengineering*. United Kingdom: Elsevier.

15 Duan, Y., Qiao, X., Xu, L. et al. (2022). Electrogenerated chemiluminescence biosensor for assay of matrix metalloproteinase-14 and protein-expressing cancer cells via inhibitory peptides-based sandwich assay. *Microchem. J.* 181: 107829. https://doi.org/10.1016/j.microc.2022.107829.

16 Yang, X., Chen, P., Zhang, X. et al. (2023). An electrochemical biosensor for HER2 detection in complex biological media based on two antifouling materials of designed recognizing peptide and PEG. *Anal. Chim. Acta* 1252: 341075. https://doi.org/10.1016/j.aca.2023.341075.

17 Chen, B., Kiely, J., Williams, I., and Luxton, R. (2023). A non-faradaic impedimetric biosensor for monitoring of caspase 9 in mammalian cell culture. *Bioelectrochemistry* 153: 108456. https://doi.org/10.2139/ssrn.4290463.

18 da Fonseca Alves, R., Martins, I.C., Franco, D.L. et al. (2022). A novel peptide-based electrochemical biosensor for breast cancer characterization over a poly 3-(3-aminophenyl) propionic acid matrix. *Biosens. Bioelectron.* 205: 114081. https://doi.org/10.1016/j.bios.2022.114081.

19 da Silva-Junio, A.G., Frias, I.A., Lima-Neto, R.G. et al. (2022). Electrochemical biosensor based on Temporin-PTA peptide for detection of microorganisms. *J. Pharm. Biomed. Anal.* 216: 114788. https://doi.org/10.1016/j.jpba.2022.114788.

20 El-Said, W.A. and Choi, J.w. (2019). High selective spectroelectrochemical biosensor for HCV-RNA detection based on a specific peptide nucleic acid. *Spectrochim. Acta - Part A Mol. Biomol. Spectrosc.* 217: 288–293. https://doi.org/10.1016/j.saa.2019.03.115.

21 Meng, F., Sun, H., Huang, Y. et al. (2019). Peptide cleavage-based electrochemical biosensor coupling graphene oxide and silver nanoparticles. *Anal. Chim. Acta* 1047: 45–51. https://doi.org/10.1016/j.aca.2018.09.053.

22 Wang, Y., Li, X., Waterhouse, G.I.N. et al. (2019). Photoelectrochemical biosensor for protein kinase a detection based on carbon microspheres, peptide functionalized au-ZIF-8 and TiO2/g-C3N4. *Talanta* 196: 197–203. https://doi.org/10.1016/j.talanta.2018.12.035.

23 Fu, P., Xing, S., Xu, M. et al. (2020). Peptide nucleic acid-based electrochemical biosensor for simultaneous detection of multiple microRNAs from cancer cells with catalytic hairpin assembly amplification. *Sensors Actuators B Chem.* 305: 127545. https://doi.org/10.1016/j.snb.2019.127545.

24 Zheng, Y. and Ma, Z. (2018). Dual-reaction triggered sensitivity amplification for ultrasensitive peptide-cleavage based electrochemical detection of matrix metalloproteinase-7. *Biosens. Bioelectron.* 108: 46–52. https://doi.org/10.1016/j.bios.2018.02.045.

25 Palomar, Q., Xu, X.X., Selegård, R. et al. (2020). Peptide decorated gold nanoparticle/carbon nanotube electrochemical sensor for ultrasensitive detection of matrix metalloproteinase-7. *Sensors Actuators B Chem.* 325: 128789. https://doi.org/10.1016/j.snb.2020.128789.

26 Malvano, F., Pilloton, R., and Albanese, D. (2020). A novel impedimetric biosensor based on the antimicrobial activity of the peptide nisin for the detection of salmonella spp. *Food Chem.* 325: 126868. https://doi.org/10.1016/j.foodchem.2020.126868.

27 Sun, L., Chen, Y., Chen, F., and Ma, F. (2020). Peptide-based electrochemical biosensor for matrix metalloproteinase-14 and protein-overexpressing cancer cells based on analyte-induced cleavage of peptide. *Microchem. J.* 157: 105103. https://doi.org/10.1016/j.microc.2020.105103.

28 Moccia, M., Caratelli, V., Cinti, S. et al. (2020). Paper-based electrochemical peptide nucleic acid (PNA) biosensor for detection of miRNA-492: a pancreatic ductal adenocarcinoma biomarker. *Biosens. Bioelectron.* 165: 112371. https://doi.org/10.1016/j.bios.2020.112371.

29 Shahbazmohammadi, H., Sardari, S., and Omidinia, E. (2020). An amperometric biosensor for specific detection of glycated hemoglobin based on recombinant engineered fructosyl peptide oxidase. *Int. J. Biol. Macromol.* 142: 855–865. https://doi.org/10.1016/j.ijbiomac.2019.10.025.

30 Xu, Y., Wang, Z., Ding, C., and Luo, X. (2020). Ratiometric antifouling electrochemiluminescence biosensor based on bi-functional peptides and low toxic quantum dots. *Sensors Actuators B Chem.* 322: 128613. https://doi.org/10.1016/j.snb.2020.128613.

31 Ye, Z., Li, G., Xu, L. et al. (2020). Peptide-conjugated hemin/G-quadruplex as a versatile probe for 'signal-on' electrochemical peptide biosensor. *Talanta* 209: 120611. https://doi.org/10.1016/j.talanta.2019.120611.

32 Chen, M., Song, Z., Han, R. et al. (2021). Low fouling electrochemical biosensors based on designed Y-shaped peptides with antifouling and recognizing branches for the detection of IgG in human serum. *Biosens. Bioelectron.* 178: 113016. https://doi.org/10.1016/j.bios.2021.113016.

33 Li, W., Cai, Y., Yang, Y. et al. (2021). Novel electrochemical nuclear factorkappa B biosensor via analyte-restrained peptide nucleic acid displacement reaction constructed on different gold nanoparticle-deposited carbon electrodes. *Sensors Actuators B Chem.* 335: 129702. https://doi.org/10.1016/j.snb.2021.129702.

34 Liu, X., Wang, Q., Chen, J. et al. (2021). Ultrasensitive electrochemiluminescence biosensor for the detection of tumor exosomes based on peptide recognition and luminol-AuNPs@g-C3N4 nanoprobe signal amplification. *Talanta* 221: 121379. https://doi.org/10.1016/j.talanta.2020.121379.

35 Yin, N., Zhao, R., Zhang, J. et al. (2021). A lable-free SPR biosensor based on one peptide sequence with three recognition sites for O-GlcNAc transferase detection. *Talanta* 222: 121664. https://doi.org/10.1016/j.talanta.2020.121664.

36 Li, Y., Song, Z., Chen, M. et al. (2022). Designed multifunctional peptides with two recognizing branches specific for one target to achieve highly sensitive and low fouling electrochemical protein assay in human serum. *Anal. Chim. Acta* 1208: 339841. https://doi.org/10.1016/j.aca.2022.339841.

37 Wang, Y., Kong, L., Shu, G. et al. (2023). Development of sensitive and stable electrochemical impedimetric biosensor based on T1R1 receptor and its application to detection of umami substances. *Food Chem.* 423: 136233. https://doi.org/10.1016/j.foodchem.2023.136233.

38 Zheng, J., Zhao, H., Ning, G. et al. (2021). A novel affinity peptide–antibody sandwich electrochemical biosensor for PSA based on the signal amplification of MnO2-functionalized covalent organic framework. *Talanta* 233: 122520. https://doi.org/10.1016/j.talanta.2021.122520.

39 Liu, J., Zhang, N., Li, J. et al. (2022). A novel umami electrochemical biosensor based on AuNPs@ZIF-8/Ti3C2 MXene immobilized T1R1-VFT. *Food Chem.* 397: 133838. https://doi.org/10.1016/j.foodchem.2022.133838.

40 Fedacı, C., Ertuğrul Uygun, H.D., Uygun, Z.O., and Akçay, Y. (2022). A novel biorecognition receptor Citropin-a modified impedimetric biosensor for detection of LNCaP prostate cancer cells. *Anal. Biochem.* 652: 114772. https://doi.org/10.1016/j.ab.2022.114772.

41 Soto, D. and Orozco, J. (2022). Peptide-based simple detection of SARS-CoV-2 with electrochemical readout. *Anal. Chim. Acta* 1205: 339739. https://doi.org/10.1016/j.aca.2022.339739.

42 Wang, W. et al. (2022). A peptide aptamer based electrochemical amperometric sensor for sensitive L-glutamate detection. *Bioelectrochemistry* 146: 108165. https://doi.org/10.1016/j.bioelechem.2022.108165.

43 Zhang, Z., Xu, Y., Zhang, Y. et al. (2022). Antifouling and sensitive biosensor based on multifunctional peptide and urease@ZIFs for metal matrix protease-7. *Sensors Actuators B Chem.* 364: 131844. https://doi.org/10.1016/j.snb.2022.131844.

44 Liang, Q., Huang, Y., Wang, M. et al. (2023). An electrochemical biosensor for SARS-CoV-2 detection via its papain-like cysteine protease and the protease inhibitor screening. *Chem. Eng. J.* 452 (P4): 139646. https://doi.org/10.1016/j.cej.2022.139646.

45 Filippova, T.A., Masamrekh, R.A., Shumyantseva, V.V. et al. (2023). Electrochemical biosensor for trypsin activity assay based on cleavage of immobilized tyrosine-containing peptide. *Talanta* 257: 124341. https://doi.org/10.1016/j.talanta.2023.124341.

46 Zhang, K., Yang, M., Sun, H. et al. (2023). Novel strategy to inhibit CRISPR/Cas13a activity by PNA/crRNA duplex and its application in MMP-2 biosensor. *Sensors Actuators B Chem.* 376: 133023. https://doi.org/10.1016/j.snb.2022.133023.

47 Zhao, S., Zhang, Y., Xu, Z. et al. (2023). A low-fouling electrochemical biosensor for biomarker detection in serum based on designed α/β-peptides with anti-enzymolysis and antifouling capabilities. *Anal. Chim. Acta* 1263: 341244. https://doi.org/10.1016/j.aca.2023.341244.

48 Vo, T., Paul, A., Kumar, A. et al. (2019). Biosensor-surface plasmon resonance: a strategy to help establish a new generation RNA-specific small molecules. *Methods* 167: 15–27. https://doi.org/10.1016/j.ymeth.2019.05.005.

49 Qian, H., Huang, Y., Duan, X. et al. (2019). Fiber optic surface plasmon resonance biosensor for detection of PDGF-BB in serum based on self-assembled aptamer and antifouling peptide monolayer. *Biosens. Bioelectron.* 140: 111350. https://doi.org/10.1016/j.bios.2019.111350.

50 Zhu, H., Mao, Z., Chen, J. et al. (2021). Cucurbit[7]urils induced bimetallic nanoparticles network for ultra-sensitive detection of Caspase-3 based on surface plasmon resonance. *Microchem. J.* 171: 106792. https://doi.org/10.1016/j.microc.2021.106792.

51 Guo, P., Wang, Y., and Zhuang, Q. (2019). Highly sensitive and selective biosensor for heparin detection with rhodamine B-labelled peptides as fluorescent bioreceptors. *Sensors Actuators B Chem.* 299, no. July: 126873. https://doi.org/10.1016/j.snb.2019.126873.

52 Nangare, S., and Patil, P. (2022). Chitosan mediated layer-by-layer assembly based graphene oxide decorated surface plasmon resonance biosensor for highly sensitive detection of β-amyloid. *International Journal of Biological Macromolecules*, 214: 568–582. https://doi.org/10.1016/j.ijbiomac.2022.06.129.

53 Zhang, K., Yang, Q., Fan, Z. et al. (2019). Platelet-driven formation of interface peptide nano-network biosensor enabling a non-invasive means for early detection of Alzheimer's disease. *Biosens. Bioelectron.* 145, no. August: 111701. https://doi.org/10.1016/j.bios.2019.111701.

54 Chang, P.H., Weng, C.C., Li, B.R., and Li, Y.K. (2020). An antifouling peptide-based biosensor for determination of streptococcus pneumonia markers in human serum. *Biosens. Bioelectron.* 151: 111969. https://doi.org/10.1016/j.bios.2019.111969.

55 Fournel, A., Mantel, M., Pinger, M. et al. (2020). An experimental investigation comparing a surface plasmon resonance imaging-based artificial nose with natural olfaction. *Sensors Actuators B Chem.* 320: https://doi.org/10.1016/j.snb.2020.128342.

56 Gaggiotti, S., Hurot, C., Weerakkody, J.S. et al. (2020). Development of an optoelectronic nose based on surface plasmon resonance imaging with peptide and hairpin DNA for sensing volatile organic compounds. *Sensors Actuators B Chem.* 303: 127188. https://doi.org/10.1016/j.snb.2019.127188.

57 Liu, X., Zhang, Y., Wang, S. et al. (2020). Performance comparison of surface plasmon resonance biosensors based on ultrasmall noble metal nanoparticles templated using bovine serum albumin. *Microchem. J.* 155: 104737. https://doi.org/10.1016/j.microc.2020.104737.

58 Bai, L., Gu, C., Liu, J. et al. (2023). Photofuel cell-based self-powered biosensor for HER2 detection by integration of plasmonic-metal/conjugated molecule hybrids and electrochemical sandwich structure. *Biosens. Bioelectron.* 220: 114850. https://doi.org/10.1016/j.bios.2022.114850.

59 Rauf, S., Luo, J., Qazi, H.I.A. et al. (2023). A novel leaky surface acoustic wave biosensor for detection of PKA activity in cell lysates based on peptide biomineralized metal nanoclusters. *Sensors Actuators A Phys.* 351: 114107. https://doi.org/10.1016/j.sna.2022.114107.

60 O'Connell, L., Poirier, B., Bratash, O. et al. (2023). Rapid fabrication of interdigitated electrodes by laser ablation with application to electrokinetically enhanced surface plasmon resonance imaging. *Opt. Laser Technol.* 161: 109167. https://doi.org/10.1016/j.optlastec.2023.109167.

61 Jiang, Y., Zhu, P., Zhao, J. et al. (2023). Sensitive biosensors based on topological insulator Bi2Se3 and peptide. *Anal. Chim. Acta* 1239: 340655. https://doi.org/10.1016/j.aca.2022.340655.

62 Toma, K., Satomura, Y., Iitani, K. et al. (2023). Long-range surface plasmon aptasensor for label-free monitoring of vancomycin. *Biosens. Bioelectron.* 222: 114959. https://doi.org/10.1016/j.bios.2022.114959.

63 Ham, Y., Cho, N.C., Kim, D. et al. (2023). The SpACE-CCM: a facile and versatile cell culture medium-based biosensor for detection of SARS-CoV-2 spike-ACE2 interaction. *Biosens. Bioelectron.* 227: 115169. https://doi.org/10.1016/j.bios.2023.115169.

64 Qi, M., Lv, D., Zhang, Y. et al. (2022). Development of a surface plasmon resonance biosensor for accurate and sensitive quantitation of small molecules in blood samples. *J. Pharm. Anal.* 12 (6): 929–936. https://doi.org/10.1016/j.jpha.2022.06.003.

65 Lai, Y.S., Chen, Y.L., Lin, C.C., and Su, Y.H. (2022). Ultrafast chiral peptides purification via surface plasmon enhanced spin selectivity. *Biosens. Bioelectron.* 211: 114339. https://doi.org/10.1016/j.bios.2022.114339.

66 Tu, Y., Wu, J., Chai, K. et al. (2023). A turn-on unlabeled colorimetric biosensor based on aptamer-AuNPs conjugates for amyloid-β oligomer detection. *Talanta* 260: 1–8. https://doi.org/10.1016/j.talanta.2023.124649.

67 Khattab, T.A., Fouda, M.M.G., Abdelrahman, M.S. et al. (2019). Co-encapsulation of enzyme and tricyanofuran hydrazone into alginate microcapsules incorporated onto cotton fabric as a biosensor for colorimetric recognition of urea. *React. Funct. Polym.* 142 (June): 199–206. https://doi.org/10.1016/j.reactfunctpolym.2019.06.016.

68 Ling, Z., Xu, F., Edwards, J.V. et al. (2019). Nanocellulose as a colorimetric biosensor for effective and facile detection of human neutrophil elastase. *Carbohydr. Polym.* 216: 360–368. https://doi.org/10.1016/j.carbpol.2019.04.027.

69 Kumar, N., Bhatia, S., Pateriya, A.K. et al. (2020). Label-free peptide nucleic acid biosensor for visual detection of multiple strains of influenza a virus suitable for field applications. *Anal. Chim. Acta* 1093: 123–130. https://doi.org/10.1016/j.aca.2019.09.060.

70 Nguyen, Q.H. and Il Kim, M. (2020). Nanomaterial-mediated paper-based biosensors for colorimetric pathogen detection. *TrAC - Trends Anal. Chem.* 132: 116038. https://doi.org/10.1016/j.trac.2020.116038.

71 Zhao, V.X.T., Wong, T.I., Zheng, X.T. et al. (2020). Colorimetric biosensors for point-of-care virus detections. *Mater. Sci. Energy Technol.* 3: 237–249. https://doi.org/10.1016/j.mset.2019.10.002.

72 Xu, M., Xing, S., Zhao, Y., and Zhao, C. (2021). Peptide nucleic acid-assisted colorimetric detection of single-nucleotide polymorphisms based on the intrinsic peroxidase-like activity of hemin-carbon nanotube nanocomposites. *Talanta* 232: 122420. https://doi.org/10.1016/j.talanta.2021.122420.

73 Coşkuner Filiz, B., Basaran Elalmis, Y., Bektaş, S., and Kantürk Figen, A. (2021). Fabrication of stable electrospun blended chitosan-poly(vinyl alcohol) nanofibers for designing naked-eye colorimetric glucose biosensor based on GOx/HRP. *Int. J. Biol. Macromol.* 192: 999–1012. https://doi.org/10.1016/j.ijbiomac.2021.10.048.

74 Korkmaz, N., Hwang, C., Kessler, K.K. et al. (2021). A novel copper (II) binding peptide for a colorimetric biosensor system design. *Talanta* 232: 122439. https://doi.org/10.1016/j.talanta.2021.122439.

75 Lee, J.I., Jang, S.C., Chung, J. et al. (2021). Colorimetric allergenic fungal spore detection using peptide-modified gold nanoparticles. *Sensors Actuators B Chem.* 327: 128894. https://doi.org/10.1016/j.snb.2020.128894.

76 Li, X.Y., Zhang, M.M., Zhou, X.D., and Hu, J.M. (2021). A functional peptide-mediated colorimetric assay for mercury ion based on dual-modified gold nanoparticles. *Anal. Biochem.* 631: 114369. https://doi.org/10.1016/j.ab.2021.114369.

77 Kong, Y., Liu, F., Liu, Z. et al. (2022). Synthesis of globotriose-modified peptides for the preparation of a colorimetric biosensor to detect Shiga toxins. *Talanta* 243: 123353. https://doi.org/10.1016/j.talanta.2022.123353.

78 Zhu, Q. and Zhou, X. (2022). A colorimetric sandwich-type bioassay for SARS-CoV-2 using a hACE2-based affinity peptide pair. *J. Hazard. Mater.* 425: 127923. https://doi.org/10.1016/j.jhazmat.2021.127923.

79 Geleta, G.S. (2023). A colorimetric aptasensor based on two dimensional (2D) nanomaterial and gold nanoparticles for detection of toxic heavy metal ions: a review. *Food Chem. Adv.* 2: 100184. https://doi.org/10.1016/j.focha.2023.100184.

80 Liu, P., Han, L., Wang, F. et al. (2018). Sensitive colorimetric immunoassay of: Vibrio parahaemolyticus based on specific nonapeptide probe screening from a phage display library conjugated with MnO2 nanosheets with peroxidase-like activity. *Nanoscale* 10 (6): 2825–2833. https://doi.org/10.1039/c7nr06633c.

81 Li, X., Li, Y., Qiu, Q. et al. (2019). Efficient biofunctionalization of MoS 2 nanosheets with peptides as intracellular fluorescent biosensor for sensitive detection of caspase-3 activity. *J. Colloid Interface Sci.* 543: 96–105. https://doi.org/10.1016/j.jcis.2019.02.011.

82 Tang, Y.Y., Kang, A., Yang, X.T. et al. (2019). A robust OFF-ON fluorescent biosensor for detection and clearance of bacterial endotoxin by specific peptide based aggregation induced emission. *Sensors Actuators B Chem.* 304: 2020. https://doi.org/10.1016/j.snb.2019.127300.

83 Feng, T., Yan, S., Hou, S., and Fan, X. (2022). Novel fluorescence biosensor custom-made for protein tyrosine phosphatase 1B detection based on titanium dioxide-decorated single-walled carbon nanohorn nanocomposite. *Spectrochim. Acta - Part A Mol. Biomol. Spectrosc.* 280: 121548. https://doi.org/10.1016/j.saa.2022.121548.

84 Ruan, Q., Lin, X., Wang, L. et al. (2023). An engineered (CAGA)12-EGFP cell-based biosensor for high-content and accurate detection of active TGF-β. *Biosens. Bioelectron.* 220: 114884. https://doi.org/10.1016/j.bios.2022.114884.

85 Xie, Y., Si, S., Deng, C., and Wu, H. (2023). A sensitive 'turn-on' fluorescent biosensor for the detection of biomarkers based on three-dimensional DNA walker fluorescent biosensor. *Talanta* 253: 124071. https://doi.org/10.1016/j.talanta.2022.124071.

86 Ren, X., Tao, M., Liu, X. et al. (2023). Caspase-1-responsive fluorescence biosensors for monitoring endogenous inflammasome activation. *Biosens. Bioelectron.* 219: 114812. https://doi.org/10.1016/j.bios.2022.114812.

87 Wells, P.K., Smutok, O., Guo, Z. et al. (2023). Fluorometric biosensing of α-amylase using an artificial allosteric biosensor immobilized on nanostructured interface. *Talanta* 255: 124215. https://doi.org/10.1016/j.talanta.2022.124215.

88 Akinloye, O., Krishnamurthy, R., Wishart, D., and Goss, G.G. (2017). Peptide-based fluorescence biosensors for detection/measurement of nanoparticles. *Anal. Bioanal. Chem.* 409 (4): 903–915. https://doi.org/10.1007/s00216-016-0042-7.

89 Pan, J., Deng, F., and Chen, J. (2023). A fluorescent biosensor for Cd2+ detection in water samples based on Cd2+–fueled wheel DNAzyme walker and its logic gate applications. *Sci. Total Environ.* 864: 161046. https://doi.org/10.1016/j.scitotenv.2022.161046.

90 Shumeiko, V., Paltiel, Y., Bisker, G. et al. (2020). A paper-based near-infrared optical biosensor for quantitative detection of protease activity using peptide-encapsulated swcnts. *Sensors* 20 (18): 1–14. https://doi.org/10.3390/s20185247.

91 Shen, Y., Huang, Z., Huang, F. et al. (2022). A self-reference interference sensor based on coherence multiplexing. *Front. Chem.* 10: 1–8. https://doi.org/10.3389/fchem.2022.880081.

92 Zaraee, N., Kanik, F.E., Bhuiya, A.M. et al. (2020). Highly sensitive and label-free digital detection of whole cell E. Coliwith interferometric reflectance imaging. *Biosens. Bioelectron.* 162: 112258. https://doi.org/10.1016/j.bios.2020.112258.

93 Kaur, H., Shorie, M., and Sabherwal, P. (2020). Biolayer interferometry-SELEX for Shiga toxin antigenic-peptide aptamers & detection via chitosan-WSe2 aptasensor. *Biosens. Bioelectron.* 167: 112498. https://doi.org/10.1016/j.bios.2020.112498.

94 Cheng, X.R., Daaboul, G.G., Ünlü, M.S., and Kerman, K. (2014). LED-based interferometric reflectance imaging sensor for the detection of amyloid-β aggregation. *Analyst* 139 (1): 59–65. https://doi.org/10.1039/c3an01307c.

95 Ravikumar, R., Chen, L.H., Jayaraman, P. et al. (2018). Chitosan-nickel film based interferometric optical fiber sensor for label-free detection of histidine tagged proteins. *Biosens. Bioelectron.* 99: 578–585. https://doi.org/10.1016/j.bios.2017.08.012.

96 Barth, I., Conteduca, D., Reardon, C. et al. (2020). Common-path interferometric label-free protein sensing with resonant dielectric nanostructures. *Light Sci. Appl.* 9 (1): https://doi.org/10.1038/s41377-020-0336-6.

97 Layouni, R., Cao, T., Coppock, M.B. et al. (2021). Peptide-based capture of chikungunya virus E2 protein using porous silicon biosensor. *Sensors* 21 (24): 1–10. https://doi.org/10.3390/s21248248.

98 Murillo, A.M.M., Tomé-Amat, J., Ramírez, Y. et al. (2021). Developing an optical interferometric detection method based biosensor for detecting specific SARS-CoV-2 immunoglobulins in serum and saliva, and their corresponding ELISA correlation. *Sensors Actuators B Chem.* 345: https://doi.org/10.1016/j.snb.2021.130394.

99 Gao, S., Li, Q., Zhang, S. et al. (2023). Peptide–nucleic acid aptamer pair biosensor for disease biomarker detection in clinical samples. *Chem. Eng. J.* 458: 141499. https://doi.org/10.1016/j.cej.2023.141499.

100 Effah, C.Y., Ding, L., Tan, L. et al. (2023). A SERS bioassay based on vancomycin-modified PEI-interlayered nanocomposite and aptamer-functionalized SERS tags for synchronous detection of Acinetobacter baumannii and Klebsiella pneumoniae. *Food Chem.* 423: 136242. https://doi.org/10.1016/j.foodchem.2023.136242.

101 Shu, Y., Zhi, S., Li, S. et al. (2022). A new peptide-mediated COF nanocatalytic amplification SERS quantitative assay for ultratrace Cu2+. *J. Ind. Eng. Chem.* 113: 196–205. https://doi.org/10.1016/j.jiec.2022.05.046.

102 Yadav, S., Khanam, R., and Singh, J.P. (2022). A purview into highly sensitive magnetic SERS detection of hemozoin biomarker for rapid malaria diagnosis. *Sensors Actuators B Chem.* 355: 131303. https://doi.org/10.1016/j.snb.2021.131303.

103 Zhong, Q., Zhang, K., Huang, X. et al. (2022). In situ ratiometric SERS imaging of intracellular protease activity for subtype discrimination of human breast cancer. *Biosens. Bioelectron.* 207: 114194. https://doi.org/10.1016/j.bios.2022.114194.

104 Gholami, M.D., Sonar, P., Ayoko, G.A., and Izake, E.L. (2020). A highly sensitive SERS quenching nanosensor for the determination of tumor necrosis factor alpha in blood. *Sensors Actuators B Chem.* 310: 127867. https://doi.org/10.1016/j.snb.2020.127867.

105 Bhattacharjee, G., Majumder, S., Senapati, D. et al. (2020). Core-shell gold @silver hollow nanocubes for higher SERS enhancement and non-enzymatic biosensor. *Mater. Chem. Phys.* 239: 122113. https://doi.org/10.1016/j.matchemphys.2019.122113.

106 Wang, X.Y., Yang, J.Y., Wang, Y.T. et al. (2021). M13 phage-based nanoprobe for SERS detection and inactivation of Staphylococcus aureus. *Talanta* 221: 121668. https://doi.org/10.1016/j.talanta.2020.121668.

107 Wei, C., Sun, R., Jiang, Y. et al. (2021). Protease-protection strategy combined with the SERS tags for detection of O-GlcNAc transferase activity. *Sensors Actuators B Chem.* 345: 130410. https://doi.org/10.1016/j.snb.2021.130410.

108 Huang, Q. et al. (2023). SERS-based self-calibrating aptamer sensor for selective detection of IL-6. *Sensors Actuators B Chem.* 374: 132828. https://doi.org/10.1016/j.snb.2022.132828.

109 Li, J., Li, C., and Jiang, Z. (2023). TbMOF@au catalytic determination of trace malathion with aptamer SERS/RRS/abs assay. *Spectrochim. Acta Part A Mol. Biomol. Spectrosc.* 294: 122581. https://doi.org/10.1016/j.saa.2023.122581.

110 Ahi, E.E., Torul, H., Zengin, A. et al. (2022). A capillary driven microfluidic chip for SERS based hCG detection. *Biosens. Bioelectron.* 195: 113660. https://doi.org/10.1016/j.bios.2021.113660.

111 Ouhibi, A., Raouafi, A., Lorrain, N. et al. (2021). Functionalized SERS substrate based on silicon nanowires for rapid detection of prostate specific antigen. *Sensors Actuators B Chem.* 330: 129352. https://doi.org/10.1016/j.snb.2020.129352.

8

Synthetic BREs and Smart Nanomaterial-Based Biosensors

8.1 MIPs as Bioreceptors and Their Applications

Molecularly imprinted polymers (MIPs) are synthesized in lab and are synthetic in nature that can be designed and tailored according to areas of application. MIPs possess the following properties: they are stable; they mimic other bioreceptors; they can be reused multiple times, which reduces costs and saves resources; they are robust; and there is high selectivity and affinity toward the template molecule [1]. MIPs have been explored in different areas that include the target isolation from complex mixtures, drug delivery, biosensing applications and catalyzing chemical reactions. MIP synthesis is done mainly through four steps: (i) template molecule selection, (ii) functional monomer choice, (iii) polymerization process, (iv) template removal [1]. All the steps for MIP synthesis are depicted in Figure 8.1.

The selection of template molecule or target is dependent on the type of application, while functional-monomers upon the interaction ability interact with the template molecule. These interactions are covalent, hydrogen bonding, semicovalent electrostatic interactions, and hydrophobic interactions [2]. After the selection of functional monomer and template molecule, fabrication involves the polymerization of functional monomers using a cross-linker to the form a 3D polymer network with imprinted cavities. Commonly used functional monomers are carboxylic acids, sulfonic acids, heteroaromatic bases, and dimethacrylate esters of diols as cross-linkers and azo-compounds and peroxides for initiator purposes. The next step involves the separation of template molecule 3D polymer matrix, leaving behind cavities that can bind the target molecule in a specific way [3]. This can be achieved by washing the polymer in appropriate solvents or by methods like heat or pH treatment.

Biosensors: Nanomaterials, Approaches, and Performance-Enhancement Strategies,
First Edition. Baljinder Kaur, Santosh Kumar, and Brajesh Kumar Kaushik.

Published 2025 by John Wiley & Sons, Inc.
Companion website: www.wiley.com/go/kaur

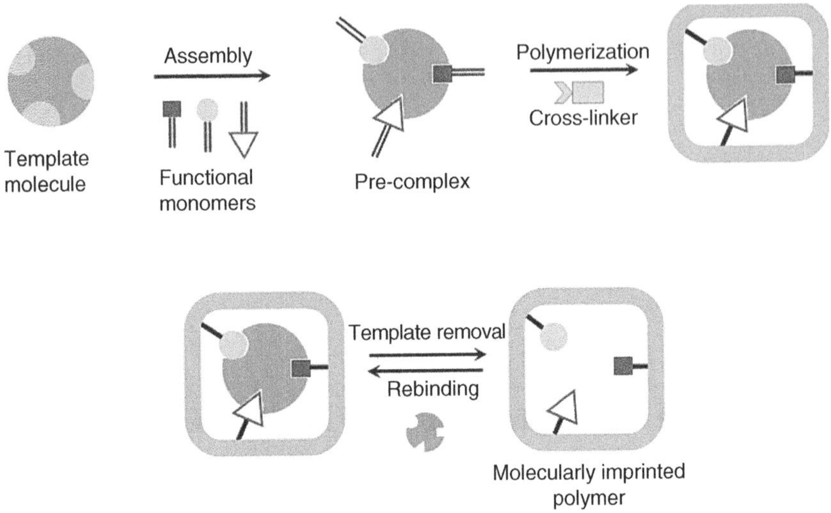

Figure 8.1 Schematic of fabrication and stepwise details of MIP. *Source:* [1]/MDPI/CC BY 4.0.

Further polymerization can be done in two ways (i.e. free and controlled radical polymerization). Controlled radical polymerization that includes techniques such as addition-fragmentation chain transfer via degenerative chain transfer, atom transfer radical polymerization, and nitroxide-mediated polymerization has capability to synthesize precise molecular-weight copolymers. These techniques offer precise control over polymer chain length, structure, and functionality, leading to MIPs with well-defined properties [4]. MIPs offer several advantages over other bioreceptors such as antibodies, aptamers, and nucleic acids (Nas). These advantages include stability under harsh conditions (temperature, pH, or organic solvents), robustness, low cost, broader target molecule range, high selectivity, and tailored binding for specific target molecules. Compared to antibodies or natural receptors, the synthesis of MIPs can be scaled up, allowing for large-scale production at a relatively low cost. MIPs also suffer from several drawbacks that include synthesis optimization due to its complex and time-consuming process, lack of dynamic binding, slower binding kinetics compared to other receptors, and low affinity toward target molecules. The rigid structure of the polymer matrix and fixed binding sites restrict the ability of MIPs to undergo the conformational changes required for rapid and dynamic binding.

Finding the ideal combination of monomers, cross-linkers, and polymerization conditions to achieve the desired selectivity can be challenging, especially for complex target molecules. MIP synthesis can also have batch-to-batch variability, leading to variations in performance and selectivity that require careful quality control and optimization. After synthesis, MIPs lack adaptability to changes in the target molecule structure, necessitating modifications or adaptations to recognize different analogs or variants. Despite these limitations, ongoing research aims to address these challenges and enhance the performance of MIPs in various applications [5].

MIPs can be prepared using bulk polymerization, solution polymerization, dispersion polymerization, controlled or living polymerization, suspension polymerization, and emulsion polymerization. Bulk, suspension emulsion is the type of free-radical polymerization. Each polymerization technique has different morphologies, activity, cost, and adsorption effects. Bulk polymerization is used at large scale for medical and industrial applications. In case of bulk polymerization using functional monomers, a cross-linkers polymer matrix is created and a template monomer is printed inside this matrix. Then this monomer is removed using a solvent-washing process [6]. With bulk polymerization, it is difficult to remove the template completely, requiring pulverization and grinding due to blocking of MIP, asymmetrical morphology, random distribution of binding sites, and nonuniform size of polymers [7].

Emulsion polymerization is generally used in the synthesis of MIP nanoparticles that involve polymerization within droplets dispersed in an aqueous medium. The functional monomers, molecule fixer cross-linkers, and template molecule are emulsified in the presence of a surfactant, and polymerization is initiated, resulting in spherical nanoparticles that can be easily separated from the aqueous phase. In emulsion polymerization, MIPs of uniform size and particular shape (i.e., spherical) can be generated without complex treatments of grinding and screening. In this technique, recognition sites can be easily accessed with favorable binding kinetics. Imprinted sites can be created on solid support surfaces, such as silica particles or polymer films. The template molecule is immobilized onto the support, and functional monomers and cross-linkers are polymerized around it. As the polymerization process is completed, the template is removed that generates imprinted sites on the surface of support. This technique uses a reduced number of imprinted sites due to fewer template molecules, which produces low sensitivity as compared to bulk polymerization. An Au metal imprinted with sialic acid–based QCM sensor can detect sialic acid, diabetes, cancer, and heart-diseases biomarkers in urine samples. Sialic acid can be detected in the concentration range of 0.025–0.5 mol/l with lowest concentration of 1.0 nmol/l [8]. An ECL biosensor imprinted with poly (glycidylmethacrylate-co-ethylene glycol dimethacrylate), PDMS, CNT, and cellulose nanocrystals for cortisol detection was reported. It can detect cortisol with LOD of 2.0 ng/ml and shows linear response in the range of 10–66 ng/ml, and reproducibility of 2.6% RSD. It was stored for 1 month, and then performance was evaluated; no performance change was noted [9].

An organic ECL transistors using PEDOT-poly(styrenesulfonate) polymer, a noncovalent imprinting method coated on the flexible substrate surface of styrene-ethylene-butylene-styrene, was developed as a skin patch to detect the cortisol biomarker for stress. Gate, source, and drain were constructed using Ag/AgCl paste. The selected polymer has high mechanical strength and is deformation resistant and stable at room temperature. The device showed high sensitivity and selectivity for cortisol, with a limit of detection of 0.5 ng/ml and a dynamic range of 1–100 ng/ml [10]. Table 8.1 lists different types of biosensors using MIP methods.

8.2 Nanomaterials-Based Sensors

Materials having a minimum one dimension on the nanoscale (less than 100 nm) can be either natural or synthetic. Fullerenes are examples of natural nanomaterials that occur in nature, and synthetic nanomaterials are created by humans; for example, CNT made up of graphene sheets. Nanoparticles (Nps) can be classified into nano-crystalline, polymeric, nonpolymeric, and lipid-based classes based on their properties, morphology, and composition [9]. Based on composition, inorganic nanomaterials include metals, metal oxides, and semiconductors, for example, quantum dots (QDs), carbon nanotubes, and titanium dioxide nanoparticles as shown in Figure 8.2. It also discusses the dimensionality and shape-based different reported nanomaterials such as solid, hollow NPs, nanorods, nano-shells, and QDs. Organic nanomaterials are made up of organic materials that include carbon, polymers, and proteins such as graphene, fullerenes, and dendrimers [10]. Based on morphology, nanomaterials can be zero-, one-, two-, or three-dimensional, depending on the number of directions on the nanoscale. Based on properties, they can be optical, electrical, magnetic, or mechanical nanomaterials. These nanomaterials exhibit distinct characteristics at the nanoscale, which makes them attractive for various fields of research and technological advancements. Various metals – Ag, Au, Cu, Fe, TiO_2 – have been explored for applications in different areas. Metal oxides (iron oxide: FeO, silver dioxide: Ag_2O, zinc oxide: ZnO) NPs possesses antimicrobial properties that include killing of microorganisms and stop their growth. Nanomaterial structure is small in size and offers a large surface area that enhances the enzyme-like and catalytic activities. AuNPs have been explored on a large scale due to their anti-oxidant, inert and stable nature in industrial and medical applications [25, 26].

8.2.1 Metals and Metal-Oxide-Based Nanomaterials

These nanomaterials have been explored in catalytic, miniaturization of devices, molecular functionalization, and water pollutants removal. Nanomaterials can store and convert energy efficiently, be used as a coating or protective layer, and transport drugs and imaging contrast agents. Numerous nanomaterials based on

Table 8.1 Summary of recently reported biosensors using different MIP methods.

S. No.	Sensor structure	MIP	LOD	Range	Refs.
1.	Boron nitride QDs-based ECL sensor for cardiac troponin-I	Polymerization method	5×10^{-4} ng/ml	0.01–5 ng/ml	[11]
2.	Polydopamine encapsulated surface-enhanced Raman spectroscopy (SERS) CEA sensor	Surface molecularly imprinted	0.064 pg/ml	0.1 pg/ml–10 μg/ml	[12]
3.	Poly(Toluidine) blue-based ECL sensor for PSA	Trapping on the cavity	1 μg/l	1–60 μg/l	[13]
4.	SiO_2@Ag and aptamer-based ECL sensor to detect Amyloid-β Oligomer in Alzheimer's	Polymerization method	1.22 pg/ml	5 pg/ml–10 ng/ml	[14]
5.	Chemiluminescence sensor for acetylcholinesterase detection	Dual-recognized strategy	0.86 μg/kg	2.5–200 μg/kg	[15]
6.	Enzyme-free MIP ECL sensor for L-hydroxyproline	Laser scanning confocal microscopy	0.1 μg/ml	0.4–25 μg/ml	[16]
7.	SERS-based boronate affinity biosensor for glycoproteins	Surface-imprinted magnetic polymers	0.078 ng/ml	0.1~100 mg/ml	[17]
8.	Si and CdTe QDs-coated MIP fluorescence sensor	Cross-linked MIP	3.2 μg/ml	10–120 μg/ml	[18]
9.	Dual-responsive ECL sensor for CD44 biomarker	Artificial protein imprinted polymers	10^{-5} ng/ml	10^{-6}–10^{-2} ng/ml	[19]
10.	Au@3-mpa and dopamine functional monomer-based surface plasmon resonance (SPR) sensor detection of lysozyme	Surface imprinting	0.19 μg/ml	0.50–2.0 μg/ml	[20]
11.	Electrodeposited MIP modified screen printed carbon electrode detection of creatinine	ECL polymerization	22 nM	0–75 nM	[21]
12.	Paper-based fluorometric sensor for detection of malachite green	Aptamer-MIPs	0.06 ng/ml	0.1–10 ng/ml	[22]
13.	Two different MIP-based sensors for Ribavirin detection	Photo-polymerization	n.r.[a]	10^{-12}–10^{-11} M	[23]

[a] not reported.

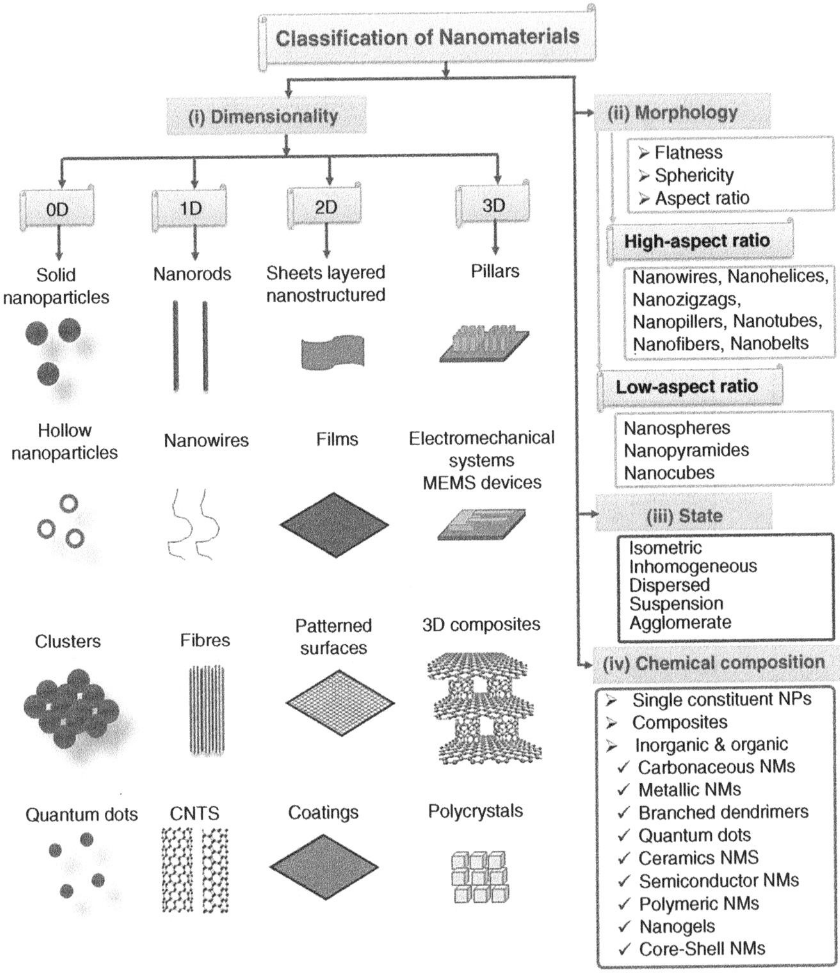

Figure 8.2 Classification of nanomaterials used in optical platforms to detect various diseases. *Source:* [24]/with permission of Elsevier.

metal and their oxides have been reported so far. Table 8.2 shows the details of metal and metal-oxide nanomaterial-based biosensors that include magnetic materials, carbon and metal complexes, 2D materials, and nanocomposites.

8.2.2 Carbon-Based Nanomaterials

An ECL biosensor that consists of GO, Ag, and Ag-Fe_3O_4 hybrid on a glassy carbon electrode was developed to detect ascorbic acid in the blood. The sensor structure involved the coupling of GO with Ag and its hybrid nanoparticles. The biosensing

Table 8.2 Summary of various metal and metal-oxide nanomaterial-based sensors.

Sr. No.	NPs-based sensor	Analyte	LOD	Linear range	Refs.
1	Fe_3O_4@Au core-shell NPs based LSPR sensor	Catechol	2 μM	5.0–70.0 μM	[27]
2	Au nanorod@SiO_2 NPs based ECL sensor	Organophosphate pesticides	5.3 nM	0.018–13.6 μM	[28]
3	ds-DNA/Au-NPs/pencil graphite electrode-based ECL sensor	Temodal	1.0 nM	5.0 nM–45.0 μM	[29]
4	Left- and right-handed double helix CNT, polypyrrole, AuNPs and cysteine-based ECL sensor	L-tyrosine	0.012 L-tyrosine%	0–310 μM	[30]
5	Lysine oxidase nanoparticles	Lysine	10 μM	10–800 μM	[31]
6	Au NPs-ZnO nanocone arrays/graphene-based ECL sensor	Dopamine	0.04 μM	0–80 μM	[32]
7	AuNPs-MoS_2-reduced GO – polyimide-based surface acoustic wave biosensor	Carcinoembryonic antigen	0.084 ng/ml	0–80 ng/ml	[33]
8	Au@CDs nanoflowers-based ECL sensor	p53 DNA	0.34 fM	1 fM to 10 pM	[34]
9	Au@Pt/MIL-53-based ECL sensor	SARS-CoV-2	8.3 pg/ml	0.025–50 ng/ml	[35]
10	DNA acid-Au-Pt bimetallic NPs-GO-chitosan on pencil graphite electrode ECL sensor	Zidovudine	0.003 pM	0.01 pM to 10.0 nM	[36]
11	AuNPs-based SPR sensor	Pb^{2+} ion	8.56 pM	10^{-11} M to 10^{-6} M	[37]
12	Fe_2O_3 and AuNPs-based ECL sensor	Permethrin	8.7×10^{-10} mol/l	2.6×10^{-9}–4.3×10^{-5} mol/l	[38]
13	AuNPs and polydopamine co-modified SPR biosensor	IgG	50 ng/ml	50 ng/ml	[39]

(*Continued*)

Table 8.2 (Continued)

Sr. No.	NPs-based sensor	Analyte	LOD	Linear range	Refs.
14	AuNPs and porous anodic aluminum oxide Microfluidic-based SERS biosensor	MicroRNA-21	10 fM	10 fM–10 nM	[40]
15	Au NPs/CNTs hybrid-based ECL sensor	Recombinant human erythropoietin	1 ng/l	0–22 000 ng/l	[41]
16	Magnetic beads aptamers bound nanoparticles	Carcinoembryonic antigen	0.092 pg/ml	0.001–8 ng/ml	[42]
17	Fe_3O_4@Au-Teicoplanin and aptamer functionalized Au@AgNPs-based SERS sensor	*Staphylococcus aureus*	1.09 CFU/ml	7.6×10^1–10^7 CFU/ml	[43]
18	Au NPs/SnO_2/$ZnIn_2S_4$	Ribonuclease A	0.2 pg/ml	10 to 5×10^3 pg/ml	[44]
19	pyruvate oxidase Au@CNTs/glassy carbon electrode-based ECL sensor	Pyruvate	5 nM	10–480 μM	[45]
20	AuNPs zinc selenide quantum dots-based ECL sensor	DNA	0.33 fM	1 fM to 10 nM	[46]
21	AuNPs/MoS_2 nanosheets – Chitosan modified screen-printed electrode ECL sensor	Chlorpyrifos	5.6 nM	0.004–28.52 μM	[47]
22	Urchin-like Au and Ag nanoparticles LSPR-ECL biosensor	*S. aureus*	52 CFU/ml	10^2–10^8 CFU/ml	[48]
23	DNAzyme-based opto-fluidic colorimetric biosensor	L-histidine	5×10^{-16} M	1–50 nM	[49]
24	MXene-Au nanocomposite-based ECL sensor	microRNA-377	1.35 aM	10 aM–100 pM	[50]
25	Aptamer-nanoparticle biosensor Colorimetric	*Salmonella serovars* *S. minnesota*	10^3–10^4 CFU/ml	100 μM	[51]

26	Ball resonator with AuNPs-based LSPR fiber biosensor to detect cancer biomarker	CD44	0.111 pM	42.9 aM to 100 nM	[52]
27	MXene Ti_3C_2-reduced GO-Au nanocomposites-based ECL sensor	microRNA-21	0.42 fM	1 fM to 1 nM	[53]
28	Cu_7S_4-Au-MIP-based ECL sensor	SARS-CoV-2	17×10^{-2} ng/ml	10^{-2}–10^{3} ng/ml	[54]
29	Bi_2S_3@Au nanoflowers-based Electrochemiluniscence sensor	Cd (II) and ampicillin	3.42×10^{-4} ng/l	10^{-3}–10^{6} ng/l	[55]
30	AuNPs APTES multimer-based LSPR sensor	Deoxynivalenol	0.04 ng/ml	0–20 µM	[56]
31	AuNPs/CNT-based ECL sensor	HER2 biomarker	4.4 pg/ml	10^{-3}–25 ng/ml	[57]
31	Ultrasmall Fe_3O_4-Au core-shell NPs-based ECL sensor	Human papillomavirus type 16	0.1 nM	1–10 µM	[58]
32	Bimetallic Au-Pt NPs-based ECL sensor	Glycated albumin	0.1 nM	0.1 nM to 500 mM	[59]
33	Dual-gated locked mesoporous silica-NPs-based SERS sensor	Aflatoxin B1	0.133 pg/ml	0.001–100 ng/ml	[60]
34	Nd-MOF nanosheets functionalized with ionic liquid and AuNPs-based photo-ECL and ECL sensor	ctDNA	0.63 fmol/l	1 fmol/l–10 nmol/l Photo ECL 1 fmol/l–1.0 nmol/l ECL	[61]
35	Au-$BaTiO_3$-FeGa alloy and PDMS magneto-strictive sensor	BSA	n.r.[a]	10–50 µg/ml	[62]
36	Ferrite NPs-based ECL sensor	Urea	0.17 µM	0.5–45.0 µM	[63]
37	Reduced GO/ palladium NPs/ polymer nanocomposite-based ECL sensor	Interaction of mitomycin C-DNA and acyclovir-DNA	0.0513 µM	0.1–0.5 µM.	[64]
38	MOFs@Au NPs showed based ECL sensor	Autism	78.9 fM	200 fM ~ 2.00 nM	[65]

(Continued)

Table 8.2 (Continued)

Sr. No.	NPs-based sensor	Analyte	LOD	Linear range	Refs.
39	SAM Au@MXene liver microsome-based ECL sensor	Aflatoxin B1	2.8 nM	0.01 μM to 50 μM	[66]
40	MXene@Au-GCE-based ECL sensor	Methicillin-resistant *S. aureus*	3.8×10^1 CFU/m	3.8×10^1–10^7 CFU/ml	[66]
41	AuNP-rGO-poly-(methylene blue)/poly(ionic liquids)-based ECL sensor	SARS-CoV-2	38 pg/ml	0.1–1000 ng/ml	[67]
42	MXenes-Au NPs-based ECL sensor	Multiple exosome surface proteins	10^6 particles/μl	10^2 to 5×10^6 particles/μl	[68]
43	Bismuth vanadate: $BiVO_4$, Au-NPs and electrode of florin tin oxide-based photo-ECL sensor	miRNA-25 biomarker	3.4 fM	10^{-14}–10^{-6} M	[69]
44	Bismuth-rich bromide oxides ($Bi_4O_5Br_2$)-Au-CdS based photo-ECL sensor	DNA demethylase	0.09 ng/ml	0.3–200 ng/ml	[70]
45	DNA-Avidin-iridium NPs bilayer-based ECL sensor	*Aphanizomenon flos-aquae*	9.99 pg/ml	0.1–10^3 ng/ml	[71]
46	Fe_3O_4 @ SiO_2-Au and angiotensin-converting enzyme 2 on graphite carbon electrode-based ECL sensor	SARS-CoV-2 spike protein	4.78 pg/ml	10^{-4}–10 μg/ml	[72]
47	Poly-L-methionine, Au, and platinum bimetallic NPs coating-based ECL sensor	Imatinib and Erlotinib	0.18, 0.009 nM	2.33–80 nM 0.032–1.0 nM	[73]

process involves the oxidation of target acid on the electrode surface that produces a measurable electric signal. The ascorbic acid shows linear response for the concentrations of 0.2–60 μM, with a LOD of 74 nM and a sensitivity of 1147 $\mu Am/M/cm^2$ [74]. A duplex DNA-based SERS biosensor was constructed using GO and AuNPs and a Raman tag for the simultaneous detection of two food adulterants. The sensor reported the 10^{-14} M, LOD values for ascorbic acid target and showed the linear response for 10^{-14}–10^{-13} M concentration ranges [75]. An Au and platinum with metal–organic frameworks −53, HRP, G-quadruplex DNAzyme-based ECL aptamer biosensor was developed to detect the protein associated with SARS-CoV-2 virus (Figure 8.3). The sensor structure involved the use of metal–organic frameworks as a support matrix and combination of nanomaterials to enhance the response of the biosensor, enabling efficient detection of the target protein. It relied on the dual-aptamer strategy modified with thiols N48 and N61, which were utilized to selectively capture the nucleocapsid protein. The captured protein then facilitated the catalytic reaction of the enzymes, resulting in an amplified electrochemical signal that could be measured and correlated with the protein concentration. COVID-19 nucleocapsid showed the linear response

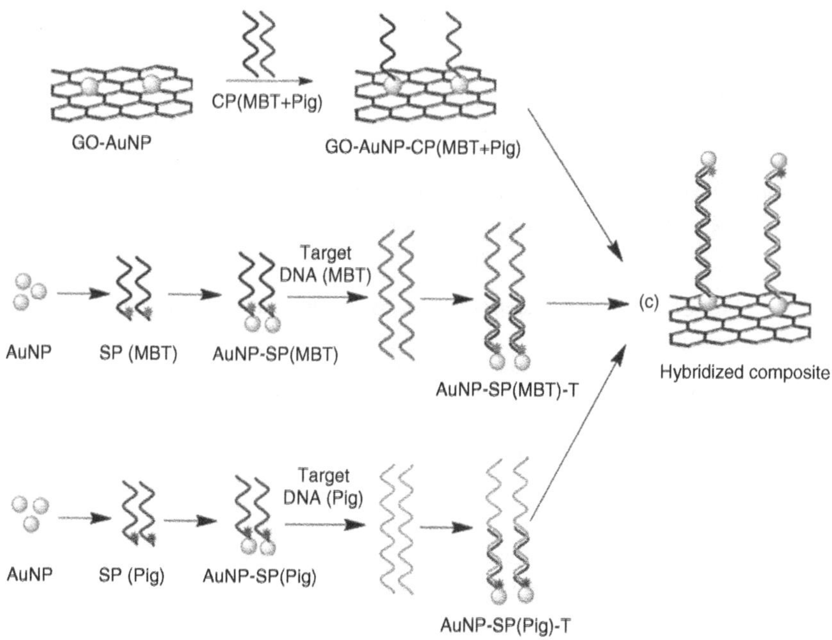

Figure 8.3 Schematic illustration of Au and platinum with metal-organic frameworks −53, HRP, G-quadruplex DNAzyme based ECL aptameric-biosensor. *Source:* [75]/with permission of Elsevier.

for the concentrations of 0.025–50 ng/ml and minimum value of 8.33 pg/ml [35]. An ITO NPs, chitosan, hexaammineruthenium (III) chloride, was deposited on a carbon electrode-based ECL biosensor to sense the lead, nickel, cadmium metal ions. LOD of lead, cadmium, nickel ions were 8, 1, and 3 nM. The sensitivity and linear concentration ranges of the biosensor in case of lead, cadmium, nickel ions were found to be 11.97, 10.99, 10.84 μA/μM/cm^2, and 0.009–0.301 mM, 0.008–0.372 μM, 0.011–0.368 μM [76]. An ITO, hairpin DNA, AuNPs-based ECL biosensor was developed to detect antibiotic-resistance genes. DNA probe became hybridized in the presence of target genes. The detection limit and correlation of target with ECL signal was found to be 30 pg/μl and 0.987 [77]. Table 8.3 discusses the carbon-nanomaterial-based biosensor used to detect analytes such as blood cholesterol, enzyme, glucose, and disease biomarkers.

A glucose biosensor was reported using a carbon activated to produce carbon paste for electrode with shells of coconut composite, nickel ferrite ($NiFe_2O_4$) NPs, glucose oxidase enzyme electrode made of activated carbon and nanoparticles. Glucose was detected with the help of its electrochemical oxidation on carbon paste electrode. The biosensors provide the linear response for 2–10 mM with detection limit of 1.1 mM [95]. A microfluidic-based SERS biosensor using Au and Ag core-shell structure nano-tag, AuNPs on aluminum oxide as substrate material, and a DNA strand (single) was found to detect miRNA-21 in linear range of 10 fM–10 nM with the lowest detectable concentration of 10 fM and RSD of 17% [40]. An amperometric biosensor was prepared from zirconium oxide NPs, glutaraldehyde, and tyrosinase to detect phenol. ZrO_2 NPs were synthesized with the help of 1-butyl-3-methylimidazolium trifluoroacetate and then modified with a phenol-selective polymer. Phenol can be detected in the range and was found to be 10–90 μM and 10.522 μA/mM, 9.468 μM [96].

8.2.3 Magnetic, 2D Nanomaterials, Quantum Dots, and Polymer-Based Nanomaterials

A polymeric magnetic NPs-based SERS immunosensor with two Raman reporter molecules was demonstrated to detect the *S. typhimurium* (Figure 8.4). *S. typhimurium* was detected in concentrations of 100 and 10 cells/ml and 10–10^7 cells/ml with 4-mercapto benzoic acid and 5,50-dithiobis (succinimidyl-2-nitrobenzoate) [97]. An Au-polypyrrole-chitosan and Ni-ferrite NPs based composite layer based SPR biosensor was used to detect various metal ions that include nickel, iron, cobalt, aluminum, manganese, mercury, and lead. Ferromagnetic ions were detected with LOD of 0.001 ppm and 0.5 ppm in case of diamagnetic ions [99]. A hollow Au nanospheres polydopamine-Ag@Fe_3O_4-reduce GO-antibody is a novel biosensor that can be used to capture rabbit IgG. Large surface area hollow Au nanospheres couples the light into Au layer, and binding of IgG to antibody

Table 8.3 Summary of various carbon-nanomaterial-based sensors.

S. No.	Nanomaterials and structures	Analyte	LOD	Linear range	Refs.
1.	AgNPs@MOF-based SERS sensor	Blood cholesterol	0.36 μM	1.0–100 μM	[78]
2.	3D Ag-nanoparticle/graphene aerogel composites-based ECL sensor	Sulfite oxidase enzyme	0.007 mg/l	0.025–40 mg/l	[79]
3.	Pomegranate-inspired bi-functional electrode materials-based ECL sensor	Acetylcholinesterase	3.5×10^{-15} g/ml	10^{-14}–10^{-8} g/ml	[80]
4.	CaF_2 nanocrystals in mesoporous Si nanotemplets-based Fluorescent biosensor	microRNAs	0.145 nM	10 pM–10 μM	[81]
5.	GOx AuNPs/Tannic acid-3-aminopropyltriethoxysilane (TA-APTES) on activated carbon cloth-based ECL sensor	Glucose	3.3 μM	0.01–18 μM	[82]
6.	CuO-colloid NPs and graphene-modified nanocomposite electrode based	Glucose	1 μmol/l	1–850 μM	[83]
7.	miR-25/BSA/ss-DNA/MPA/AuNPs/ 3-Mercaptopropionic acid, bismuth vanadate, fluorine doped tin oxide-based sensor	miR-25	3.4 fM	1.0×10^{-14}–10^{-6} M	[69]
8.	ECL biosensor made up of DNA-AuPt and poly-L- methionine	Imatinib Erlotinib	32×10^{-3}–1.0 nM Adenine 0.23–1.0 nM Guanine	0.009 nM Adenine 0.07 nM Guanine	[84]
9.	Graphene-poly (3-aminobenzoic acid)-Ag-Au NPs	PSA	0.13 pg	0.01–80 ng/ml	[85]
10.	rGO (Mg/Zn) bimetallic strip-based sensor	Folic acid	25 nM	0.9–8.52 μM	[86]

(Continued)

Table 8.3 (Continued)

S. No.	Nanomaterials and structures	Analyte	LOD	Linear range	Refs.
11.	GO-ferrocene nanofilm polyethyleneimine-based sensor	Cystatin C	0.03 ng/ml	0.1–1000 ng/ml	[87]
12.	Carboxyl-functionalized GO on Au chip	Cytokeratin 19 for lung cancer	1 fg/ml	1 fg/ml–1 ng/ml	[88]
13.	GO-AgNPs-antibody-based sensor	PSA	0.000 23 ng/ml	0.5–500 pg/ml	[89]
14.	MWCNTs carbonized silk fabric–based sensor	Glucose	0.05 mM	0–1.5 mM	[90]
15.	MWCNT and polyethyleneimine dispersion–based sensor	Zearalenone	0.000 15 ng/ml	0.001–0.1 ng/ml	[91]
16.	Au nanocage /MWCNT-NH_2-decorated screen-printed carbon electrode-based sensor	RNA	42.8 fM	10^{-14}–10^{-7} M	[92]
17.	SWCNTs-based sensor	Hydrogen peroxide	n.r.	5×10^{-6}–5×10^{-3}	[93]
18.	MWCNT/Au nanocomposites–based sensor	MicroRNA 155	3.34×10^{-14}	10^{-13}–10^{-9}	[94]

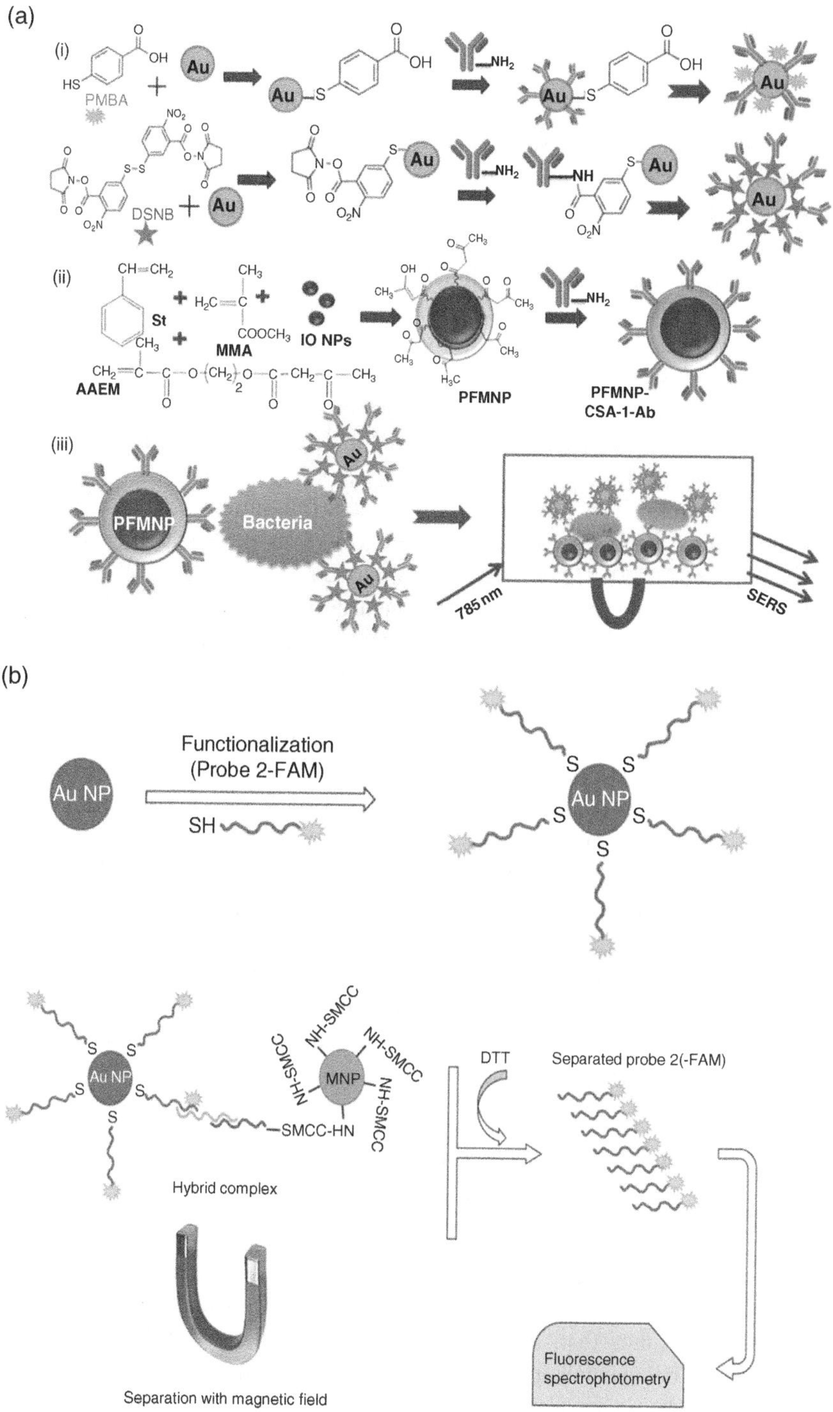

Figure 8.4 Schematic of (a) AuNPs modified SERS sensor to detect the S. typhimurium. *Source:* [97]/with permission of Elsevier. (b) AuNPs and MNP-based fluorescent biosensor for Vibrio cholera detection. *Source:* [98]/with permission of Elsevier.

causes change in the SPR curve with high sensitivity. Rabbit IgG was detected with LOD and range of the sensor 0.019 μg/ml, 0.019–40 μg/ml [100]. An AuNPs, magnetic NPs, decomposer dithiothreitol based fluorescent biosensor was investigated to detect the Vibrio cholera O1 OmpW gene. Tetraethoxysilane, sulfo-succinimidyl 4-Nmaleimidomethyl cyclohexane-1-carboxylate and 3-aminopropyl-triethoxysilane were used to functionalize the magnetic NPs. LOD of the sensor were determined to be 2.34 ng/ml and linear response for the concentrations of 5–250 ng/ml was observed [98]. $BiFeO_3$ possesses the properties of ferroelectric and ferromagnetic materials i.e. a multiferroic material. it responds to both electric as well as magnetic fields of the SPR signal. An BK7-Ag-$BiFeO_3$-monolayer-graphene-based biosensor was demonstrated to detect the biomolecules in the RI range of 1.33–1.38 RIU.

Different thickness of $BiFeO_3$ and three metals (aluminum, copper, and silver) were explored, with the increase of thickness (5–9 nm) sensitivity increases. The sensitivity of 303, 321, 412 Deg./RIU was reported in case of Ag-$BiFeO_3$-graphene, Al-$BiFeO_3$-graphene and Cu-$BiFeO_3$-graphene at $\lambda = 633$ nm [101]. A $Fe@Fe_2O_3$/g-C_3N_4 nanocomposites-based photo-electrochemical sensor was reported to detect the rhodamine B and phenol contaminants from wastewater. The composite material has better catalytic activity rather than pure g-C_3N_4 or $Fe@Fe_2O_3$ [102]. A bismuth ferrite oxide: $Bi_2Fe_4O_9$ nanoparticles and chromogenic peroxidase substrate-based colorimetric sensor was for dopamine detection. Dopamine showed the linear response in the range of 0.15–50 μM and lowest concentration of 51 nM [103]. A glutathione-capped MXene-derived QD was immobilized on a magnetic bio-mimic vesicle-based ECL biosensor to detect miRNA-221. MXene QDs have excellent luminescent properties that are capped with glutathione to improve stability. A LOD of 10 fM for miRNA concentrations in the 10 fM–10 nM range was achieved. MXene QD suffers from the drawback of complex synthesis steps that limit its further use in various applications [104]. Tables 8.4 and 8.5 summarize the recently reported magnetic, 2D nanomaterials, quantum dots, and polymer nanomaterials-based biosensors.

8.2.4 Nanomaterials for Wearable Biosensors

Wearable biosensors can be fixed to the body to monitor activity, heart rate, temperature sensors, respiratory rate, blood pressure, and blood glucose levels. Wearable sensors are gaining attention due to various advantages that include (i) continuous monitoring of physiological signals that provide more accurate and comprehensive data than traditional devices that only collect data at periodic intervals; (ii) being small and lightweight, making them easy to wear and transport; and (iii) being inexpensive and affordable, making them more accessible to people of all income levels. Additionally, use in harsh conditions, electromagnetic

Table 8.4 Magnetic, 2D nanomaterials, quantum dots, and polymer nanomaterials-based sensors.

Sensor structure	Transduction	Analyte	LOD	Linear range	Refs.
Copper ferrite inverse spinel NPs-based gas sensor	chemi-resistive	formalin	3 ppm	5–30 ppm	[105]
$CuFe_2O_4$-based sensor	Fluorescence	*E. coli*	5.8×10^2 CFU/ml	10^3–10^6 CFU/ml	[106]
Quartz@Au-layer-antibody biosensor	QCM	Morphine	0.25 ng/ml	0.25–2500 ng/ml	[107]
Au-PolyPyrrole nanocomposite sensor	ECL	Morphine	0.1 ng/ml	800–2500 ng/ml	[108]
Ag/$BiFeO_3$/Ni/perovskite $MAPbBr_3$	SPR	Not specified	n.r.[a]	1.3–1.35 RIU	[109]
Hollow CuO and TiO_2 polyhedra	QCM	Protein tyrosine phosphatase 1B	0.009 pM	0.01–10^5 pM	[110]
AuNPs and CNTs α-Fe_2O_3 nano-flowers	ECL	Organophosphorus pesticides	1.9×10^{-15} M	10^{-13}–10^{-7} M	[111]
Carbon spheres decorated with Fe_2O_3/Fe_3C/Fe composite NPs	ECL	Nitrite	0.06 μM	1–2540 μM	[112]
Fe_2O_3–CuO nanocomposite	ECL	Amiprofos-methyl herbicide	0.0065 μg/mL	0.05–30 μg/ml	[113]
Fe_3O_4/α-Fe_2O_3@Au magnetic nanocomposites	ECL	TP53 gene	0.26 pM	1 pM–1 μM	[114]
Geobacter sulfurreducens biofilms on Fe_2O_3/FTO support-electrodes-based ECL sensor	ECL	Sodium acetate	5.9 mM	10–110 mM	[115]
Ag–Ag_2S decorated hematite photoanode	Photo ECL	Thrombin	40.2 fM	0.0001–50 nM	[116]
Zr–Fe_2O_3/In_2O_3 photocatalyst	Photo ECL	*E. coli* and *S. aureus*	n.r.[a]	20–90 μg/ml	[117]

(*Continued*)

Table 8.4 (Continued)

Sensor structure	Transduction	Analyte	LOD	Linear range	Refs.
α-Fe_2O_3 nanorods deposited on carbon yarn immunosensor	ECL	Interleukin-6 cancer	0.26 pg/ml	0.001–100 ng/ml	[118]
GOQDs/ITO using EDC-NHS cross-linker	ECL	Aflatoxin B1	0.05 ng/g	0.1–2 ng/ml	[119]
CuInZnS/ZnS quantum dots sensor	ECL	Thrombin	1.82 fM	10 fM to 1 nM	[120]
Nitrogen-doped carbonized polymer dots	ECL	*E. coli*	3.33×10^{-20} mol/l	10^{-19}–10^{-6} mol/l	[121]
CdS QD/WS_2 nanosheet heterostructure	Photo ECL	DNA	2.29 fM	5 fM to 50 pM	[122]
CdSeTeS QDs and AuNPs	LSPR	Dengue virus	11.4–39.7 fM	10^{-15} to 10^{-10} M	[123]
QDs beads@SiO_2-COOH nanobead-based sensor	Lateral flow immunoassay	cTnI Creatine kinase- Myoglobin	0.036 ng/ml	0.12–125 ng/ml	[124]
Zn–Ag–In–S QD-based sensor	ECL	Hg^{2+}	0.11 pM	10 pM to 1 mM	[125]
Polymer QD and nanocomposites of C60 fullerene, multi-walled CNTs- and polyethylenimine-based sensor	ECL	Thrombin	6 fmol/l	50 fmol/l–20 nmol/l	[126]
Iron oxide NPs Aptamer conjugated CdTe-MPA QDS-based sensor	Fluorescence	*E. coli*	10^2 cells	10–100 μg	[127]

[a] not reported.

Table 8.5 Sensor design with target for magnetic, 2D nanomaterials, quantum dots, and polymer nanomaterials-based sensors.

S. No.	Sensor design with target	Linear range	LOD	Refs.
1.	AuNPs-Fe_3O_4Au enzyme free cleavage-based ECL sensor to detect thrombin	0.01 pM–10 nM	8.6 fM	[128]
2.	AuNPs and iron NPs based-fluorescent biosensor for *Shigella bacteria*	10^2–10^7 CFU/ml	90 CFU/ml	[129]
3.	Fe_3O_4, Au, chondroitin sulfate, polyethylene glycol NPs ECL sensor to detect *Mycoplasma pneumoniae*	10 aM–0.1 nM	3.3 aM	[130]
4.	Fe_3O_4/SiO_2/AgNPs/Ab_1 – human carboxylesterase 1–Ab_2/AgNPs SERS sensor for human carboxylesterase 1	0.1–10^6 μg/l	0.1 μg/l	[131]
5.	$CoFe_2O_4$ magnetic substrate, Ag, single-walled CNT-based SERS sensor to detect the Hg^{2+} detection	1 pM–100 nM	0.84 pM	[132]
6.	Platinum-Fe_3O_4-based ECL sensor for sarcosine detection	0.5–60 μM	0.4×10^{-6} M	[133]
7.	Fe_3O_4@Pt core shell-based immunoassay for human chorionic gonadotropin	0.01–1.0 ng/ml	0.025 ng/ml	[134]
8.	Fe_3O_4- GO-platinum NPs and aptamer-based ECL sensor for *Mycobacterium tuberculosis*	5 fg/ml–1.0 ng/ml	0.34 fg/ml	[135]
9.	Penicillin detection using graphene-Fe_3O_4 and multi-walled CNTs-based ECL sensor	0.05–10^2 ng/ml	25.3 pg/ml	[136]
10.	Fe_3O_4 metal organic framework and NiCd-QDs ECL sensor to detect PSA biomarker	10^{-3}–10^2 ng/ml	0.45 pg/ml	[137]
11.	Fe_3O_4 antibody and CdTe-CdS QDs based ECL immunosensor for hepatitis B virus	3 fg/ml–0.3 ng/ml	0.80 fg/ml	[138]
12.	Acetylcholine detection using Fe_2O_3 magnetic NPs-based ECL sensor	2.5–60 μM	1 μM	[139]

(*Continued*)

Table 8.5 (Continued)

S. No.	Sensor design with target	Linear range	LOD	Refs.
13.	Thiadiazol and carboxyl group NPs-based ECL sensor for paraoxon and trichlorfon pesticide	0–10 μg/l	6.7×10^{-6} μM	[140]
14.	Aptamer-antibody and toluidine blue O-based biosensor for thrombin detection	1–500 nM	4.9 nM	[141]
15.	ITO, covalent organic polymer, palladium NPs and aptamer-based ECL sensor for A549 cancer cell detection	$10–10^6$ cells/ml	8 cells/ml	[142]
16.	GO, Fe_3O_4 carbon QDs chemiluminescence-based aptasensor for adenosine	$10^{-13}–10^{-9}$ mol/l	2.1×10^{-13} mol/l	[143]
17.	Fe_3O_4·magnetic mesoporous silica, graphite oxide-based chemiluminescence aptasensor for dopamine	$10^{-9}–2 \times 10^{-13}$ mol/l	3.9×10^{-14} mol/l	[144]
18.	Fe_3O_4 NPs-based aptasensor detect gamma-interferon protein	$10^{-18}–10^{-8}$ M	1.54 fM	[145]
19.	Triglycerides detection using lipase, magnetite-chitosan, CuO NPs, multiwalled CNT, and pectin nanocomposite-based ECL sensor	$10^3–10^5$ μg/l	3.2×10^3 μg/l	[146]
20.	Nitrogen doped CNTs, Fe_3O_4, and Au-based ECL sensor to detect H_2O_2	0.35–8.8 μM	0.3 μM	[147]
21.	Multiwalled CNTs, MnO_2 AgNPs-based ECL sensor for CEA biomarker	0.5–10 μg/l	0.03 pg/ml	[148]
22.	*Salmonella typhimurium* detection multiwalled CNT-based ECL immunosensor structure in PBS and milk	$10–10^6$ CFU/ml	7.9 and 17.3 CFU/ml	[149]
23.	ITO, polystyrene sheets-thiolated carbon, and/Au-based ECL detect *Leishmania* species	0.1–98 fg/ml	15 fM	[150]
24.	Polyaniline, magnetic graphene-based ECL sensor for hydroquinone	0.4–337.2 μmol/l	2.94 μM	[151]
25.	Glucose oxidase, Fe_3O_4 NPs, reduce GO self-assembly-based ECL glucose sensor	0.05–1 mM	0.1 μM	[152]
26.	HRP reduced GO-based H_2O_2 ECL sensor	0–100 μM	n.r	[153]

27.	Glutamate dehydrogenase, Fe_3O_4, graphene, chitosan nano-composite-based ECL sensor to detect NH_4^+	0.4–2 μM	0.08 μM	[154]
28.	Fe_3O_4-AuNPs-antibody-luminol-based ECL biosensor for tetrodotoxin detection	0.01–10^2 μg/l	0.01 ng/ml	[155]
29.	AuNPs, antibody, GO, Fe_3O_4 NPs-based ECL CEA sensor	0.01–100 ng/ml	6.9×10^{-5} μg/l	[156]
30.	ITO, Au nanorod, polydopamine, and GO-based ECL sensor to detect microcystin-LR toxin detection	0.01–50 μg/l	0.007 μg/l	[157]
31.	Rabbit IgG detection using polydopamine, Ag, Fe_3O_4, and reduced GO based SPR sensor	0.019–40 μg/ml	0.019 μg/ml	[100]
32.	Nafion, Fe_3O_4, reduced GO, AuNPs, antibody ECL sensor for cortisol detection	0.1–10^3 μg/l	0.05 μg/l	[158]
33.	GO, Fe_3O_4 NPs, chitosan, aptamer-based chemiluminescence for thrombin detection	10^{-15}–2.5×10^{-10} mol/l	10^{-15} mol/l	[159]
34.	GO, Fe_3O_4, chitosan, aptamer chemiluminescence for tetracycline detection	0.16 pM–2.0 nM	21 fM	[160]
35.	GO, Fe_3O_4NPs, QDs-luminol, aptamer, and HKUST-1 metal organic framework chemiluminescence biosensor for adenosine	10^{-12}–2.2×10^{-10} mol/l	2.1×10^{-13} mol/l	[161]
36.	Fe_3O_4, AuNPs, hemin-functionalized reduced GO-based colorimetric sensor to detect Nopaline synthase	0.5–100 nM	0.19 nM	[162]
37.	Double hydroxides, GO, cobalt ferrite, chitosan ECL sensor on fluorine tin oxide substrate to detect etoposide	0.2–10 μM	0.0010 μM	[163]
38.	Reduced GO, nickel, platinum NPs-based fluorescent sensor for mycotoxin detection	0.01–1 μg/ml	0.70 ng/ml	[164]

interference immunity, miniaturization, small volumes (nano) detection, fiber integration, better sensitivity at low cost, and resistant against corrosion make it an emerging biosensing technology. Some uses of commercially available nanomaterials-based wearable sensors are listed in Table 8.6.

Table 8.6 Summary of commercially available nanomaterials-based wearable sensors.

Structure details with target	Linear range	LOD	Refs.
AuNPs and super absorbent polymer-based colorimetric sensor to detect chloride	0–125 mM	n.r.[a]	[165]
CRISPR and freeze-dried, cell-free-based colorimetric and fluorescence biosensor to detect sars-cov-2	n.r.[a]	2.7 fM	[166]
AuNPs and glucose oxidase-based glucose measurement colorimetric sensor	0.01–0.15 mM	0.01 mM	[167]
AuNPs and lactate oxidase colorimetric lactate sensor	10–30 mM	0.06 mM	[168]
AuNPs- PDMS microfluidic colorimetric sensor to measure chloride, glucose, lactate, pH, temperature	25–100 mM 25–100 mM 5–20 mM 5–6.5 25–37 °C	0.06 mM	[169]
Glucose and nitrite detection using glucose oxidase-HRP paper-based colorimetric	0–2.0 to 0–400 μM	27 μM 7 μM	[170]
Fluorescence biosensor for glucose, lactate, chloride monitoring	10–250 μM 1.0–12.5 mM 10–100 mM	7 μM 0.4 mM 5 mM	[171]
Glucose detection using fluorescent-based smart contact lens using 2-hydroxyethyl methacrylate	23 μM–1.0 mM	9.3 μM	[172]
Fluorescence chloride sensor	0–200 mM	0.1 mM	[173]
A549 cancer cells AuNPs LSPR sensor	n.r.[a]	n.r.[a]	[174]
AuNPs SERS for glucose detection	100–10 000 μM	16.8 μM	[175]
Au nano-islands SERS to detect para-amino-thiophenol	200 nM–10 μM	11.4 μM	[176]
$Ti_3C_2T_x$ MXenes SERS biosensor to detect 4-mercaptobenzoic acid	5–500 μM	1000 μM	[177]

Table 8.6 (Continued)

Structure details with target	Linear range	LOD	Refs.
Ag nano-cube SERS biosensor to detect nicotine	10–100 nM	0.01 nM	[178]
Ag and MoS_2 SERS biosensor to detect rhodamine 6 g	1000–10 000 μM	10^{-13} M	[179]
Ag nano-mushroom SERS for urea, lactate, pH	1–10 mM, 1–10 mM, 5.5–7.0	n.r.[a]	[180]
Photonic microstructure for glucose detection	0–50 mM	n.r.[a]	[181]

[a] not reported.

8.3 Summary

MIPs technique can be covalent, semicovalent, and noncovalent; among the three, noncovalent MIPs are widely used for synthesis purpose. Free radical polymerization is a commonly used process as compared to controlled radical polymerization. The advancement and advent of new nanomaterials has improved the performance that include figure of merit, sensitivity, selectivity, and overall performance of biosensors. One notable area of progress is the application of nanomaterials like carbon nanotubes, graphene, metal nanoparticles, and quantum dots in biosensor platforms. The biocompatibility, lower toxicity, large surface-to-volume ratio, and good electrical and optical properties have made nanomaterials an excellent candidate in the sensing applications. Researchers have explored diverse strategies to integrate nanomaterials into biosensors, including the use of nanocomposite films, nanowires, and nanoscale patterns. The integration of nanomaterials with biosensors holds significant potential for advancing personalized medicine, early disease detection, and real-time monitoring of biological processes.

Notably, recent work in this field has focused on the development of wearable biosensors capable of continuously monitoring biomolecules within the human body. Utilizing nanomaterials like graphene, carbon nanotubes, quantum dots, and nanoparticles, these sensors offer smaller sizes, increased sensitivity, and enhanced versatility compared to traditional sensors. They have the capability to transform health monitoring, disease detection, and treatment tracking by providing real-time feedback and early detection. Moreover, they can contribute to improvements in athletic performance and fitness tracking. Although the growth of nanomaterial-based biosensors is still in its early stages, the potential benefits are substantial. As technology advances, these sensors are expected to become more accessible and affordable, ultimately impacting many aspects of our lives. Continued research in this area will drive the development of next-generation biosensors with even greater performance and expanded applications.

References

1 Saylan, Y., Akgönüllü, S., Yavuz, H. et al. (2019). Molecularly imprinted polymer based sensors for medical applications. *Sensors* 19 (6): 1279. https://doi.org/10.3390/s19061279.

2 El-Schich, Z., Zhang, Y., Feith, M. et al. (2020). Molecularly imprinted polymers in biological applications. *Biotechniques* 69 (6): 407–420. https://doi.org/10.2144/btn-2020-0091.

3 Bakhtiar, S., Bhawani, S.A., and Shafqat, S.R. (2019). Synthesis and characterization of molecular imprinting polymer for the removal of 2-phenylphenol from spiked blood serum and river water. *Chem. Biol. Technol. Agric.* 6 (1): 1–10. https://doi.org/10.1186/s40538-019-0152-5.

4 Zhao, G., Liu, J., Liu, M. et al. (2020). Synthesis of molecularly imprinted polymer via emulsion polymerization for application in solanesol separation. *Appl. Sci.* 10 (8): https://doi.org/10.3390/APP10082868.

5 Rajpal, S. and Mishra, P. (2022). Next generation biosensors employing molecularly imprinted polymers as sensing elements for in vitro diagnostics. *Biosens. Bioelectron.: X* 11 (July): 100201. https://doi.org/10.1016/j.biosx.2022.100201.

6 Ertürk, G. and Mattiasson, B. (2017). Molecular imprinting techniques used for the preparation of biosensors. *Sensors* 17 (2): 1–17. https://doi.org/10.3390/s17020288.

7 Adumitrăchioaie, A., Tertiş, M., Cernat, A. et al. (2018). Electrochemical methods based on molecularly imprinted polymers for drug detection. A review. *Int. J. Electrochem. Sci.* 13 (3): 2556–2576. https://doi.org/10.20964/2018.03.75.

8 Qiu, X., Xu, X.Y., Chen, X. et al. (2018). Preparation of a molecularly imprinted sensor based on quartz crystal microbalance for specific recognition of sialic acid in human urine. *Anal. Bioanal.Chem.* 410 (18): 4387–4395. https://doi.org/10.1007/s00216-018-1094-7.

9 Chenthamara, D., Subramaniam, S., Ramakrishnan, S.G. et al. (2019). Therapeutic efficacy of nanoparticles and routes of administration. *Biomater. Res.* 23 (1): 1–29. https://doi.org/10.1186/s40824-019-0166-x.

10 Abdellatif, A.A.H. and Alsowinea, A.F. (2021). Approved and marketed nanoparticles for disease targeting and applications in COVID-19. *Nanotechnol. Rev.* 10 (1): 1941–1977. https://doi.org/10.1515/ntrev-2021-0115.

11 Yola, M.L. and Atar, N. (2019). Development of cardiac troponin-I biosensor based on boron nitride quantum dots including molecularly imprinted polymer. *Biosens. Bioelectron.* 126: 418–424. https://doi.org/10.1016/j.bios.2018.11.016.

12 Lin, X., Wang, Y., Wang, L. et al. (2019). Interference-free and high precision biosensor based on surface enhanced Raman spectroscopy integrated with surface molecularly imprinted polymer technology for tumor biomarker detection in human blood. *Biosens. Bioelectron.* 143 (June): 111599. https://doi.org/10.1016/j.bios.2019.111599.

13 Abbasy, L., Mohammadzadeh, A., Hasanzadeh, M., and Razmi, N. (2020). Development of a reliable bioanalytical method based on prostate specific antigen trapping on the cavity of molecular imprinted polymer towards sensing of PSA using binding affinity of PSA-MIP receptor: a novel biosensor. *J. Pharm. Biomed. Anal.* 188: 113447. https://doi.org/10.1016/j.jpba.2020.113447.

14 You, M., Yang, S., An, Y. et al. (2020). A novel electrochemical biosensor with molecularly imprinted polymers and aptamer-based sandwich assay for determining amyloid-β oligomer. *J. Electroanal. Chem.* 862: 114017. https://doi.org/10.1016/j.jelechem.2020.114017.

15 Qi, J.f., Tan, D., Wang, X.J. et al. (2021). A novel acetylcholinesterase biosensor with dual-recognized strategy based on molecularly imprinted polymer. *Sens. Actuators, B* 337: 129760. https://doi.org/10.1016/j.snb.2021.129760.

16 Jesadabundit, W., Jampasa, S., Patarakul, K. et al. (2021). Enzyme-free impedimetric biosensor-based molecularly imprinted polymer for selective determination of L-hydroxyproline. *Biosens. Bioelectron.* 191 (April): 113387. https://doi.org/10.1016/j.bios.2021.113387.

17 Hu, C., Peng, F., Mi, F. et al. (2022). SERS-based boronate affinity biosensor with biomimetic specificity and versatility: surface-imprinted magnetic polymers as recognition elements to detect glycoproteins. *Anal. Chim. Acta* 1191: 339289. https://doi.org/10.1016/j.aca.2021.339289.

18 Wang, L., Wang, H., Tang, X., and Zhao, L. (2022). Molecularly imprinted polymers-based novel optical biosensor for the detection of cancer marker lysozyme. *Sens. Actuators, A* 334: 113324. https://doi.org/10.1016/j.sna.2021.113324.

19 Cui, M., Sun, X., Liu, R. et al. (2022). A dual-responsive electrochemical biosensor based on artificial protein imprinted polymers and natural hyaluronic acid for sensitive recognition towards biomarker CD44. *Sens. Actuators, B* 371: 132554. https://doi.org/10.1016/j.snb.2022.132554.

20 Zhu, L., Hu, Z., Shen, Y., and Wang, Y. (2023). Preparation and application of lysozyme molecularly imprinted surface plasmon resonance biosensors. *Microchem. J.* 190 (March): 108665. https://doi.org/10.1016/j.microc.2023.108665.

21 Nur Ashakirin, S., Zaid, M.H.M., Haniff, M.A.S.M. et al. (2023). Sensitive electrochemical detection of creatinine based on electrodeposited molecular imprinting polymer modified screen printed carbon electrode. *Measurement* 210: 112502. https://doi.org/10.1016/j.measurement.2023.112502.

22 Duan, N., Chen, X., Lin, X. et al. (2023). Paper-based fluorometric sensing of malachite green using synergistic recognition of aptamer-molecularly imprinted polymers and luminescent metal–organic frameworks. *Sens. Actuators, B* 384 (February): 133665. https://doi.org/10.1016/j.snb.2023.133665.

23 Cetinkaya, A., Unal, M.A., Nazır, H. et al. (2023). Two different molecularly imprinted polymeric coating techniques for creating sensitive and selective electrochemical sensors for the detection of Ribavirin. *Sens. Actuators, B* 389 (April): 133914. https://doi.org/10.1016/j.snb.2023.133914.

24 Saleh, T.A. (2020). Nanomaterials: classification, properties, and environmental toxicities. *Environ. Technol. Innovation* 20: 101067. https://doi.org/10.1016/j.eti.2020.101067.

25 Maduraiveeran, G., Sasidharan, M., and Jin, W. (2019). Earth-abundant transition metal and metal oxide nanomaterials: synthesis and electrochemical applications. *Prog. Mater Sci.* 106 (June): 100574. https://doi.org/10.1016/j.pmatsci.2019.100574.

26 Liu, B. and Liu, J. (2019). Sensors and biosensors based on metal oxide nanomaterials. *TrAC – Trends Anal. Chem.* 121: 115690. https://doi.org/10.1016/j.trac.2019.115690.

27 Karami, C. and Taher, M.A. (2019). A catechol biosensor based on immobilizing laccase to Fe_3O_4@Au core-shell nanoparticles. *Int. J. Biol. Macromol.* 129: 84–90. https://doi.org/10.1016/j.ijbiomac.2019.02.015.

28 Cui, H.F., Zhang, T.T., Lv, Q.Y. et al. (2019). An acetylcholinesterase biosensor based on doping Au nanorod@SiO_2 nanoparticles into TiO_2-chitosan hydrogel for detection of organophosphate pesticides. *Biosens. Bioelectron.* 141 (June): 111452. https://doi.org/10.1016/j.bios.2019.111452.

29 Jahandari, S., Taher, M.A., Karimi-Maleh, H. et al. (2019). A powerful DNA-based voltammetric biosensor modified with Au nanoparticles, for the determination of Temodal; an electrochemical and docking investigation. *J. Electroanal. Chem.* 840 (March): 313–318. https://doi.org/10.1016/j.jelechem.2019.03.049.

30 Zhang, Q., Fu, M., Lu, H. et al. (2019). Novel potential and current type chiral amino acids biosensor based on L/D-handed double helix carbon nanotubes@polypyrrole@Au nanoparticles@L/D-cysteine. *Sens. Actuators, B* 296 (June): 126667. https://doi.org/10.1016/j.snb.2019.126667.

31 Nohwal, B., Chaudhary, R., Kumar, P., and Pundir, C.S. (2020). Fabrication and application of an amperometric lysine biosensor based on covalently immobilized lysine oxidase nanoparticles onto Au electrode. *Int. J. Biol. Macromol.* 146: 907–915. https://doi.org/10.1016/j.ijbiomac.2019.09.213.

32 Yue, H.Y., Zhang, H.J., Huang, S. et al. (2020). Highly sensitive and selective dopamine biosensor using Au nanoparticles-ZnO nanocone arrays/graphene foam electrode. *Mater. Sci. Eng., C* 108 (October 2019): 110490. https://doi.org/10.1016/j.msec.2019.110490.

33 Jandas, P.J., Luo, J., Prabakaran, K. et al. (2020). Highly stable, love-mode surface acoustic wave biosensor using Au nanoparticle-MoS_2-rGO nano-cluster doped polyimide nanocomposite for the selective detection of carcinoembryonic antigen. *Mater. Chem. Phys.* 246: 122800. https://doi.org/10.1016/j.matchemphys.2020.122800.

34 Wang, L., Liu, P., Liu, Z. et al. (2021). A dual-potential ratiometric electrochemiluminescence biosensor based on Au@CDs nanoflowers,

Au@luminol nanoparticles and an enzyme-free DNA nanomachine for ultrasensitive p53 DNA detection. *Sens. Actuators, B* 327: 128890. https://doi.org/10.1016/j.snb.2020.128890.

35 Tian, J., Liang, Z., Hu, O. et al. (2021). An electrochemical dual-aptamer biosensor based on metal-organic frameworks MIL-53 decorated with Au@Pt nanoparticles and enzymes for detection of COVID-19 nucleocapsid protein. *Electrochim. Acta* 387: 138553. https://doi.org/10.1016/j.electacta.2021.138553.

36 Akbari Hasanjani, H.R. and Zarei, K. (2021). DNA/Au-Pt bimetallic nanoparticles/graphene oxide-chitosan composites modified pencil graphite electrode used as an electrochemical biosensor for sub-picomolar detection of anti-HIV drug zidovudine. *Microchem. J.* 164: 106005. https://doi.org/10.1016/j.microc.2021.106005.

37 Wang, F., Zhang, Y., Lu, M. et al. (2021). Near-infrared band gold nanoparticles-Au film 'hot spot' model based label-free ultratrace lead (II) ions detection via fiber SPR DNAzyme biosensor. *Sens. Actuators, B* 337: 129816. https://doi.org/10.1016/j.snb.2021.129816.

38 Zhao, Y., Tian, L., Wu, S. et al. (2021). Ultrasensitive electrochemiluminescence biosensor for permethrin based on iron oxide nanomaterials and Au nanoparticles. *Microchem. J.* 168: 106487. https://doi.org/10.1016/j.microc.2021.106487.

39 Du, B., Mu, X., Xu, J. et al. (2022). A Au nanoparticle and polydopamine co-modified biosensor: a strategy for in situ and label-free surface plasmon resonance immunoassays. *Arabian J. Chem.* 15 (10): 104158. https://doi.org/10.1016/j.arabjc.2022.104158.

40 Ma, W., Liu, L., Zhang, X. et al. (2022). A microfluidic-based SERS biosensor with multifunctional nanosurface immobilized nanoparticles for sensitive detection of MicroRNA. *Anal. Chim. Acta* 1221: 1–10. https://doi.org/10.1016/j.aca.2022.340139.

41 Peng, C., Ji, H., and Wang, Z. (2022). An electrochemical biosensor based on gold nanoparticles/carbon nanotubes hybrid for determination of recombinant human erythropoietin in human blood plasma. *Int. J. Electrochem. Sci.* 17 (11): 221127. https://doi.org/10.20964/2022.11.28.

42 Shu, Q., Zhu, Y., Xiao, Y. et al. (2022). A novel chemiluminescence biosensor based on dual aptamers bound nanoparticles with multi-site signal amplification for sensitive detection of carcinoembryonic antigen. *Microchem. J.* 179: 107482. https://doi.org/10.1016/j.microc.2022.107482.

43 Qi, X., Ye, Y., Wang, H. et al. (2022). An ultrasensitive and dual-recognition SERS biosensor based on Fe_3O_4@Au-Teicoplanin and aptamer functionalized Au@Ag nanoparticles for detection of Staphylococcus aureus. *Talanta* 250: 123648. https://doi.org/10.1016/j.talanta.2022.123648.

44 Ying, Y., Zhou, M., Dai, S. et al. (2022). Au nanoparticles/SnO_2/$ZnIn_2S_4$-based biosensor for photoelectrochemical/electrochemical dual-signal detection of RNase A by combining the enzymolysis of DNA probe and the generation of molybdophosphate precipitate. *Sens. Actuators, B* 354: 131251. https://doi.org/10.1016/j.snb.2021.131251.

45 Shao, M., Shi, Z., Pu, S. et al. (2022). Development of nanostructured enzymic amperometric biosensor based on gold nanoparticles for detection of pyruvate in natural samples. *Int. J. Electrochem. Sci.* 17 (4): 220423. https://doi.org/10.20964/2022.04.47.

46 Tu, Y.P., Wang, H.H., Long, D. et al. (2022). Highly sensitive photoelectrochemical biosensor based on Au nanoparticles sensitized zinc selenide quantum dots for DNA detection. *Sens. Actuators, B* 357: 131255. https://doi.org/10.1016/j.snb.2021.131255.

47 W. Li, Z. Zhao, W. Yang et al., "Immobilization of bovine hemoglobin on Au nanoparticles/MoS2 nanosheets – chitosan modified screen-printed electrode as chlorpyrifos biosensor," *Enzyme Microb. Technol.*, vol. 154, p. 109959, 2022, https://doi.org/10.1016/j.enzmictec.2021.109959.

48 Han, D., Li, X., Bian, X. et al. (2022). Localized surface plasmon-enhanced electrochemiluminescence biosensor for rapid, label-free, and single-step detection of broad-spectrum bacteria using urchin-like Au and Ag nanoparticles. *Sens. Actuators, B* 355: 131120. https://doi.org/10.1016/j.snb.2021.131120.

49 Wang, Z., Liu, Y., Wang, H. et al. (2022). Ultra-sensitive DNAzyme-based optofluidic biosensor with liquid crystal-Au nanoparticle hybrid amplification for molecular detection. *Sens. Actuators, B* 359: 131608. https://doi.org/10.1016/j.snb.2022.131608.

50 Wu, Q., Li, Z., Liang, Q. et al. (2022). Ultrasensitive electrochemical biosensor for microRNA-377 detection based on MXene-Au nanocomposite and G-quadruplex nano-amplification strategy. *Electrochim. Acta* 428: 140945. https://doi.org/10.1016/j.electacta.2022.140945.

51 Wisineski, V., Neta, V., Valério, A. et al. (2023). Development of a novel, efficient and fast method for colorimetric detection of multiple Salmonella serovars based on aptamer-nanoparticle biosensor. *Cleaner Chem. Eng.* 7: 100113. https://doi.org/10.1016/j.clce.2023.100113.

52 Ashikbayeva, Z., Bekmurzayeva, A., Myrkhiyeva, Z. et al. (2023). Green-synthesized gold nanoparticle-based optical fiber ball resonator biosensor for cancer biomarker detection. *Opt. Laser Technol.* 161 (December 2022): 109136. https://doi.org/10.1016/j.optlastec.2023.109136.

53 Guo, S., Lin, Y., Lian, Z. et al. (2023). A label-free ultrasensitive microRNA-21 electrochemical biosensor based on MXene (Ti_3C_2)-reduced graphene oxide-Au nanocomposites. *Microchem. J.* 190: 1–8. https://doi.org/10.1016/j.microc.2023.108656.

54 Yin, Z.Z., Liu, Z., Zhou, M. et al. (2023). A surface molecularly imprinted electrochemical biosensor for the detection of SARS-CoV-2 spike protein by using Cu_7S_4-Au as built-in probe. *Bioelectrochemistry* 152: 108462. https://doi.org/10.1016/j.bioelechem.2023.108462.

55 Zhai, H., Wang, Y., Geng, L. et al. (2023). Bipotential-resolved electrochemiluminescence biosensor based on Bi_2S_3@Au nanoflowers for simultaneous detection of Cd(II) and ampicillin in aquatic products. *Food Chem.* 414 (266): 135708. https://doi.org/10.1016/j.foodchem.2023.135708.

56 Lei, H., Zhu, S., Liu, C. et al. (2023). Constructing the Au nanoparticle multimer on optical fiber end face to enhance the signal of localized surface plasmon resonance biosensors: a case study for deoxynivalenol detection. *Sens. Actuators, B* 380: 133380. https://doi.org/10.1016/j.snb.2023.133380.

57 Makableh, Y., Athamneh, T., Ajlouni, M. et al. (2023). Enhanced response and selective gold nanoparticles/carbon nanotubes biosensor for the early detection of HER2 biomarker. *Sens. Actuators Rep.* 5: 100158. https://doi.org/10.1016/j.snr.2023.100158.

58 Rasouli, E., Jefrey, W., Rafie, M. et al. (2023). Sensing and bio-sensing research electrochemical DNA-nano biosensor for the detection of cervical cancer-causing HPV-16 using ultrasmall Fe_3O_4-Au core-shell nanoparticles. *Sens. Bio-Sensing Res.* 40: 100562. https://doi.org/10.1016/j.sbsr.2023.100562.

59 Kumar, S., Balayan, S., Chauhan, N., and Rosario, W. (2023). Advances fabricating a rapid and low-cost electrochemical biosensor with imprints of glycated albumin molecules to detect diabetes using bimetallic Au-Pt nanoparticles on μ SPE. *Appl. Surf. Sci. Adv.* 16: 100425. https://doi.org/10.1016/j.apsadv.2023.100425.

60 Wu, Z., Sun, D.W., Pu, H., and Wei, Q. (2023). A dual signal-on biosensor based on dual-gated locked mesoporous silica nanoparticles for the detection of Aflatoxin B1. *Talanta* 253: 124027. https://doi.org/10.1016/j.talanta.2022.124027.

61 Zha, R., Wu, R., Zong, Y. et al. (2023). A high performance dual-mode biosensor based on Nd-MOF nanosheets functionalized with ionic liquid and gold nanoparticles for sensing of ctDNA. *Talanta* 258: 124377. https://doi.org/10.1016/j.talanta.2023.124377.

62 Zhang, Q., Xu, M., Liu, Y. et al. (2023). A magnetostrictive self-powered biosensor based on Au-$BaTiO_3$-FeGa & PDMS. *J. Ind. Eng. Chem.* 117: 247–254. https://doi.org/10.1016/j.jiec.2022.10.012.

63 Sanko, V., Şenocak, A., Tümay, S.O., and Demirbas, E. (2023). A novel comparative study for electrochemical urea biosensor design: effect of different ferrite nanoparticles (MFe_2O_4, M: Cu, Co, Ni, Zn) in urease immobilized composite system. *Bioelectrochemistry* 149: 108324. https://doi.org/10.1016/j.bioelechem.2022.108324.

64 Yanik, S., Emre, D., Alp, M. et al. (2023). A novel electrochemical biosensor based on palladium nanoparticles decorated on reduced graphene oxide-polyaminophenol matrix for the detection and discrimination of mitomycin C-DNA and acyclovir-DNA inter. *J. Pharm. Biomed. Anal.* 234: 115524. https://doi.org/10.1016/j.jpba.2023.115524.

65 Shan, H.Y., Shen, K.Y., Song, S.S. et al. (2023). In situ synthesis of Au nanoparticles confined in 2D sheet-like metal organic frameworks to construct competitive PEC biosensor for sensitive analysis of autism spectrum disorder miRNA. *Sens. Actuators, B* 375: 132849. https://doi.org/10.1016/j.snb.2022.132849.

66 Sun, X., Sun, J., Ye, Y. et al. (2023). Metabolic pathway-based self-assembled Au@MXene liver microsome electrochemical biosensor for rapid screening of aflatoxin B1. *Bioelectrochemistry* 151: 108378. https://doi.org/10.1016/j.bioelechem.2023.108378.

67 Yang, X., Yin, Z.Z., Zheng, G. et al. (2023). Molecularly imprinted miniature electrochemical biosensor for SARS-CoV-2 spike protein based on Au nanoparticles and reduced graphene oxide modified acupuncture needle. *Bioelectrochemistry* 151: 108375. https://doi.org/10.1016/j.bioelechem.2023.108375.

68 Wang, Z., Zhang, Z., Zhang, Y. et al. (2023). MXenes-Au NPs modified electrochemical biosensor for multiple exosome surface proteins analysis. *Talanta* 265: 124848. https://doi.org/10.1016/j.talanta.2023.124848.

69 Koohi, F., Zare, H.R., and Shekari, Z. (2023). Photoelectrochemical biosensor based on FTO modified with $BiVO_4$ film and gold nanoparticles for detection of miRNA-25 biomarker and single-base mismatch. *J. Electroanal. Chem.* 929: 117099. https://doi.org/10.1016/j.jelechem.2022.117099.

70 Cao, L.L., Zhou, Y., Gao, L. et al. (2023). Photoelectrochemical biosensor for DNA demethylase detection based on enzymatically induced double-stranded DNA digestion by endonuclease-exonuclease system and $Bi_4O_5Br_2$–Au/CdS photoactive material. *Talanta* 262: 124670. https://doi.org/10.1016/j.talanta.2023.124670.

71 Seo, Y., Yoon, Y., Lee, M. et al. (2023). Rapid electrochemical biosensor composed of DNA probe/iridium nanoparticle bilayer for Aphanizomenon flos-aquae detection in fresh water. *Colloids Surf., B* 225 (February): 113218. https://doi.org/10.1016/j.colsurfb.2023.113218.

72 You, X., Liu, Y., Li, Y. et al. (2023). Sensitive detection of SARS-CoV-2 spike protein based on electrochemical impedance spectroscopy of Fe_3O_4 @ SiO_2 – Au/GCE biosensor. *Adv. Sens. Energy Mater.* 2 (3): 100067. https://doi.org/10.1016/j.asems.2023.100067.

73 Eskiköy Bayraktepe, D., Yıldız, C., and Yazan, Z. (2023). The development of electrochemical DNA biosensor based on poly-L-methionine and bimetallic AuPt nanoparticles coating: Picomolar detection of Imatinib and Erlotinib. *Talanta* 257: 124361. https://doi.org/10.1016/j.talanta.2023.124361.

74 Hashemi, S.A., Mousavi, S.M., Bahrani, S. et al. (2020). Coupled graphene oxide with hybrid metallic nanoparticles as potential electrochemical biosensors for precise detection of ascorbic acid within blood. *Anal. Chim. Acta* 1107: 183–192. https://doi.org/10.1016/j.aca.2020.02.018.

75 Khalil, I., Yehye, W.A., Muhd Julkapli, N. et al. (2021). Simultaneous detection of dual food adulterants using graphene oxide and gold nanoparticle based surface enhanced Raman scattering duplex DNA biosensor. *Vib. Spectrosc.* 116: 103293. https://doi.org/10.1016/j.vibspec.2021.103293.

76 Dalkıran, B. (2020). Amperometric determination of heavy metal using an HRP inhibition biosensor based on ITO nanoparticles-ruthenium (III) hexamine trichloride composite: central composite design optimization. *Bioelectrochemistry* 135: 107569. https://doi.org/10.1016/j.bioelechem.2020.107569.

77 Wan, C., Qu, A., Deng, L. et al. (2022). Preparation of an electrochemical biosensor based on indium tin oxide and its performance in detecting antibiotic resistance genes. *Microchem. J.* 182 (July): 107953. https://doi.org/10.1016/j.microc.2022.107953.

78 Wu, Y., Chen, J.Y., and He, W.M. (2022). Surface-enhanced Raman spectroscopy biosensor based on silver nanoparticles@metal-organic frameworks with peroxidase-mimicking activities for ultrasensitive monitoring of blood cholesterol. *Sens. Actuators, B* 365: 131939. https://doi.org/10.1016/j.snb.2022.131939.

79 Sroysee, W., Kongsawatvoragul, K., Phattharaphuti, P. et al. (2022). Enzyme-immobilized 3D silver nanoparticle/graphene aerogel composites towards biosensors. *Mater. Chem. Phys.* 277: 125572. https://doi.org/10.1016/j.matchemphys.2021.125572.

80 Wei, W., Tang, H., Dong, S. et al. (2022). A novel pomegranate-inspired bifunctional electrode materials design for acetylcholinesterase biosensor and methanol oxidation reaction. *Bioelectrochemistry* 145: 108094. https://doi.org/10.1016/j.bioelechem.2022.108094.

81 Gu, T., Zhong, J., Wang, Z., and Bai, P. (2023). A membrane biosensor based on colour differences encoded upconversion silica nanoparticles for multiplex nucleic acids detection. *Chem. Eng. J.* 469: 144022. https://doi.org/10.1016/j.cej.2023.144022.

82 Zhu, Y., Qi, Y., Xu, M., and Luo, J. (2023). Flexible biosensor based on signal amplification of gold nanoparticles-composite flower clusters for glucose detection in sweat. *Colloids Surf., A* 661: 130908. https://doi.org/10.1016/j.colsurfa.2022.130908.

83 Mubarakali, A., Gopinath, S., Parthasarathy, P. et al. (2023). Highly efficient and sensitive non-enzymatic glucose biosensor based on flower-shaped CuO-colloid nanoparticles decorated with graphene-modified nanocomposite electrode. *Measurement* 217: 113145. https://doi.org/10.1016/j.measurement.2023.113145.

84 Aydın, E.B., Aydın, M., and Sezgintürk, M.K. (2023). A label-free electrochemical biosensor for highly sensitive detection of GM2A based on gold nanoparticles/conducting amino-functionalized thiophene polymer layer. *Sens. Actuators, B* 392: 134025. https://doi.org/10.1016/j.snb.2023.134025.

85 Pothipor, C., Wiriyakun, N., Putnin, T. et al. (2019). Highly sensitive biosensor based on graphene–poly (3-aminobenzoic acid) modified electrodes and porous-hollowed-silver-gold nanoparticle labelling for prostate cancer detection. *Sens. Actuators, B* 296: 126657. https://doi.org/10.1016/j.snb.2019.126657.

86 Senthilkumar, E., Shanmugharaj, A.M., Suresh Babu, R. et al. (2019). Development of constructed nanoporous graphene-modified electrode for electrical detection of folic acid. *J. Mater. Sci.: Mater. Electron.* 30 (14): 13488–13496. https://doi.org/10.1007/s10854-019-01716-z.

87 Trindade, E.K.G., Silva, B.V.M., and Dutra, R.F. (2019). A probeless and label-free electrochemical immunosensor for cystatin C detection based on ferrocene functionalized-graphene platform. *Biosens. Bioelectron.* 138: 111311. https://doi.org/10.1016/j.bios.2019.05.016.

88 Chiu, N.F., Lin, T.L., and Kuo, C.T. (2018). Highly sensitive carboxyl-graphene oxide-based surface plasmon resonance immunosensor for the detection of lung cancer for cytokeratin 19 biomarker in human plasma. *Sens. Actuators, B* 265: 264–272. https://doi.org/10.1016/j.snb.2018.03.070.

89 Yang, L., Zhen, S.J., Li, Y.F., and Huang, C.Z. (2018). Silver nanoparticles deposited on graphene oxide for ultrasensitive surface-enhanced Raman scattering immunoassay of cancer biomarker. *Nanoscale* 10 (25): 11942–11947. https://doi.org/10.1039/c8nr02820f.

90 Chen, C., Ran, R., Yang, Z. et al. (2018). An efficient flexible electrochemical glucose sensor based on carbon nanotubes/carbonized silk fabrics decorated with Pt microspheres. *Sens. Actuators, B* 256: 63–70. https://doi.org/10.1016/j.snb.2017.10.067.

91 Riberi, W.I., Tarditto, L.V., Zon, M.A. et al. (2018). Development of an electrochemical immunosensor to determine zearalenone in maize using carbon screen printed electrodes modified with multi-walled carbon nanotubes/polyethyleneimine dispersions. *Sens. Actuators, B* 254: 1271–1277. https://doi.org/10.1016/j.snb.2017.07.113.

92 Chen, M., Wu, D., Tu, S. et al. (2021). A novel biosensor for the ultrasensitive detection of the lncRNA biomarker MALAT1 in non-small cell lung cancer. *Sci. Rep.* 11 (1): 1–11. https://doi.org/10.1038/s41598-021-83244-7.

93 Safaee, M.M., Gravely, M., and Roxbury, D. (2021). A wearable optical microfibrous biomaterial with encapsulated nanosensors enables wireless monitoring of oxidative stress. *Adv. Funct. Mater.* 31 (13): 1–14. https://doi.org/10.1002/adfm.202006254.

94 Ma, H., Xue, N., Li, Z. et al. (2018). Ultrasensitive detection of miRNA-155 using multi-walled carbon nanotube-gold nanocomposites as a novel fluorescence quenching platform. *Sens. Actuators, B* 266: 221–227. https://doi.org/10.1016/j.snb.2018.03.071.

95 Fatoni, A., Widanarto, W., Anggraeni, M.D., and Dwiasi, D.W. (2022). Glucose biosensor based on activated carbon – $NiFe_2O_4$ nanoparticles composite modified carbon paste electrode. *Results Chem.* 4: 100433. https://doi.org/10.1016/j.rechem.2022.100433.

96 Tapak, N.S., Nawawi, M.A., Tjih, E.T.T. et al. (2022). The synthesis of zirconium oxide (ZrO2) nanoparticles (NPs) in 1-butyl-3-methylimidazolium trifluoroacetate (BMIMCF3COO) for an amperometry phenol biosensor. *Mater. Today Commun.* 33: 104142. https://doi.org/10.1016/j.mtcomm.2022.104142.

97 Chattopadhyay, S., Sabharwal, P.K., Jain, S. et al. (2019). Functionalized polymeric magnetic nanoparticle assisted SERS immunosensor for the sensitive detection of S. typhimurium. *Anal. Chim. Acta* 1067: 98–106. https://doi.org/10.1016/j.aca.2019.03.050.

98 Narmani, A., Kamali, M., Amini, B. et al. (2018). Highly sensitive and accurate detection of Vibrio cholera O1 OmpW gene by fluorescence DNA biosensor based on gold and magnetic nanoparticles. *Process Biochem.* 65: 46–54. https://doi.org/10.1016/j.procbio.2017.10.009.

99 Sadrolhosseini, A.R., Naseri, M., and Rashid, S.A. (2017). Polypyrrole-chitosan/nickel-ferrite nanoparticle composite layer for detecting heavy metal ions using surface plasmon resonance technique. *Opt. Laser Technol.* 93: 216–223. https://doi.org/10.1016/j.optlastec.2017.03.008.

100 Li, S., Wu, Q., Ma, P. et al. (2018). A sensitive SPR biosensor based on hollow gold nanospheres and improved sandwich assay with PDA-Ag@Fe_3O_4/rGO. *Talanta* 180: 156–161. https://doi.org/10.1016/j.talanta.2017.12.051.

101 Li, C., Li, Z., Guo, S. et al. (2021). Sensitivity enhancement by employing $BiFeO_3$ and graphene hybrid structure in surface plasmon resonance biosensors. *Opt. Mater.* 121: 111618. https://doi.org/10.1016/j.optmat.2021.111618.

102 Instruments, A. and Science, E. (2021). Synergistic photocatalytic performance of Fe@Fe_2O_3 core-shell nanostructures supported on g-C_3N_4 nanosheets for RhB and phenol decolorization: fabrication, characterization, and mechanistic insights. *J. Water Process Eng.* 169 (3): 1–10. https://doi.org/10.1016/j.jwpe.2023.103866.

103 Razavi, M., Barras, A., Ifires, M. et al. (2022). Colorimetric assay for the detection of dopamine using bismuth ferrite oxide ($Bi_2Fe_4O_9$) nanoparticles as an efficient peroxidase-mimic nanozyme. *J. Colloid Interface Sci.* 613: 384–395. https://doi.org/10.1016/j.jcis.2022.01.041.

104 Li, Z., Wang, Z., Nie, Y. et al. (2022). A novel GSH-capping MXene QD-based ECL biosensor for the detection of miRNA221 in triple-negative breast cancer tumor. *Chem. Eng. J.* 448: 137636. https://doi.org/10.1016/j.cej.2022.137636.

105 Mahapatra, P.L., Das, S., Keasberry, N.A. et al. (2022). Copper ferrite inverse spinel-based highly sensitive and selective chemiresistive gas sensor for the detection of formalin adulteration in fish. *SSRN Electron. J.* 960: 170792. https://doi.org/10.2139/ssrn.4241868.

106 Fu, L., Chen, Q., Deng, S., and Jia, L. (2022). $CuFe_2O_4$ magnetic particles assisted construction of a label-free fluorescent sensor for detection of

Escherichia coli. *Microchem. J.* 183: 1–8. https://doi.org/10.1016/j.microc.2022.107993.

107 Soltanabadi, Z., Esmaeili, A., and Bambai, B. (2022). Fabrication of morphine detector based on quartz@Au-layer biosensor. *Microchem. J.* 175: 107127. https://doi.org/10.1016/j.microc.2021.107127.

108 Soltanabadi, Z. and Esmaeili, A. (2022). Invention of a fast response biosensor based on Au-polypyrrole nanocomposite-modified quartz ceramic to detect morphine concentration. *J. Photochem. Photobiol., A* 429: 113919. https://doi.org/10.1016/j.jphotochem.2022.113919.

109 El barghouti, M., Akjouj, A., and Mir, A. (2022). Modeling of surface plasmon resonance biosensor based on Ag/$BiFeO_3$/Ni using 2D nanomaterial perovskite $MAPbBr_3$. *Mater. Today Commun.* 33: 104591. https://doi.org/10.1016/j.mtcomm.2022.104591.

110 Xiao, K., Fu, Y., Zhu, R. et al. (2022). Photoelectrochemical and quartz crystal microbalance dual-mode assay of protein tyrosine phosphatase 1B activity based on hollow CuO and TiO_2 polyhedra. *Sens. Actuators, B* 353: 131179. https://doi.org/10.1016/j.snb.2021.131179.

111 Zhao, C., Zhao, Y., Wang, L. et al. (2022). AuNPs and CNTs embellished three-dimensional bloom-like α-Fe_2O_3 nanocomposites for highly sensitive electrochemical pesticides detection. *Microchem. J.* 191 (November): 2023. https://doi.org/10.1016/j.microc.2023.108762.

112 Luo, L., Xu, Q.Q., Chen, K.K. et al. (2023). Carbon spheres decorated with Fe_2O_3/Fe_3C/Fe composite nanoparticles for highly sensitive and selective electrochemical determination of nitrite (NO_2-). *Sens. Actuators, B* 382: 133488. https://doi.org/10.1016/j.snb.2023.133488.

113 Puthalapattu, R.P., Punyasamudram, S., Bathinapatla, A. et al. (2023). Electrochemical non-enzymatic strategy with green synthesized Fe_2O_3–CuO nanocomposite for detection of amiprofos-methyl herbicide in industrial effluents and soils. *Chem. Phys. Impact* 6 (February): 100195. https://doi.org/10.1016/j.chphi.2023.100195.

114 Liu, R., Zhang, Y., Liu, M. et al. (2023). Electrochemical sensor based on Fe_3O_4/α-Fe_2O_3@Au magnetic nanocomposites for sensitive determination of the TP53 gene. *Bioelectrochemistry* 152: 108429. https://doi.org/10.1016/j.bioelechem.2023.108429.

115 Huerta-miranda, G.A., Rodríguez-torres, L.M., Martínez-garcía, A.L., and Ju, K. (2023). Geobacter sulfurreducens electroactive biofilms on Fe_2O_3/FTO support-electrodes for developing a sodium acetate electrochemical biosensor. *Biosens. Bioelectron.: X* 14: 100370. https://doi.org/10.1016/j.biosx.2023.100370.

116 Zhang, Q., Liu, Q., Liu, Y. et al. (2023). PEC thrombin aptasensor based on Ag–Ag_2S decorated hematite photoanode with signal-down effect of precipitation catalyzed by G-quadruplexes/hemin. *Biosens. Bioelectron.* 232 (January): https://doi.org/10.1016/j.bios.2023.115321.

117 Khan, M.A., Khan, A.U., Tahir, K. et al. (2023). Synthesis of Zr–Fe_2O_3/In_2O_3 photocatalyst by novel hydrothermal method for highly selective photo inhibition of pathogens, pollutant degradation and DPPH stabilization. *Mater. Chem. Phys.* 302: 127746. https://doi.org/10.1016/j.matchemphys.2023.127746.

118 Prabhu, K., Lakshminarayanan, M., Mohankumar, G. et al. (2023). Vertically pillared α-Fe_2O_3 nanorods on carbon yarn as a textile-based stable immunosensor electrode for selective electrochemical sensing of interleukin-6 cancer biomarker. *Sens. Actuators, A* 357: 114419. https://doi.org/10.1016/j.sna.2023.114419.

119 Bhardwaj, H., Singh, C., Kotnala, R.K., and Sumana, G. (2018). Graphene quantum dots-based nano-biointerface platform for food toxin detection. *Anal. Bioanal.Chem.* 410 (28): 7313–7323. https://doi.org/10.1007/s00216-018-1341-y.

120 Xu, Y., Wang, Z., Ding, C., and Luo, X. (2020). Ratiometric antifouling electrochemiluminescence biosensor based on bi-functional peptides and low toxic quantum dots. *Sens. Actuators, B* 322: 128613. https://doi.org/10.1016/j.snb.2020.128613.

121 Shi, F., Wang, B., Yan, L. et al. (2022). In-situ growth of nitrogen-doped carbonized polymer dots on black phosphorus for electrochemical DNA biosensor of Escherichia coli O157: H7. *Bioelectrochemistry* 148: 108226. https://doi.org/10.1016/j.bioelechem.2022.108226.

122 Ju, Y., Hu, X., Zang, Y. et al. (2019). Amplified photoelectrochemical DNA biosensor based on a CdS quantum dot/WS2 nanosheet heterojunction and hybridization chain reaction-mediated enzymatic hydrolysis. *Anal. Methods* 11 (16): 2163–2169. https://doi.org/10.1039/c9ay00166b.

123 Chowdhury, A.D., Takemura, K., Khorish, I.M. et al. (2020). The detection and identification of dengue virus serotypes with quantum dot and AuNP regulated localized surface plasmon resonance. *Nanoscale Adv.* 2 (2): 699–709. https://doi.org/10.1039/c9na00763f.

124 Li, J., Lv, Y., Li, N. et al. (2021). Chemical dual protecting encapsulation synthesis of ultrastable quantum-dot nanobeads for sensitive and accurate detection of cardiac biomarkers. *Sens. Actuators, B* 344: 130275. https://doi.org/10.1016/j.snb.2021.130275.

125 Zhang, W., Zhang, P., Liang, Y. et al. (2022). Rapid electrochemical quantification of trace Hg^{2+} using a hairpin DNA probe and quantum dot modified screen-printed gold electrodes. *RSC Adv.* 12 (21): 13448–13455. https://doi.org/10.1039/d2ra01817a.

126 Jamei, H.R., Rezaei, B., and Ensafi, A.A. (2021). Ultra-sensitive and selective electrochemical biosensor with aptamer recognition surface based on polymer quantum dots and C60/MWCNTs- polyethylenimine nanocomposites for analysis of thrombin protein. *Bioelectrochemistry* 138: 107701. https://doi.org/10.1016/j.bioelechem.2020.107701.

127 Pandit, C., Alajangi, H.K., Singh, J. et al. (2022). Development of magnetic nanoparticle assisted aptamer-quantum dot based biosensor for the detection of Escherichia coli in water samples. *Sci. Total Environ.* 831: 154857. https://doi.org/10.1016/j.scitotenv.2022.154857.

128 Zhong, X., Lv, J., Xue, S. et al. (2018). An electrochemical assay based on acid-induced dissolution of nanoparticles to trigger enzyme-free cleavage for target detection. *J. Electrochem. Soc.* 165 (5): B223–B226. https://doi.org/10.1149/2.1151805jes.

129 Elahi, N., Kamali, M., Baghersad, M.H., and Amini, B. (2019). A fluorescence Nano-biosensors immobilization on iron (MNPs) and gold (AuNPs) nanoparticles for detection of Shigella spp. *Mater. Sci. Eng., C* 105: 110113. https://doi.org/10.1016/j.msec.2019.110113.

130 Zhao, S., Zhou, Y., Wei, L., and Chen, L. (2020). Low fouling strategy of electrochemical biosensor based on chondroitin sulfate functionalized gold magnetic particle for voltammetric determination of mycoplasma ovipneumonia in whole serum. *Anal. Chim. Acta* 1126: 91–99. https://doi.org/10.1016/j.aca.2020.06.015.

131 Feng, J., Xu, Y., Huang, W. et al. (2020). A magnetic SERS immunosensor for highly sensitive and selective detection of human carboxylesterase 1 in human serum samples. *Anal. Chim. Acta* 1097 (268): 176–185. https://doi.org/10.1016/j.aca.2019.11.004.

132 Yang, X., He, Y., Wang, X., and Yuan, R. (2017). A SERS biosensor with magnetic substrate $CoFe_2O_4$ @Ag for sensitive detection of Hg^{2+}. *Appl. Surf. Sci.* 416: 581–586. https://doi.org/10.1016/j.apsusc.2017.04.106.

133 Yang, Q., Li, N., Li, Q. et al. (2019). Amperometric sarcosine biosensor based on hollow magnetic Pt–Fe_3O_4@C nanospheres. *Anal. Chim. Acta* 1078: 161–167. https://doi.org/10.1016/j.aca.2019.06.031.

134 Kim, M.S., Kweon, S.H., Cho, S. et al. (2017). Pt-decorated magnetic nanozymes for facile and sensitive point-of-care bioassay. *ACS Appl. Mater. Interfaces* 9 (40): 35133–35140. https://doi.org/10.1021/acsami.7b12326.

135 Gou, D., Xie, G., Li, Y. et al. (2018). Voltammetric immunoassay for Mycobacterium tuberculosis secretory protein MPT64 based on a synergistic amplification strategy using rolling circle amplification and a gold electrode modified with graphene oxide, Fe_3O_4 and Pt nanoparticles. *Microchim. Acta* 185 (9): https://doi.org/10.1007/s00604-018-2972-6.

136 Guo, W., Umar, A., Alsaiari, M.A. et al. (2020). Ultrasensitive and selective label-free aptasensor for the detection of penicillin based on nanoporous PtTi/graphene oxide-Fe_3O_4/MWCNT-Fe_3O_4 nanocomposite. *Microchem. J.* 158 (May): 105270. https://doi.org/10.1016/j.microc.2020.105270.

137 Ehzari, H., Amiri, M., and Safari, M. (2020). Enzyme-free sandwich-type electrochemical immunosensor for highly sensitive prostate specific antigen based on conjugation of quantum dots and antibody on surface of modified glassy carbon electrode with core–shell magnetic metal-organic frameworks. *Talanta* 210 (November 2019): 120641. https://doi.org/10.1016/j.talanta.2019.120641.

138 Babamiri, B., Hallaj, R., and Salimi, A. (2018). Ultrasensitive electrochemiluminescence immunosensor for determination of hepatitis B virus surface antigen using CdTe@CdS-PAMAM dendrimer as luminescent labels and Fe_3O_4 nanoparticles as magnetic beads. *Sens. Actuators, B* 254: 551–560. https://doi.org/10.1016/j.snb.2017.07.016.

139 da Silva, W. and Brett, C.M.A. (2020). Novel biosensor for acetylcholine based on acetylcholinesterase/poly(neutral red) – deep eutectic solvent/Fe_2O_3 nanoparticle modified electrode. *J. Electroanal. Chem.* 872: 114050. https://doi.org/10.1016/j.jelechem.2020.114050.

140 Dzudzevic Cancar, H. et al. (2016). A novel acetylcholinesterase biosensor: core-shell magnetic nanoparticles incorporating a conjugated polymer for the detection of organophosphorus pesticides. *ACS Appl. Mater. Interfaces* 8 (12): 8058–8067. https://doi.org/10.1021/acsami.5b12383.

141 Chung, S., Moon, J.M., Choi, J. et al. (2018). Magnetic force assisted electrochemical sensor for the detection of thrombin with aptamer-antibody sandwich formation. *Biosens. Bioelectron.* 117 (May): 480–486. https://doi.org/10.1016/j.bios.2018.06.068.

142 Cui, L., Shen, J., Ai, S. et al. (2020). In-situ synthesis of covalent organic polymer thin film integrates with palladium nanoparticles for the construction of a cathodic photoelectrochemical cytosensor. *Biosens. Bioelectron.* 168 (August): 112545. https://doi.org/10.1016/j.bios.2020.112545.

143 Sun, Y., Ding, C., Lin, Y. et al. (2018). Highly selective and sensitive chemiluminescence biosensor for adenosine detection based on carbon quantum dots catalyzing luminescence released from aptamers functionalized graphene@magnetic β-cyclodextrin polymers. *Talanta* 186 (April): 238–247. https://doi.org/10.1016/j.talanta.2018.04.068.

144 Sun, Y., Lin, Y., Ding, C. et al. (2018). An ultrasensitive and ultraselective chemiluminescence aptasensor for dopamine detection based on aptamers modified magnetic mesoporous silica @ graphite oxide polymers. *Sens. Actuators, B* 257: 312–323. https://doi.org/10.1016/j.snb.2017.10.171.

145 Wen, D., Liu, Q., Li, L. et al. (2019). Ultrasensitive aptamer fluorometric detection of IFN-Γ by dual atom transfer radical polymerization amplification. *Sens. Actuators, B* 295 (December 2018): 40–48. https://doi.org/10.1016/j.snb.2019.05.036.

146 Di Tocco, A., Robledo, S.N., Osuna, Y. et al. (2018). Development of an electrochemical biosensor for the determination of triglycerides in serum samples based on a lipase/magnetite-chitosan/copper oxide nanoparticles/multiwalled carbon nanotubes/pectin composite. *Talanta* 190 (May): 30–37. https://doi.org/10.1016/j.talanta.2018.07.028.

147 Zhang, M., Zheng, J., Wang, J. et al. (2019). Direct electrochemistry of cytochrome c immobilized on one dimensional Au nanoparticles functionalized magnetic N-doped carbon nanotubes and its application for the detection of H_2O_2. *Sens. Actuators, B* 282 (October 2018): 85–95. https://doi.org/10.1016/j.snb.2018.11.005.

148 Han, J., Li, Y., Feng, J. et al. (2017). A novel sandwich-type immunosensor for detection of carcino-embryonic antigen using silver hybrid multiwalled carbon nanotubes/manganese dioxide. *J. Electroanal. Chem.* 786: 112–119. https://doi.org/10.1016/j.jelechem.2017.01.021.

149 Ngoensawat, U., Rijiravanich, P., Surareungchai, W., and Somasundrum, M. (2018). Electrochemical immunoassay for salmonella typhimurium based on an immuno-magnetic redox label. *Electroanalysis* 30 (1): 146–153. https://doi.org/10.1002/elan.201700568.

150 Frias, I.A.M., Andrade, C.A.S., Balbino, V.Q., and de Melo, C.P. (2017). Use of magnetically disentangled thiolated carbon nanotubes as a label-free impedimetric genosensor for detecting canine Leishmania spp. infection. *Carbon* 117: 33–40. https://doi.org/10.1016/j.carbon.2017.02.031.

151 Lou, C., Jing, T., Zhou, J. et al. (2020). Laccase immobilized polyaniline/magnetic graphene composite electrode for detecting hydroquinone. *Int. J. Biol. Macromol.* 149: 1130–1138. https://doi.org/10.1016/j.ijbiomac.2020.01.248.

152 Pakapongpan, S. and Poo-arporn, R.P. (2017). Self-assembly of glucose oxidase on reduced graphene oxide-magnetic nanoparticles nanocomposite-based direct electrochemistry for reagentless glucose biosensor. *Mater. Sci. Eng., C* 76: 398–405. https://doi.org/10.1016/j.msec.2017.03.031.

153 Waifalkar, P.P., Chougale, A.D., Kollu, P. et al. (2018). Magnetic nanoparticle decorated graphene based electrochemical nanobiosensor for H_2O_2 sensing using HRP. *Colloids Surf., B* 167: 425–431. https://doi.org/10.1016/j.colsurfb.2018.04.042.

154 Yu, L., Zhang, Q., Jin, D. et al. (2019). A promising voltammetric biosensor based on glutamate dehydrogenase/Fe_3O_4/graphene/chitosan nanobiocomposite for sensitive ammonium determination in PM2.5. *Talanta* 197 (November 2018): 622–630. https://doi.org/10.1016/j.talanta.2018.12.090.

155 Shang, F., Liu, Y., Wang, S. et al. (2017). Electrochemiluminescence immunosensor based on functionalized graphene/Fe_3O_4-Au magnetic capture probes for ultrasensitive detection of tetrodotoxin. *Electroanalysis* 29 (9): 2098–2105. https://doi.org/10.1002/elan.201700223.

156 Li, Y., Ke, C., Liu, X. et al. (2017). Compositional depth profiles of the type 316 stainless steel undergone the corrosion in liquid lithium using laser-induced breakdown spectroscopy. *J. Nucl. Mater.* 497: 1–9. https://doi.org/10.1016/j.jnucmat.2017.06.025.

157 He, Z., Wei, J., Gan, C. et al. (2017). A rolling circle amplification signal-enhanced immunosensor for ultrasensitive microcystin-LR detection based on a magnetic graphene-functionalized electrode. *RSC Adv.* 7 (63): 39906–39913. https://doi.org/10.1039/c7ra07696g.

158 Sun, B., Gou, Y., Ma, Y. et al. (2017). Investigate electrochemical immunosensor of cortisol based on gold nanoparticles/magnetic functionalized reduced graphene oxide. *Biosens. Bioelectron.* 88: 55–62. https://doi.org/10.1016/j.bios.2016.07.047.

159 Sun, Y., Wang, Y., Li, J. et al. (2017). An ultrasensitive chemiluminescence aptasensor for thrombin detection based on iron porphyrin catalyzing luminescence desorbed from chitosan modified magnetic oxide graphene composite. *Talanta* 174 (July): 809–818. https://doi.org/10.1016/j.talanta.2017.07.001.

160 Sun, Y., Dai, Y., Zhu, X. et al. (2020). A nanocomposite prepared from bifunctionalized ionic liquid, chitosan, graphene oxide and magnetic nanoparticles for aptamer-based assay of tetracycline by chemiluminescence. *Microchim. Acta* 187 (1): 1–10. https://doi.org/10.1007/s00604-019-4012-6.

161 Lin, Y., Dai, Y., Sun, Y. et al. (2018). A turn-on chemiluminescence biosensor for selective and sensitive detection of adenosine based on HKUST-1 and QDs-luminol-aptamer conjugates. *Talanta* 182 (October 2017): 116–124. https://doi.org/10.1016/j.talanta.2018.01.065.

162 Cao, X., Xia, Z., Yan, W. et al. (2020). Colorimetric biosensing of nopaline synthase terminator using Fe_3O_4@Au and hemin-functionalized reduced graphene oxide. *Anal. Biochem.* 602 (May): 113798. https://doi.org/10.1016/j.ab.2020.113798.

163 Vajedi, F.s. and Dehghani, H. (2020). A high-sensitive electrochemical DNA biosensor based on a novel ZnAl/layered double hydroxide modified cobalt ferrite-graphene oxide nanocomposite electrophoretically deposited onto FTO substrate for electroanalytical studies of etoposide. *Talanta* 208 (September 2019): 120444. https://doi.org/10.1016/j.talanta.2019.120444.

164 Molinero-Fernández, Á., Jodra, A., Moreno-Guzmán, M. et al. (2018). Magnetic reduced graphene oxide/nickel/platinum nanoparticles micromotors for mycotoxin analysis. *Chemistry* 24 (28): 7172–7176. https://doi.org/10.1002/chem.201706095.

165 Kim, S.B., Zhang, Y., Won, S.M. et al. (2018). Super-absorbent polymer valves and colorimetric chemistries for time-sequenced discrete sampling and chloride analysis of sweat via skin-mounted soft microfluidics. *Small* 14 (12): 1–11. https://doi.org/10.1002/smll.201703334.

166 Nguyen, P.Q., Soenksen, L.R., Donghia, N.M. et al. (2021). Wearable materials with embedded synthetic biology sensors for biomolecule detection. *Nat. Biotechnol.* 39 (11): 1366–1374. https://doi.org/10.1038/s41587-021-00950-3.

167 Vaquer, A., Barãn, E., and De La Rica, R. (2021). Detection of low glucose levels in sweat with colorimetric wearable biosensors. *Analyst* 146 (10): 3273–3279. https://doi.org/10.1039/d1an00283j.

168 Vaquer, A., Barón, E., and De La Rica, R. (2021). Wearable analytical platform with enzyme-modulated dynamic range for the simultaneous colorimetric detection of sweat volume and sweat biomarkers. *ACS Sens.* 6 (1): 130–136. https://doi.org/10.1021/acssensors.0c01980.

169 Choi, J.H., Choi, M., Ho, T.S. et al. (2019). Soft, skin-integrated multifunctional microfluidic systems for accurate colorimetric analysis of sweat biomarkers and temperature. *ACS Sens.* 4 (2): 379–388. https://doi.org/10.1021/acssensors.8b01218.

170 de Castro, L.F., de Freitas, S.V., Duarte, L.C. et al. (2019). Salivary diagnostics on paper microfluidic devices and their use as wearable sensors for glucose monitoring. *Anal. Bioanal.Chem.* 411 (19): 4919–4928. https://doi.org/10.1007/s00216-019-01788-0.

171 Ardalan, S., Hosseinifard, M., Vosough, M., and Golmohammadi, H. (2020). Towards smart personalized perspiration analysis: An IoT-integrated cellulose-based microfluidic wearable patch for smartphone fluorimetric multi-sensing of sweat biomarkers. *Biosens. Bioelectron.* 168 (August): 112450. https://doi.org/10.1016/j.bios.2020.112450.

172 Deng, M., Song, G., Zhong, K. et al. (2022). Wearable fluorescent contact lenses for monitoring glucose via a smartphone. *Sens. Actuators, B* 352 (2): 131067. https://doi.org/10.1016/j.snb.2021.131067.

173 Xu, X.Y. and Yan, B. (2018). A fluorescent wearable platform for sweat Cl- analysis and logic smart-device fabrication based on color adjustable lanthanide MOFs. *J. Mater. Chem. C* 6 (7): 1863–1869. https://doi.org/10.1039/c7tc05204a.

174 Chang, C.Y., Lin, H.T., Lai, M.S. et al. (2018). Flexible localized surface plasmon resonance sensor with metal–insulator–metal nanodisks on PDMS substrate. *Sci. Rep.* 8: 11812. https://doi.org/10.1038/s41598-018-30180-8.

175 Wang, D., Xu, G., Zhang, X. et al. (2022). Dual-functional ultrathin wearable 3D particle-in-cavity SF-AAO-Au SERS sensors for effective sweat glucose and lab-on-glove pesticide detection. *Sens. Actuators, B* 359: 1–11. https://doi.org/10.1016/j.snb.2022.131512.

176 Choi, J.H., Choi, M., Ho, T.S. et al. (2022). Biological SERS-active sensor platform based on flexible silk fibroin film and gold nanoislands. *Opt. Express* 30 (5): 7782. https://doi.org/10.1364/oe.452665.

177 Liu, R., Jiang, L., Yu, Z. et al. (2021). MXene ($Ti_3C_2T_x$)-Ag nanocomplex as efficient and quantitative SERS biosensor platform by in-situ PDDA electrostatic self-assembly synthesis strategy. *Sens. Actuators, B* 333: 129581. https://doi.org/10.1016/j.snb.2021.129581.

178 Wang, Y., Zhao, C., Wang, J. et al. (2021). Wearable plasmonic-metasurface sensor for noninvasive and universal molecular fingerprint detection on biointerfaces. *Sci. Adv.* 7 (4): 1–11. https://doi.org/10.1126/sciadv.abe4553.

179 Li, X.J., Li, Y.T., Gu, H.X. et al. (2022). A wearable screen-printed SERS array sensor on fire-retardant fibre gloves for on-site environmental emergency monitoring. *Anal. Methods* 14 (8): 781–788. https://doi.org/10.1039/d1ay01981c.

180 He, X., Fan, C., Luo, Y. et al. (2022). Flexible microfluidic nanoplasmonic sensors for refreshable and portable recognition of sweat biochemical fingerprint. *npj Flexible Electron.* 6 (1): 1–10. https://doi.org/10.1038/s41528-022-00192-6.

181 Elsherif, M., Hassan, M.U., Yetisen, A.K., and Butt, H. (2018). Wearable contact lens biosensors for continuous glucose monitoring using smartphones. *ACS Nano* 12 (6): 5452–5462. https://doi.org/10.1021/acsnano.8b00829.

9

Advancement in Optical Biosensors to Detect Malignant Tumors

9.1 Introduction

Human cancer or malignant tumors is a heterogeneous group of diseases almost 277 different types, caused by uncontrolled multiplication of anomalous cells and specific alteration of the molecules [30, 31]. Every year millions of individuals are diagnosed with malignant tumors [32]. In men, liver, prostate, colon, stomach, and lung are the most common types of cancer, while in women colorectal, malignant neoplasm of breast, squamous cell carcinoma, lung, and thyroid carcinoma have been reported [33–37].

The high mortality rate for the roughly 10 million cancer patients diagnosed each year can be reduced with early diagnosis [38]. Currently used conventional methods that include tissue biopsies, computed tomography, enzyme-linked immunosorbent assays, positron emission tomography, magnetic resonance imaging, ultrasound, endoscopy that analyze the phenotypic features of the malignant tissue could not detect the disease at an early stage [39–42]. These techniques are also hindered by several drawbacks, including the need for skilled technicians, large sample volumes, long detection times, and costly equipment [35]. There are several ongoing efforts for earlier diagnosis of the diseases, out of which biosensors are the most promising candidates as they can detect the analyte with better sensitivity, lower detection limit, and less cost. The biosensor structure comprises a bioreceptor that recognize the target, and a transducer element to convert the signal into readable output form [43–45]. Bioreceptors have been reported for various cancers, depending on the nature of the target molecule. Each bioreceptor has its own cons and pros and there is no existence of perfect receptor to detect the

Biosensors: Nanomaterials, Approaches, and Performance-Enhancement Strategies, First Edition. Baljinder Kaur, Santosh Kumar, and Brajesh Kumar Kaushik.

Published 2025 by John Wiley & Sons, Inc.
Companion website: www.wiley.com/go/kaur

tumor. Antibodies, nucleic acids, enzymes, aptamers, bacteriophages, and molecular imprints are used as bioreceptors in the biosensor designs [46–50].

The onset and progression of cancer is related to some specific molecular alterations known as *biomarkers* that can indicate stage of the disease due to their concentration in the sample. A biomarker is a substance either available in tumor tissues or produced by it in the blood or serum that includes nucleic acids, protein, sugars, and enzymes [1, 51–56]. Several techniques involve the individual cell measurement to detect the cancer, as significant alteration in the output parameters can be obtained due to different composition of the diseased cell and normal cell [2–5, 37]. The interaction of cells with incident light leads to several phenomena such as absorption, reflection, and transmission, analyzed to detect the cancer with different technologies. Various optical sensing platforms based on absorption, plasmonic resonance, scattering, fluorescence, and interference have been reported to detect the type of cancer [6]. Numerous cell lines such as HeLa, CCL-224 and 228, HTB-133, MB23, HCC-827, CRL1504, THLE2, CL-188, HepG2, MCF 10A, and MDA have been explored [7–10]. Nanomaterials have been employed to diagnose the cancer-related diseases that include liposomes, quantum dots (QDs) [11, 12], CNT [13], buckyballs and nanodiamonds, metal- or oxide-based nanomaterials [14] (Au, Ag, Al), oxide-based materials [15], polymers, and ceria nanoparticles (NPs) [15–18].

Figure 9.1 shows the classification of NPs that include organic and inorganic [19, 20]. These nanomaterials have desirable characteristics that include controlled size, different shapes, and large surface area. Due to their large surface area, NPs can be functionalized with several molecules – which makes them multifunctional, ability to amplify signals [21]. These properties have been widely used in SERS, plasmonic, and colorimetric sensors for various applications [22]. QDs have been used in fluorescence biosensors, which are semiconducting fluorescent nanocrystals that have high quantum yields, broad absorption spectra, photostability, and resistance to photo-bleaching [23]. NPs can combine with imaging techniques to obtain the more information about the diseases [15]. Because they are multifunctional, nanoparticles can be used for diagnosis and therapy simultaneously as imaging and therapeutic agents can be fixed on the same nanoparticles [24, 25].

9.2 Cancer Biomarkers

Biomarkers indicate disease stage and treatment response that can be measured from different body fluids [51]. Biomarkers can be molecular, cellular, or imaging, depending on their characteristics:

- *Molecular biomarkers* consist of molecular components present in the body proteins, NA, metabolites, and peptides.

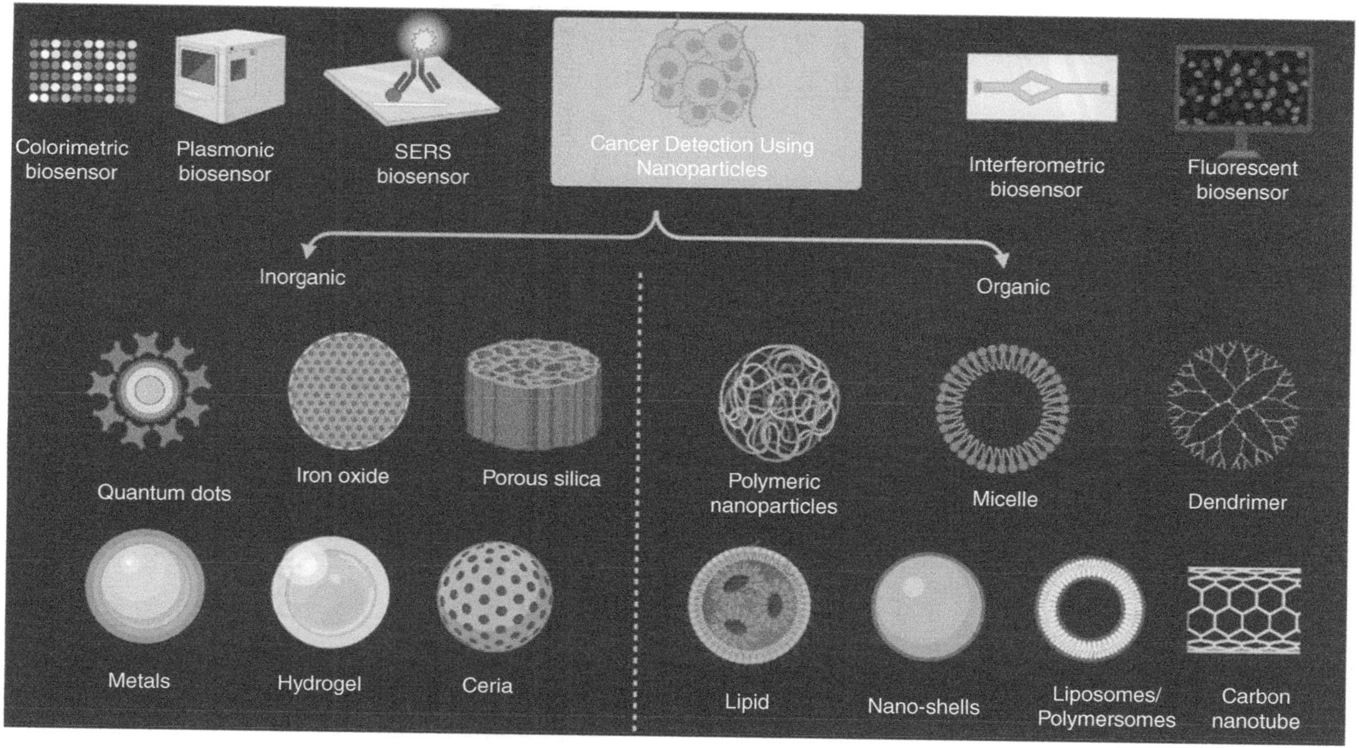

Figure 9.1 An illustration of various types of nanoparticles that include organic and inorganic with different optical platforms to detect the cancer diseases.

Table 9.1 Commonly used biomarkers associated with cancer.

Cancer types	Biomarker details	References
Liver	MicroRNA-122, microRNA-100, microRNA-223, Alpha-fetoprotein (AFP), des-γ-carboxyprot, Midkine, Golgi protein 73 (GP73), squamous cell carcinoma antigen (SCCA)	[1–5]
Lung	Cytokeratin 19, TPA, Kirsten rat sarcoma viral oncogene homolog (KRAS), ALK, HTERT, microRNA-141, microRNA-106A, CEA, CA, epidermal growth factor receptor (EGFR)	[6–11]
Breast	MicroRNA-155, miR-261, plasminogen activator inhibitor 1 (PAI-1), CA-15, CA 15–3, EGFR, HER2, BRCA1, and BRCA2, Ki-67, carcinoembryonic antigen (CEA), urokinase plasminogen activator (uPA),	[12–16]
Prostate	MicroRNA-103a, microRNA-106a, prostate specific antigen, GSTP1, PCA3	[17–21]
Stomach	MicroRNA-29c, microRNA-148a, CEA, and CA	[22–26]
Brain	Methyl guanine DNA methyl transferase (MGMT-O-6), microRNA-10b, COX2, thymosin beta-4	[27–29]

- *Cellular biomarkers* indicate the features and mechanism happening inside the cell, such as circulating tumor cells (CTCs) and CD 20. Numerous biomarkers are reported to monitor the different types and stages of the cancer.
- *Imaging biomarkers* use images to diagnose disease [52]. These biomarkers are dependent on types of cancer, heterogeneity, and reorganization element that include NA, proteins, metabolites, antibodies, and extracellular vesicles [53–56].

Table 9.1 summarized the various biomarkers reported in the literature associated with cancers of the liver, lung breast, prostate, stomach, and brain.

9.3 Types of Optical Biosensors

Optical biosensors use bioreceptor by integrating it with a transducer system that depends on phenomenon such as absorbance, reflectance, luminescence, fluorescence, and phosphorescence in the different regions of electromagnetic spectrum – i.e. ultraviolet, visible, infrared [57]. The output of optical sensor is measured in terms of wavelength shift, phase change, and intensity pattern. The next section discusses various nanomaterials-based sensing platforms to detect the cancer-related diseases.

9.3.1 SPR and LSPR Sensors

In surface plasmon resonance (SPR) phenomenon, the electron cloud is confined along a metal-dielectric interface that occurs due to coupling of incident transverse magnetic polarized electromagnetic light waves and collective oscillations of the electrons cloud moving along the interface [58, 59]. LSPR is restricted to oscillation and limited to nanoparticle having size comparable to the wavelength of light and excitable plasmons that produce more confined field. SPR has a large electric field of 250–1000 nm as compared to LSPR around 20–40 nm. In SPR, it causes a bulk effect that allows detection of both unwanted molecules that are not bonded at the surface and LSPR molecules near the surface [60–64]. Another drawback attached with SPR sensors is the need for adaptive optics to excite the surface plasmon [65].

It is reported that the concentration of exosome is higher in cancerous cells as compared to normal cells. A SPR biosensor using micro-contact imprinting due to its reusability, low cost, and easy fabrication to diagnose the prostate cancer using PSA protein. Ethylene glycol dimetharylate, methacrylic acid, and α-α′-azoisobutyronitrile are used a cross-linker, functional monomer, and initiator [66].

Figure 9.2a shows a nano-disk-based metal–insulator–metal (MIM)-based biosensor structure to detect the lung cancer using A549 cell line with LSPR effect.

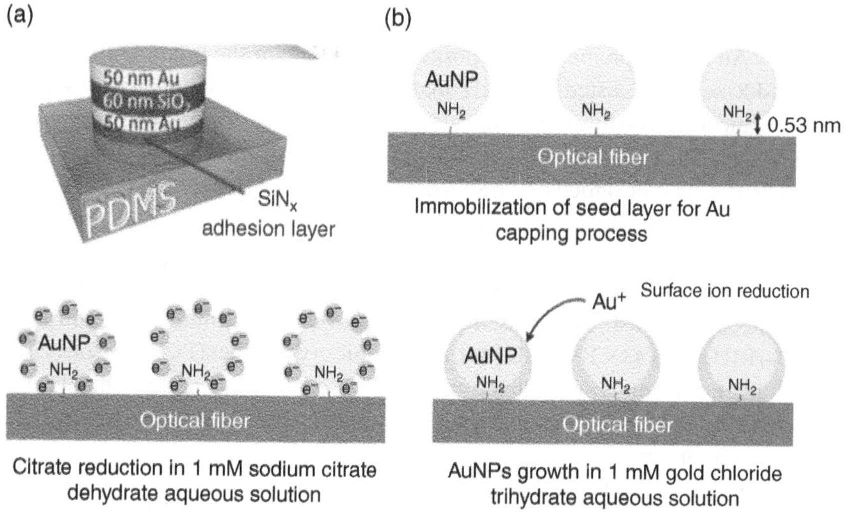

Figure 9.2 Schematic representation of (a) a MIM nano-disk-based LSPR cancer biosensor. *Source:* Adapted from [67]. (b) Immobilization of AuNPs on the fiber surface, attachment of citrate ions to AuNPs, absorption of AuNPs on the surface. *Source:* [68]/with permission of Elsevier.

Polydimethylsiloxane substrate and geometry effect of nano-disks on the sensor performance is investigated in detail. To fabricate the MIM structure, two Au disks and a SiO_2 disk of thicknesses 50 nm, 50 nm, and 60-nm, and a SiNx layer of 240 nm were used. The study was extended to single-, two-, and three-layer MIM disk-based LSPR sensors. A trilayer-based sensor structure with electric field provides a sensitivity of 1670 nm/RIU [67]. Exosomes are used to detect the cancer disease as they are available in abundance in the blood i.e. 10^9 exosomes/ml [69]. An AuNPs-based LSPR sensor using seed-mediated growth and citrate reduction methods is constructed to detect thyroid cancer, as shown in Figure 9.2b. The Turkevich method was used to deposit the nanoparticles on fiber surface, and sodium citrate was used to control the size of particles [68].

An AuNPs-based LSPR sensor to detect the survivin protein produced during bladder cancer in patients. Results are compared with enzyme-linked immunosorbent assay (ELISA) and anti-survivin antibody deposited on AuNPs. It is reported that antibody-AuNPs conjugated structure can detect bladder cancer at an early stage compared to ELISA test that detects the cancer at high grades of the disease [70]. A combination of Au film and Au-NPs has been explored for the potential to more quickly diagnose breast cancer by detecting exosomes at a lower quantity among two breast cancer cell lines (i.e. MCF7 and MCF-10A).

Figure 9.3a shows the dual AuNPs-assisted signal amplification-based SPR structure to detect breast cancer [71]. Hossain et al. numerically simulated a fiber sensor using graphene as 2D material to detect the two breast cancer genes. A high index prism of refractive index (RI) of 1.723 was fixed on a core of fiber followed by Au and graphene layer deposited on the base of the prism [74]. A fiber-based SPR sensor assisted with 2D materials has been investigated to detect various cancerous cell lines that indicate different types of cancers at $\lambda = 1550$ nm, as shown in Figure 9.3b. Results are simulated in case of three probe designs, out of which probe-I is designed using SiO_2 core, per fluorinated polymer clad, Ag and analyte layer; probe-II: SiO_2-clad of polymer material-Ag-MoS_2; and probe III: SiO_2-polymer clad-Ag-graphene. Jurkat, HeLa, PC12, MDA-MB-231, MCF7 cancerous cell lines have been investigated to detect cancers in blood, cervical, adrenal glands, and breast. MoS_2-based probe II provides maximum FOM and LoD 6654.54/RIU and 0.43×10^{-5} RIU [42]. A photonic crystal fiber (PCF) sensor-based on SPR phenomenon is simulated numerically to detect the blood plasma. ITO is used as outside layer of air clad and blood sample is introduced into this air hole for measurement purpose.

A schematic of PCF structure is shown in Figure 9.3c. PCF-based sensor design with MoS_2 is able to provide the LOD and sensitivity of detection limit (DL) of 0.0097 RIU and 6701.03 nm/RIU [72]. An AuNPs-based fiber LSPR cytosensor of Ω-shape is demonstrated to detect breast cancer using the MCF7 cells. Two structures having U-shaped and Ω-shaped fiber structure is explored

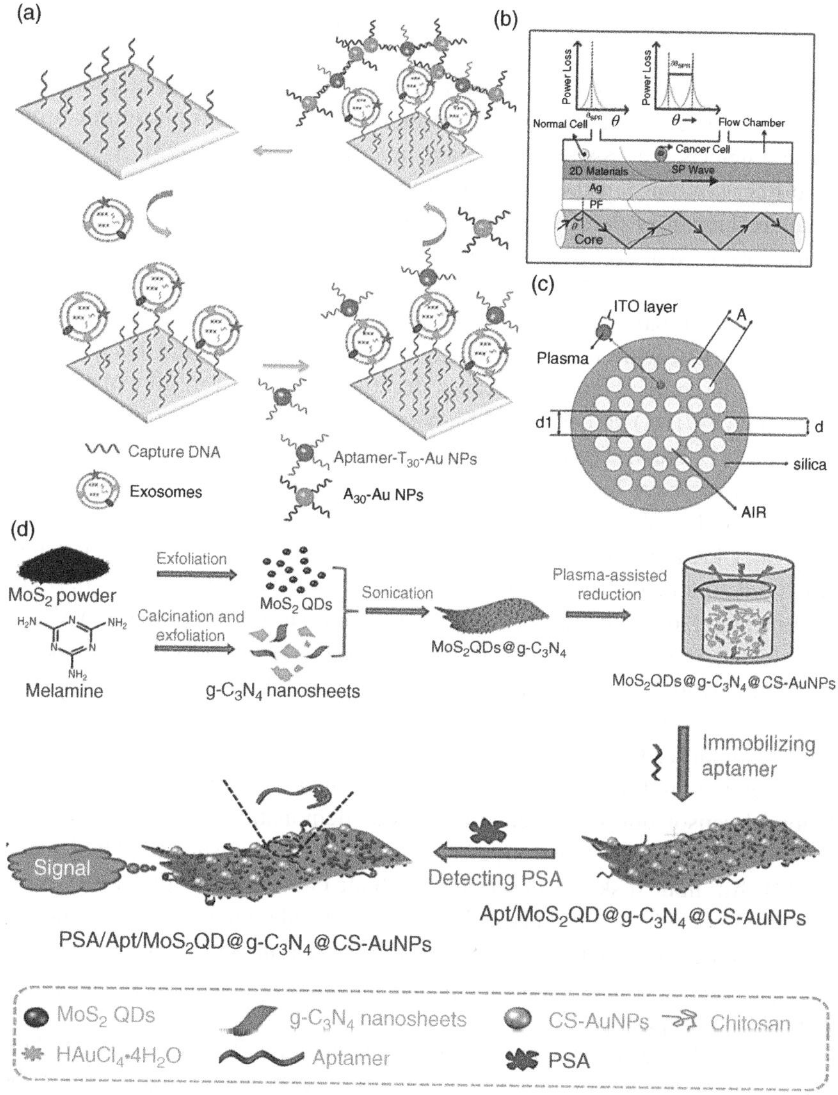

Figure 9.3 Schematic representation of (a) amplification process using dual AuNPs to detect the exosomes. *Source:* [71]/with permission of Elsevier. (b) 2D material-based fiber sensor for cancer cell detection. *Source:* [42]/with permission of IEEE. (c) ITO coated PCF sensor. *Source:* [72]/with permission of Elsevier. (d) MoS_2 and QDs based SPR aptasensor. *Source:* [73]/with permission of Elsevier.

in case of MCF-cell detection [75]. A SPR and electrochemical (ECL) process combined aptasensor is developed using AuNPs and a nanocomposite that consists of carbon nitride (g-C3N4) and MoS_2 QDs to detect the PSA biomarker as shown in Figure 9.3d. This nanocomposite has ECL as well as plasmonic property that detects the PSA with specificity and high sensitivity [73]. A MXenes-based fiber structure in the wavelength interrogation mode has been explored for colorectal cancer detection method, as reported by Kaur et al. Performance of the sensor involves the four MXenes, such as titanium carbide: Ti_3C_2 and titanium carbide with –F, –OH, –O functional groups $Ti_3C_2F_2$, $Ti_3C_2(OH)_2$, and $Ti_3C_2O_2$, are compared with Ag and Au metal to detect the cancer. Ag-MXenes-based sensors provide better sensitivity (10 766.28 nm/RIU) and FOM (76.90/RIU) value as compared to Au-MXenes structures due to lower full width at half maximum (FWHM) values. Ag-Ti_3C_2-based fiberoptic sensors provide LOD of 10^{-4} RIU [41]. AuNPs and bismuth selenide (Bi_2Se_3) nanosheets-based colorimetric sensors have been developed due to their active catalyst properties to detect cancer by using carcinoembryonic antibody (CEA) biomarkers having DL of pg/ml. CEA are glycoproteins involved in the cell adhesion process through which cells interact with each other and attach to surrounding cells [76]. A zirconium metal–organic framework and aptamer-based LSPR sensor with Ag nanoclusters was designed to detect the presence of cancer cells. This nanocomposite has strong bioaffinity, high surface area, excellent ECL properties, and high drug load ability. LOD of LSPR sensor is of order of 4.93 pg/ml for the cancer biomarker CEA having concentration range of 0.01–10 ng/ml [77]. An AuNPs and micro fluidic channel–based LSPR fiber sensor with reduced degradation of sensor due to presence of air was demonstrated for PSA detection in the linear range of 0.1–100 pg/ml [78]. An LSPR sensor fabricated using Au-SiO_2-Au- nano disk was described by Chang et al. to detect the A549 cancer cells that indicates the presence of lung cancer on substrates. The disk structure is fabricated using a SiO_2 layer of 60 nm thickness that is sandwiched between Au films of 50 nm that strongly confines the light in the structure as it can absorb the light perfectly [67].

An AuNPs-based colorimetric sensor with biotinylated BSA switchable linkers that improves the sensitivity by enhancing the signal is reported to detect the prostate-specific antigen (PSA), a biomarker for breast and prostate cancer [79]. An Au-nanoprobe-based colorimetric biosensor to detect the ovarian cancer (A2780 cell line), lung cancer (A549 cell line), breast cancer (MCF7 cell line), thyroid cancer (SW-1736 cell line), gastric cancer (AGS and MKN-45 cell line), and colon cancer (HT-29 cell line) was also reported. Sensors using ribonucleic acid biomarkers such as circulating miRNA-21 and miRNA-15. LOD of ng/μl and sensitivity of ng/μl range are effective for detecting some cancerous cell lines [80]. An elliptical air hole–based PCF-SPR sensor is demonstrated to study the analyte of RI of 1.395 RIU using the finite element method (FEM) method. It consists of more than 20 air holes in the sensor clad; the Au layer is coated on the flat plane and outer surface of the sensor structure [81].

9.3.2 Colorimetric Sensors

In colorimetric methods, a change in color is observed when an analyte binds with the surface; output can be measured in terms of either absorbance or reflected intensity with the use of chemo dyes that changes the color as sensing medium. Glucose oxidase can be used as signal amplification of the protein biomarker. A pH colorimetric sensor is developed the detect the human platelet-derived growth factor-BB biomarker as shown in Figure 9.4a. The alterations of the biomarker are detected in case of ovarian, hepatocellular, pancreatic, breast carcinoma, gastric, osteosarcoma, hematologic carcinoma [82]. A colorimetric sensor using composite of folate, Au, and iron-oxide nanoparticle was investigated to detect the HeLa cells, an indicator of cervical cancer, as shown in Figure 9.4b. Folic acid is used as recognition element and Au-iron-oxide composite nanoparticle transduces the signal. This sensor has LOD of 5 cells/ml [83]. A colorimetric sensor that consists of AuNPs and ascorbic acid was demonstrated for prostate cancer with the help of PSA biomarker. Magnetic microbeads are functionalized with peptides that selectively detect PSA and avoid the interference of various matrix components of taken biosamples [84]. A colorimetric sensor without using enzyme or other techniques for signal enhancement using hydroxy naphthol blue with AuNPs to sense the pancreatic cancer using pseudopodium-enriched atypical kinase one biomarker is demonstrated. This immunoassay can detect tyrosine kinase with 10 ng/ml LOD values with linear range of analyte 10^{-6}–10^{-8} g/ml [85]. A bifunctionalized AuNPs-based colorimetric sensor is developed to sense the four cancer biomarkers simultaneously name as cancer antigens (CA) 125, CA 15-3, CEA, and CA 19.9 in the absence of nonspecific receptors. Two different coating agents with different characteristic group, size, and electrostatic charge is used to increase the sensor performance [86].

9.3.3 Fluorescence Sensors

Fluorescence sensors involve light emission phenomenon, fluorescence, as fluorophores or labeled molecules to absorb electromagnetic light. The output signal is detected using different techniques that include fluorescence intensity measurement [87]. Figure 9.5a shows a graphitic carbon nitride QDs with Au nanoclusters-based fluorescence sensor is for CTCs detection. The fluorescence in graphitic carbon nitride can be tuned from visible to infrared wavelengths, high absorption coefficients, excellent fluorescence quantum yield, good

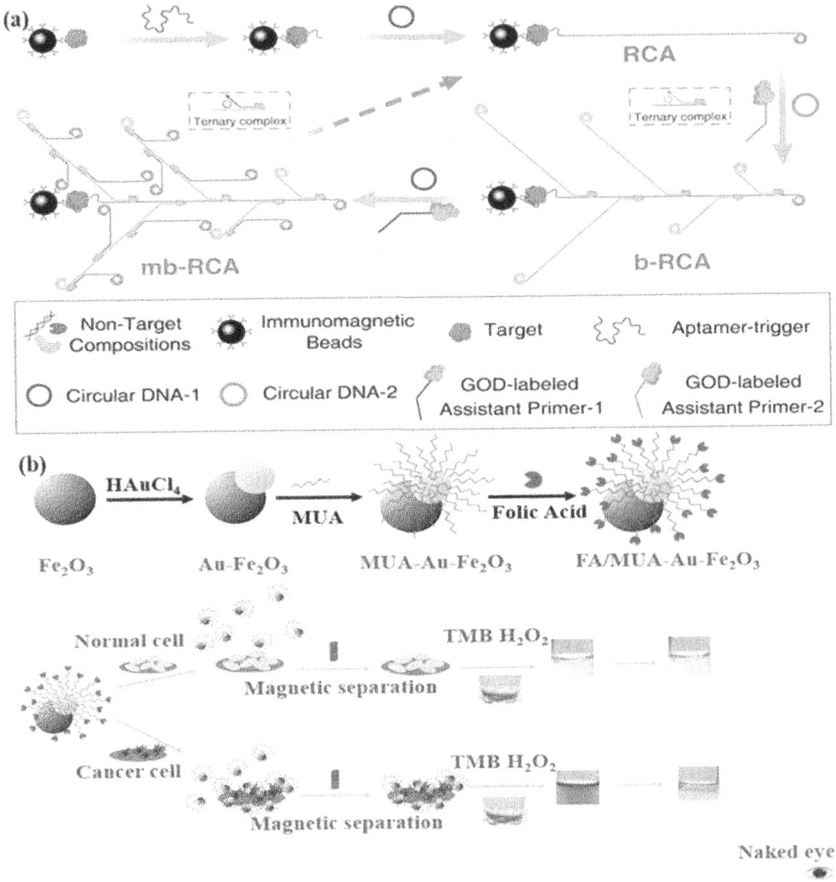

Figure 9.4 Graphic illustration of (a) pH colorimetric-based aptasensor. *Source:* [82]/ With permission of Elsevier. (b) Synthesis steps of folate-conjugated Au-iron-oxide composite nanoparticles based colorimetric sensor. *Source:* [83]/with permission of American Chemical Society.

biocompatibility and high photo-stability [88]. A TLS11a aptamers-based fluorescence sensor is reported to detect liver cancer with HepG2 cell lines. It also consists of two short nucleic acid (i.e. DNA sequences); in the presence of this sequence, aptamers have a hairpin structure that exhibit fluorophore property [91]. A graphene oxide (GO)-aptamer-based fluorescent biosensor is demonstrated by Tan et al. to detect the lymphoblastic leukemia, as shown in Figure 9.5b. GO absorbs the Sgc8 aptamer and quenches the fluorescence as it interacts with aptamer in cancer cells [89]. Zhao et al. reported a protein aptamer-based

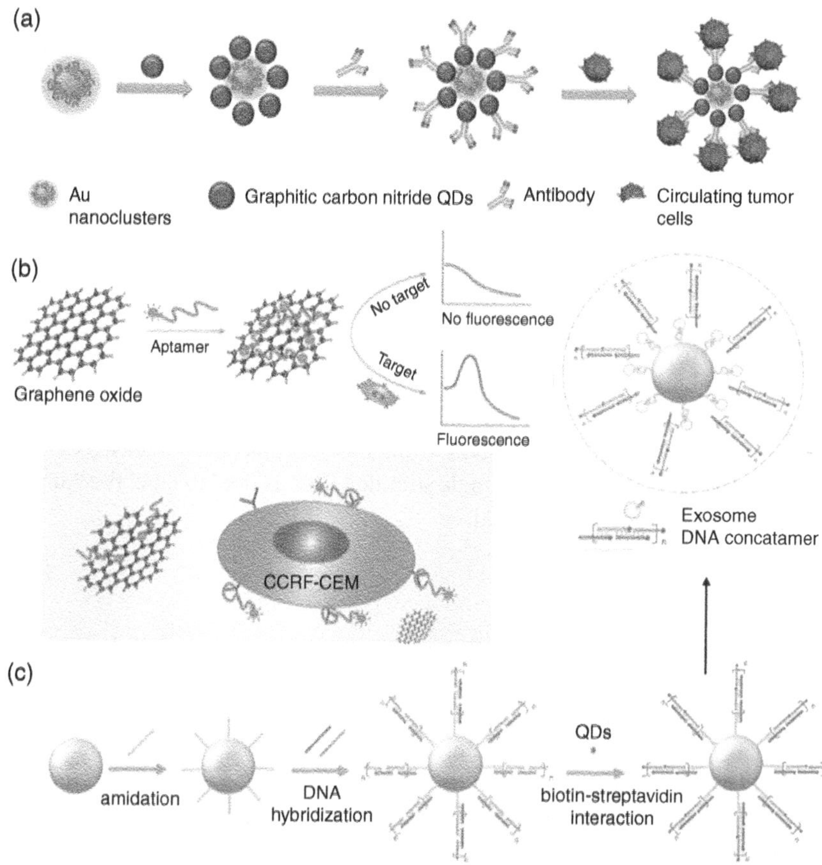

Figure 9.5 Illustration of a (a) fluorescent biosensor that consist of graphitic carbon nitride QDs for CTCs detection *Source:* [88]/with permission of American Chemical Society. (b) graphene oxide-based fluorescent aptasensor. *Source:* [89]/with permission of Springer Nature. (c) QDs-based magnetic and fluorescent biosensor for oral cancer detection using saliva exosome. *Source:* [90]/with permission of Elsevier.

fluorescent sensor that consists of nanosheets of MoS_2 to detect CEA biomarker concentrations that varies from 100 pg/ml to 100 ng/ml. MoS_2 material has high surface-to-volume ratio, high quenching efficiency, excellent stability in liquid solutions as it does not contains dangling bonds, and a tendency to load large number and variety of biomolecules [92]. A Fe_3O_4-graphene quantum dots-MoS_2 complex-based fluorescence sensor was designed to detect the CTCs. Graphene quantum dots are photo-stable, biocompatible, photo-bleaching resistant, and less toxic in nature. Aptamer-assisted complexes and MoS_2 nanosheets are used as donors and quenching purpose [93]. A nitrogen-doped graphene QD synthesized using hydrothermal method and AuNPs have been investigate to study the biosensing properties in case of lung cancer. Graphene QDs have excellent photostability, are soluble in water, and have wide-ranging excitation spectra, biocompatibility, and quantum confinement with strong edge effects as compared to semiconductor and organic dyes–based QDs. Doping of graphene QDs increases the yield, lifetime fluorescence process, and optical and electrical properties [94]. A magnetic and fluorescent biosensor (Figure 9.5c) detects oral cancer using exosomes present in the saliva. The probe is fabricated anchoring the aptamers, magnetic microspheres surface tied up with DNA concatamers that binds the bind CD63 proteins on exosomes and QDs to amplify the signal [90]. A cadmium selenide/zinc sulfide QDs due to availability of large number of holes, electrons, good fluorescence property and AuNPs to diagnose the glycoprotein based CD133 biomarker for stem cell cancer. A single stranded RNA is used to label the AuNPs and sensor has LOD of 6.99 nM [95].

9.3.4 Interferometric Sensors

Figure 9.6a shows a tilted fiber Bragg gratings and 10 nm sized AuNPs based sensor for breast disease detection. The AuNPs are functionalized with MAMA2 aptamer made up of single stranded DNA that binds the proteins present on the surface of cells [96]. An opto-fluidic interferometric sensor made up of microfiber and capillary is demonstrated for miRNA-let7a detection. Fiber structure is tapered using heat source, this tapered region acts as a light waveguide, through which distinct modes are supported. Sensor structure is fabricated using a single-mode fiber and silica capillary placed laterally [98]. Figure 9.6b shows a label free interference-based fiber sensor made up of silica microfiber to detect the EGFR 2 protein present in the breast cells. The antibodies corresponding to protein was used to specifically capture the protein. The protein molecule was measured with sensitivity of 0.1 nm/(ng/ml) [97].

9.3.5 SERS Sensors

The inelastic scattering of light as light interacts with molecules is known as Raman spectroscopy. The intensity of Raman scattering signal is quite low, making it difficult to use in applications. However, this intensity can be enhanced by placing an analyte near the metal surface, known as SERS – surfance-enhanced Raman scattering – which has the ability to detect single molecules, photobleaching resistant, small bandwidth, and excitation in near-infrared region. Due to these advances, SERS has been explored for various applications such as

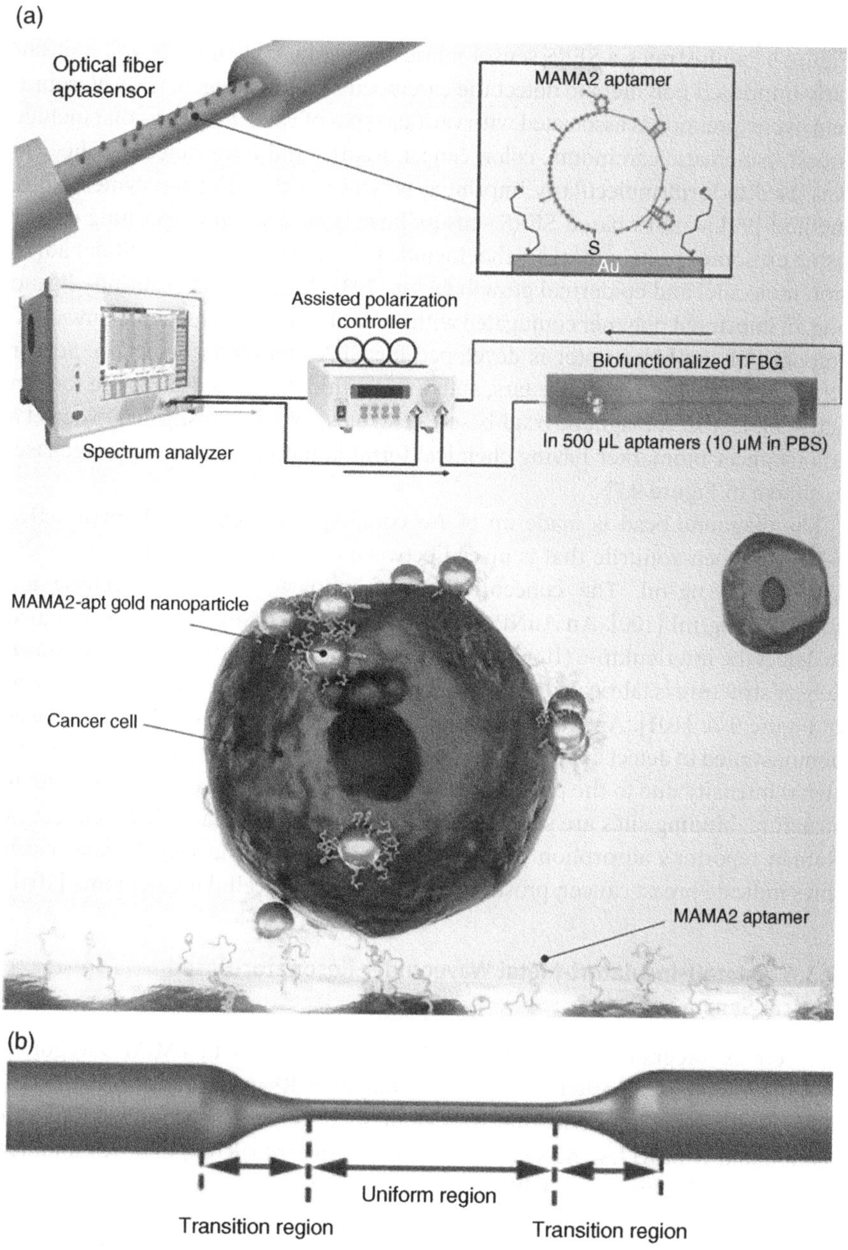

Figure 9.6 Illustration of (a) an optical fiber surface and functionalized AuNPs for breast cancer detection. *Source:* [96]/with Permission of American Chemical Society. (b) A silica microfiber-based interferometric sensor for HER2 detection. *Source:* [97]/with permission of Elsevier.

chemical, bio-sensing, and cyto-sensing that includes whole blood [102]. Figure 9.7a illustrates a SERS sensor fabricated using Au nanostars and molecularly imprinted polymers to detect the carcinoembryonic antigen. CEA glycoprotein overexpression is associated with various types of cancer diseases that include breast, pancreatic carcinoma, colon cancer, gastric, and lung cancer. Gallic acid was used to form molecularly imprinted polymer in the electro-polymerization method [99]. AuNPs-based SERS sensors have been used to detect lung cancer using exosomes protein markers that include CD9, CD81, epithelial cellular adhesion molecule, and epidermal growth factor [103]. A gallic acid as affinity ligand and an imprinted polymer conjugated with an antibody that reduces the unwanted response of the bioreceptor is developed for CEA biomarker detection. Sensor structures consist of Au nanostars, and 4-aminothiophenol is used as the Raman active molecule. A magnetic bead-based SERS biosensor is investigated to detect a colon cancer biomarker having chemical formula indoleamine-2,3-dioxygenase, as shown in Figure 9.7b.

The magnetic bead is made up of Au core, AgNPs shell, and Raman active 4-Mercaptoben-zonitrile that is placed between core and shell that provides the DL of 0.278 ng/ml. The concentrations of indoleamine-2,3-dioxygenase are 15.6–312.5 ng/ml [100]. An AuNPs and aptamer-assisted SERS sensor is designed to detect the interleukin-6 (IL-6) cytokine, a biomarker for lung and breast cancer. Sensor structure is fabricated using Au sputtering on alumina nano-tips, as shown in Figure 9.7c [101]. An Au–Ag bimetallic nanotrepangs-based SERS sensor was demonstrated to detect cancer-related exosomes. Nanotrepangs enhance the SERS signal intensity due to the presence of hotspots, and the signal is stable due to its structure; binding sites are suficient for functionalization that is independent of Raman reporter's adsorption process. SK-BR-3, LNCaP, and HepG2 cancer cell lines indicate breast cancer, prostate cancer, and hepatocellular carcinoma [104].

9.3.6 Metall-Insulatorl-Metal Waveguidel-Resonator-Based Optical Sensors

A racetrack integrated circular cavity side that is coupled with a MIM waveguide-based sensor was reported to detect the analyte in RI in the range of 1.31–1.37 RIU. The coupling of cavity and waveguide increases the light interaction with matter, and it provides the sensitivity value of 1400 nm/RIU [105]. An another MIM waveguide coupling with hexagonal ring resonator was designed using FDTD method to detect the cancer cells. The sensitivity and resolution of biosensor was found to be 2547 nm/RIU and is 3.92×10^{-6} RIU at the resonating wavelength of 2049.9 nm [106]. Another rectangular cavity coupled through nanorod and MIM-waveguide-based sensor was demonstrated to detect the cancer cells and glucose solution. Sensitivity values of 2290 and 2315 nm/RIU were obtained

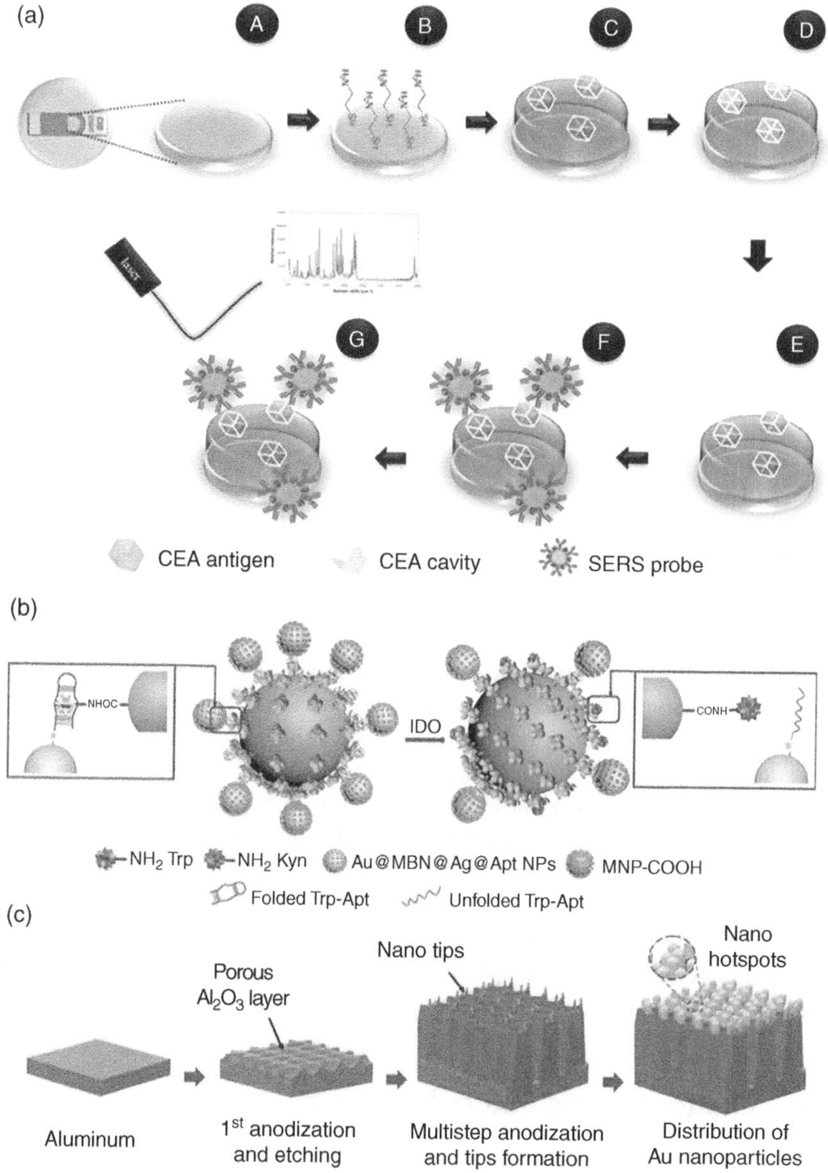

Figure 9.7 Biosensor structure of (a) a polymer imprinted SERS sensor. *Source:* [99]/with permission of Elsevier. (b) A magnetic bead-based SERS biosensor is investigated to detect a colon cancer detection mechanism of Indoleamine-2,3-dioxygenase biomarker. *Source:* [100]/with permission of Elsevier. (c) AuNPs and aptamer based SERS biosensor. *Source:* [101]/with permission of Elsevier.

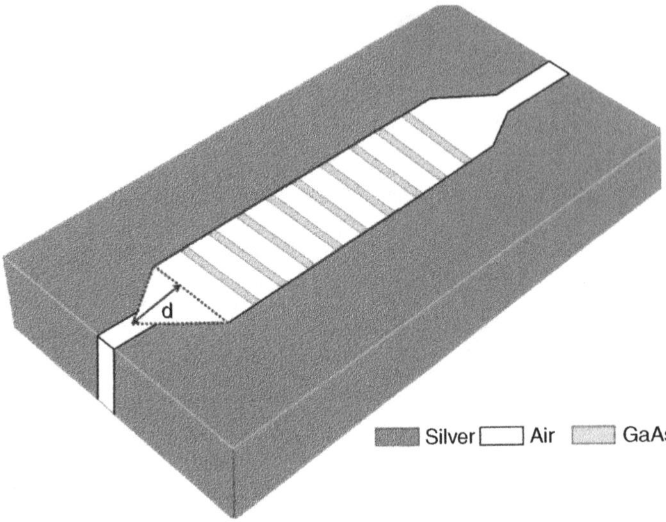

Figure 9.8 Schematic illustration of the photonic crystal and two MIM plasmonic waveguide-based cancer sensor. *Source:* [107]/with permission of Springer Nature.

in case of cancer cell and glucose solution [106]. Figure 9.8 shows a one-dimensional photonic crystal and two MIM plasmonic waveguide with sharp edges are reported to detect the basal cancer cells using FDTD. Two structures are investigated for sensing purpose one is without tapering and second design in tapered resonators are used that enhances the transmittance values. The effect of GaAs layers, lattice constant of the structure and width of the rectangular resonator on the performance of sensor is discussed in detail. GaAs layers are used for insulating layer. Sensitivity of 718.6 nm/RIU and FOM of 156.217/RIU was achieved with the MIM-based sensor [107]. Table 9.2 provides the details of various nanomaterials utilized in optical sensors designs and their performance in terms of limit of detection and linear range.

9.4 Challenges and Future Prospects

Nanomaterial-based biosensors improve signal intensity due to enhanced interaction between nanoparticles and sensing analyte medium, quantum confinement, and can detect smaller concentrations as specific bioreceptor can be attached with nanomaterials. There are several advantages and drawbacks with each technique and different nanomaterials. Currently used diagnostic methods can detect a single analyte or type of cancer at a one time; it is imperative to focus on developing

Table 9.2 Nanomaterials-based sensors.

Mechanism	Nanomaterials	Analyte	Linear range	LoD	Refs.
SPR	n.r.[a]	PSA	0.1–50 ng/ml	91 pg/ml	[66]
LSPR	AuNPs	Thyroid cell	1 pg/ml–10 ng/ml	0.19 pg/ml	[68]
Ω-shaped	AuNPs	MCF cells	$5\times10^{1}\sim1\times10^{5}$ cells/ml	12 cells/ml	[75]
Fluorescence	MoS_2 nanosheets	cancer	100–100 ng/ml	n.r.[a]	[58]
Fluorescence	CdSe/ZnSe sulfide QDs	Stem cell cancer	n.r.[a]	6.99 nM	[59]
Colorimetric	Folate-conjugated Au-iron-oxide composite nanoparticles	Cervical cancer	50–500 cells/ml	5 cells/ml	[83]
Fluorescence	Graphitic carbon nitride QDs	Epithelial cancers	2–400 cells/ml	1 cell/ml	[88]
Fluorescence	Fe_3O_4 and graphene QDs	Circulating tumor cells	2–64 nM	1.19 nM	[93]
Fluorescence	Graphene QDs and AuNPs	PSA	0.0001–1000 ng/ml	0.09 pg/ml	[94]
Fluorescence	Streptavidin- combined QDs	Oral cancer	500–105 particles/μl	500 particles/μl	[90]
Interference	AuNPs	Breast cancer cells	n.r.[a]	49 cells/ml	[96]
Interference	n.r.[a]	miRNA-let7a	2 nM–20 μM	1.43 ng/ml	[98]
SERS	Au nanostars	CEA	1–1000 ng/ml	1 ng/ml	[99]
SERS	Au and Ag NPs	Colon cancer	3.125–625 ng/ml	0.278 ng/ml	[100]
SERS	AuNPs	Lung, breast cancer	10^{-12}–10^{-7} M	0.8 pM	[101]
SERS	Bimetallic nanotrepangs	Multiple cancer	n.r.[a]	35 particles/μl	[104]
Racetrack integrated circular cavity	AuNPs	Basal cancer	1.36–1.38 RIU	n.r.[a]	[105]

[a] Not reported.

multiplexed detection techniques. In the case of fluorescent biosensors, QDs are widely explored for *in vitro* and *in vivo* measurements due to photostability and ability to excite different color QDs with the help of a single excitation light [108]. QDs have been implemented in live cell imaging to visualize multiple events simultaneously and single cell detection. QDs in combination with various organic and inorganic particle are being used for cancer diagnosis and treatment purposes [108].

Drawbacks associated with QDs include toxicity and *in vivo* cytotoxic, which can be reduced to some extent through functionalization of different molecules [108]. Toxicity and biocompatibility are associated with all types of organic and inorganic nanoparticles, so investigation for individual issues is required instead of generalization. Currently used optical techniques have low-sensitivity limited lifespan of biosensors, and high detection limits that need to improve for sensitive detection. Another challenge with nanomaterials-based biosensing techniques is detecting the cancer at an early stage, as tumors detected at 1 cm^3 indicate metastatic stage 1.

9.5 Summary

This chapter discusses various nanoparticles, technologies, and biomarkers associated with each type of cancer. Progress and improvements among various optical platforms to detect the several types of cancer are discussed in detail. Advancements in the different optical biosensors to detect the cancer are summarized in this chapter. Among all types of cancer disease, lung cancer has the highest death rate (i.e. 23% of cancer death due to all types of cancer). Therefore, there is great demand for a biomarker that is highly sensitive with lower DL for cancer-affected tissue samples. Antibodies, NA, and aptamers are used as molecular recognition unit; aptamers are a promising alternative to antibodies and are widely reported in literature for cancer detection due to easy synthesis steps, high stability, easy modification, low cost, rapid penetration in tissues, and low toxicity.

Protein biomarkers are available in low amounts and cannot be amplified like NA, as they cannot be replicated. Protein biomarkers cannot be detected at low concentrations as they are very sensitive to the surrounding environment, pH, temperature, and ion strength. In the presence of other protein in abundance, it is tedious to detect the specific type of protein directly. Among the vast variety of biomarkers, a single biomarker is not sufficient to detect one or various categories of cancer for early detection; therefore protein biomarkers exist as a complement only to current clinical technologies. The quantity of biomarkers is quite low in the different fluids of body; therefore, different amplification strategies such as dual AuNPs, 2D materials, hydroxy naphthol blue that does not require enzyme, glucose oxidase, and several nanostructures have been pursued.

References

1 Mansouri, V., Razzaghi, M., Nikzamir, A. et al. (2020). Assessment of liver cancer biomarkers. *Liver Cancer Biomarkers* 13 (6): S29–S39.

2 Chen, F., Wang, J., Wu, Y. et al. (2022). Potential biomarkers for liver cancer diagnosis based on multi-omics strategy. *Front. Oncol.* 12: 1–11. https://doi.org/10.3389/fonc.2022.822449.

3 Omar, M.A. et al. (2023). Biomarkers for hepatocellular carcinoma: from origin to clinical diagnosis. *Biomedicines* 11: 1852.

4 Chen, J., Niu, C., Yang, N. et al. (2023). Biomarker discovery and application—an opportunity to resolve the challenge of liver cancer diagnosis and treatment. *Pharmacol. Res.* 189: 106674. https://doi.org/10.1016/j.phrs.2023.106674.

5 Shahini, E., Pasculli, G., Solimando, A.G. et al. (2023). Updating the clinical application of blood biomarkers and their algorithms in the diagnosis and surveillance of hepatocellular Carcinoma: a critical review. *Int. J. Mol. Sci. Rev.* 24: 4286.

6 Melichar, B. (2023). Biomarkers in the management of lung cancer: changing the practice of thoracic oncology. *Chin. Chem. Lab. Med.* 61 (5): 906–920. https://doi.org/10.1515/cclm-2022-1108.

7 Wang, F., Su, Q., and Li, C. (2022). Identification of novel biomarkers in non - small cell lung cancer using machine learning. *Sci Rep* 12 (16693): 1–15. https://doi.org/10.1038/s41598-022-21050-5.

8 Herath, S., Rad, H.S., Radfar, P. et al. (2022). The role of circulating biomarkers in lung cancer. *Front. Oncol.* 11: 801269. https://doi.org/10.3389/fonc.2021.801269.

9 Villalobos, P. and Wistuba, I.I. (2017). Lung cancer biomarkers guideline. *Hematol. Oncol. Clin.* 31 (1): 13–29. doi: 10.1016/j.hoc.2016.08.006.

10 Lai, L., Ren, Y., Huai, Y. et al. (2023). Identification and validation of novel prognostic biomarkers and therapeutic targets for non-small cell lung cancer. *Front. Genet.* 14: 1139994. https://doi.org/10.3389/fgene.2023.1139994.

11 Davies, M.P.A., Sato, T., Ashoor, H. et al. (2023). Plasma protein biomarkers for early prediction of lung cancer. *Lancet* 93: 1–11. https://doi.org/10.1016/j.ebiom.2023.104686.

12 Zubair, M., Wang, S., and Ali, N. (2021). Advanced approaches to breast cancer classification and diagnosis. *Front. Pharmacol.* 11: 632079. https://doi.org/10.3389/fphar.2020.632079.

13 Starzer, A.M., Berghoff, A.S., and Bartsch, R. (2023). Biomarkers and translational research approaches in breast cancer – an update. *Memo* 16: 42–46.

14 Mandair, D. and Reis-filho, J.S. (2026). Biological insights and novel biomarker discovery through deep learning approaches in breast cancer histopathology. *NPJ Breast Cancer* 21: 1–11. https://doi.org/10.1038/s41523-023-00518-1.

15 Frauchiger-heuer, H. and Ring, A. (2023). Breast cancer: targets and therapy 'diagnostic and prognostic biomarkers of luminal breast cancer: where are we now?'. *Breast Cancer Targets Ther.* 15: 525–540.

16 Neves, L., Alves, R., Meira, D. et al. (2023). Biomarkers in breast cancer: an old story with a new end. *Genes* 14 (7): 1364.

17 Malode, S.J. and Shetti, N.P. (2022). New generation biomarkers for the detection of prostate cancer. *Biosens. Bioelectron.: X* 12: 100250. https://doi.org/10.1016/j.biosx.2022.100250.

18 Alarcón-zendejas, A.P., Scavuzzo, A., Jiménez-ríos, M.A. et al. (2022). The promising role of new molecular biomarkers in prostate cancer: from coding and non-coding genes to artificial intelligence approaches. *Prostate Cancer Prostatic Dis.* 25: 431–443. https://doi.org/10.1038/s41391-022-00537-2.

19 Samora, N.L., Tallman, J.E., and Tosoian, J.J. (2022). The evolving clinical use of prostate cancer biomarkers. *Prostate Cancer Prostatic Dis.* 25: 386–387. https://doi.org/10.1038/s41391-022-00567-w.

20 Singh, B., Ma, S., Hara, T.O., and Singh, S. (2023). Nanomaterials-based biosensors for the detection of prostate cancer biomarkers: recent trends and future perspective. *Adv. Mater. Technol.* 8: 2201860. https://doi.org/10.1002/admt.202201860.

21 Armstrong, A.J. (2023). Current developments in the management of prostate cancer predictive biomarkers in advanced prostate cancer. *Clin. Adv. Hematol. Oncol.* 21 (6): 290–293.

22 Sato, Y., Okamoto, K., Kawano, Y. et al. (2023). Novel biomarkers of gastric cancer: current research and future perspectives. *J. Clin. Med. Rev.* 12: 4646.

23 Hong, X. and Liu, F. (2022). Molecular biomarkers for gastric cancer. *Front. Oncol.* 12: 850373. https://doi.org/10.3389/fonc.2022.850373.

24 Zhang, Z., Wu, H., Chong, W. et al. (2022). Liquid biopsy in gastric cancer: predictive and prognostic biomarkers. *Cell Death Dis.* (May): https://doi.org/10.1038/s41419-022-05350-2.

25 Röcken, C. (2023). Predictive biomarkers in gastric cancer. *J. Cancer Res. Clin. Oncol.* 149 (1): 467–481. https://doi.org/10.1007/s00432-022-04408-0.

26 Jiang, T., Mei, L., Yang, X. et al. (2022). Heliyon biomarkers of gastric cancer: current advancement. *Heliyon* 8 (July): e10899. https://doi.org/10.1016/j.heliyon.2022.e10899.

27 Ghorbani, A., Avery, L.M., Sohaei, D. et al. (2023). Discovery of novel glioma serum biomarkers by proximity extension assay. *Clin. Proteomics* 1–12. https://doi.org/10.1186/s12014-023-09400-5.

28 Nguyen, H.D. (2023). Prognostic biomarker prediction for glioma induced by heavy metals and their mixtures: an in-silico study. *Toxicol. Appl. Pharmacol.* 459: 116356. https://doi.org/10.1016/j.taap.2022.116356.

29 Lehner, K.R., Jiang, K., Rincon-torroella, J. et al. (2023). Neoplasia cerebrospinal fluid biomarkers in pediatric brain tumors: a systematic. *Neoplasia* 35: 100852. https://doi.org/10.1016/j.neo.2022.100852.

30 Yang, G., Xiao, Z., Tang, C. et al. (2019). Recent advances in biosensor for detection of lung cancer biomarkers. *Biosens. Bioelectron.* 141: 111416. https://doi.org/10.1016/j.bios.2019.111416.

31 Chen, Y., Liu, J., Yang, Z. et al. (2019). Optical biosensors based on refractometric sensing schemes: a review. *Biosens. Bioelectron.* 144: 111693. https://doi.org/10.1016/j.bios.2019.111693.

32 Cui, F., Zhou, Z., and Zhou, H.S. (2020). Review-measurement and analysis of cancer biomarkers based on electrochemical biosensors. *J. Electrochem. Soc.* 167 (3): 037525.

33 Zhang, P.W., Chen, L., Huang, T. et al. (2015). Classifying ten types of major cancers based on reverse phase protein array profiles. *PLoS One* 10 (3): 1–16.

34 Bertozzi, C. (2022). A special virtual issue celebrating the 2022 Nobel prize in chemistry for the development of click chemistry and bioorthogonal chemistry. *ACS Cent. Sci.* I: 2–3. https://doi.org/10.1021/acscentsci.2c01430.

35 Kaur, B., Kumar, S., and Kaushik, B.K. (2022). Recent advancements in optical biosensors for cancer detection. *Biosens. Bioelectron.* 197: 113805.

36 Kaur, B., Kumar, S., and Kumar, B. (2022). Advances in photonic crystal fiber: sensing and supercontinuum generation applications. *Opt. Fiber Technol.* 72: 102982.

37 Kaur, B., Kumar, S., and Kaushik, B.K. (2023). Novel wearable optical sensors for vital health monitoring systems—a review. *Biosensors* 13 (2): 181.

38 Hassanpour, S.H. and Dehghani, M. (2017). Review of cancer from perspective of molecular. *J. Cancer Res. Pract.* 4 (4): 127–129.

39 Addanki, S., Amiri, I.S., and Yupapin, P. (2018). Review of optical fibers-introduction and applications in fiber lasers. *Results Phys.* 10 (June): 743–750. https://doi.org/10.1016/j.rinp.2018.07.028.

40 Wang, L. (2017). Early diagnosis of breast cancer. *Sensors* 17 (7): 1572.

41 Kaur, B., Kumar, S., and Kaushik, B.K. (2022). MXenes-based fiber-optic SPR sensor for colorectal cancer diagnosis. *IEEE Sens. J.* 22 (7): 6661–6668.

42 Kaur, B., Kumar, S., and Kaushik, B.K. (2021). 2D materials based fiber optic SPR biosensor for cancer detection at 1550 nm. *IEEE Sens. J.* 21 (21): 23957–23964.

43 Bellassai, N., D'Agata, R., Jungbluth, V., and Spoto, G. (2019). Surface plasmon resonance for biomarker detection: advances in non-invasive cancer diagnosis. *Front. Chem.* 7: 1–16.

44 Singh, R., Kumar, S., Liu, F.Z. et al. (2020). Etched multicore fiber sensor using copper oxide and gold nanoparticles decorated graphene oxide structure for cancer cells detection. *Biosens. Bioelectron.* 168: 112557. https://doi.org/10.1016/j.bios.2020.112557.

45 Wang, Y., Huang, Y., Bai, H. et al. (2021). Biocompatible and biodegradable polymer optical fiber for biomedical application: a review. *Biosensors* 11 (12): 1–30. https://doi.org/10.3390/bios11120472.

46 Inan, H., Poyraz, M., Inci, F. et al. (2017). Photonic crystals: emerging biosensors and their promise for point-of-care applications. *Chem. Soc. Rev.* 46 (2): 366–388. https://doi.org/10.1039/c6cs00206d.

47 Wang, Z., Zhang, W., Liu, X. et al. (2022). Novel optical fiber-based structures for plasmonics sensors. *Biosensors* 12 (11): 1–40. https://doi.org/10.3390/bios12111016.

48 Li, M., Singh, R., Wang, Y. et al. (2022). Advances in novel nanomaterial-based optical fiber biosensors—a review. *Biosensors* 12 (10): 843.

49 Chaudhary, V.S., Kumar, D., Pandey, B.P., and Kumar, S. (2022). Advances in photonic crystal fiber-based sensor for detection of physical and biochemical parameters - a review. *IEEE Sens. J.* 23 (2): 1012–1023. https://doi.org/10.1109/JSEN.2022.3222969.

50 Singh, R. and Kumar, S. (2022). Cancer targeting and diagnosis: recent trends with carbon nanotubes. *Nanomaterials* 12: 2283. https://doi.org/10.3390/nano12132283.

51 Bodaghi, A., Fattahi, N., and Ramazani, A. (2023). Biomarkers: promising and valuable tools towards diagnosis, prognosis and treatment of Covid-19 and other diseases. *Heliyon* 9 (2): e13323. https://doi.org/10.1016/j.heliyon.2023.e13323.

52 Wu, M., Zhang, M.Y., Zhang, M.Y. et al. (2019). Imaging-based biomarkers for predicting and evaluating cancer immunotherapy response. *Radiol. Imaging Cancer* 1 (2): e190031.

53 Mittal, S., Kaur, H., Gautam, N., and Mantha, A.K. (2017). Biosensors for breast cancer diagnosis: a review of bioreceptors, biotransducers and signal amplification strategies. *Biosens. Bioelectron.* 88: 217–231.

54 Mendes, I.L., das Neves, M.F., and Lopes, F.S. (2019). Biosensor applicability in breast cancer diagnosis. *Int. J. Biosens. Bioelectron.* 5 (4): 125–130. https://doi.org/10.15406/ijbsbe.2019.05.00165.

55 Venkatesan, M., Veeramuthu, L., Liang, F.C. et al. (2020). Evolution of electrospun nanofibers fluorescent and colorimetric sensors for environmental toxicants, pH, temperature, and cancer cells – a review with insights on applications. *Chem. Eng. J.* 397 (May): 125431.

56 Fukuyama, S., Kumamoto, S., Nagano, S. et al. (2021). Detection of cancer cells in whole blood using a dynamic deformable microfilter and a nucleic acid aptamer. *Talanta* 228 (February): 122239. https://doi.org/10.1016/j.talanta.2021.122239.

57 Hamola, J. (2008). Surface plasmon resonance sensors for detection of chemical and biological species. *Chem. Rev.* 108 (2): 462–493.

58 Kaur, B., Kumar, S., and Kaushik, B.K. (2023). Trends, challenges, and advances in optical sensing for pathogenic bacteria detection (PathoBactD). *Biosens. Bioelectron.: X* 14: 100352. https://doi.org/10.1016/j.biosx.2023.100352.

59 Wang, Y., Singh, R., Li, M. et al. (2023). Cardiac Troponin I detection using assisted hetro-core fiber structure. *IEEE Trans. Nanobiosci.* 22 (2): 375–382. https://doi.org/10.1109/TNB.2022.3192491.

60 Kumari, A., Member, G.S., Vyas, V. et al. (2023). Black phosphorous-based highly sensitive surface plasmonic sensor for detection of formalin. *IEEE Trans. Plasma Sci.* 51 (1): 140–147. https://doi.org/10.1109/TPS.2022.3233699.

61 Wang, Z., Singh, R., Marques, C. et al. (2021). Taper-in-taper fiber structure-based LSPR sensor for alanine aminotransferase detection. *Opt. Express* 29 (26): 43793. https://doi.org/10.1364/oe.447202.

62 He, Y.J. (2014). High-performance LSPR fiber sensor based on nanometal rings. *IEEE Photonics J.* 6 (2): https://doi.org/10.1109/JPHOT.2014.2306828.

63 He, Y.J. (2013). Novel D-shape LSPR fiber sensor based on nano-metal strips. *Opt. Express* 21 (20): 23498. https://doi.org/10.1364/oe.21.023498.

64 Semwal, V. and Gupta, B.D. (2018). LSPR- and SPR-based fiber-optic cholesterol sensor using immobilization of cholesterol oxidase over silver nanoparticles coated graphene oxide nanosheets. *IEEE Sens. J.* 18 (3): 1039–1046. https://doi.org/10.1109/JSEN.2017.2779519.

65 Gupta, B.D., Srivastava, S.K., and Verma, R. (2015). *Fiber Optic Sensors Based on Plasmonics*. Singapore: World Scientific Publishing.

66 Ertürk, G., Özen, H., Tümer, M.A. et al. (2016). Microcontact imprinting based surface plasmon resonance (SPR) biosensor for real-time and ultrasensitive detection of prostate specific antigen (PSA) from clinical samples. *Sens. Actuators, B* 224: 823–832.

67 Chang, C.Y., Lin, H.T., Lai, M.S. et al. (2018). Flexible localized surface plasmon resonance sensor with metal–insulator–metal nanodisks on PDMS substrate. *Sci. Rep.* 8: 11812. https://doi.org/10.1038/s41598-018-30180-8.

68 Kim, H.M., Hong Jeong, D., Lee, H.Y. et al. (2019). Improved stability of gold nanoparticles on the optical fiber and their application to refractive index sensor based on localized surface plasmon resonance. *Opt. Laser Technol.* 114: 171–178. https://doi.org/10.1016/j.optlastec.2019.02.002.

69 Dilsiz, N. (2020). Role of exosomes and exosomal microRNAs in cancer. *Future Sci. OA* 6 (4): FSO465. https://doi.org/10.2144/fsoa-2019-0116.

70 Jazayeri, M.H., Aghaie, T., Nedaeinia, R. et al. (2020). Rapid noninvasive detection of bladder cancer using survivin antibody-conjugated gold nanoparticles (GNPs) based on localized surface plasmon resonance (LSPR). *Cancer Immunol., Immunother.* 69 (9): 1833–1840. https://doi.org/10.1007/s00262-020-02559-y.

71 Wang, Q., Zou, L., Yang, X. et al. (2019). Direct quantification of cancerous exosomes via surface plasmon resonance with dual gold nanoparticle-assisted signal amplification. *Biosens. Bioelectron.* 135: 129–136.

72 Rajeswari, D. and Revathi, A.A. (2022). Highly sensitive SPR-based PCF bio sensor for plasma cell detection in human blood for the detection of early stage cancer. *Optik (Stuttg)* 258: 168897.

73 Duan, F., Zhang, S., Yang, L. et al. (2018). Bifunctional aptasensor based on novel two-dimensional nanocomposite of MoS_2 quantum dots and g-C3N4 nanosheets decorated with chitosan-stabilized Au nanoparticles for selectively detecting prostate specific antigen. *Anal. Chim. Acta* 1036: 121–132.

74 Hossain, M.B., Islam, M.M., Abdulrazak, L.F. et al. (2020). Graphene-coated optical fiber SPR biosensor for BRCA1 and BRCA2 breast cancer biomarker detection: a numerical design-based analysis. *Photonic Sensors* 10 (1): 67–79.

75 Luo, Z., Xu, Y., He, L. et al. (2021). Development of a rapid and ultra-sensitive cytosensor: Ω-shaped fiber optic LSPR integrated with suitable AuNPs coverage. *Sens. Actuators, B* 336: 129706. https://doi.org/10.1016/j.snb.2021.129706.

76 Xiao, L., Zhu, A., Xu, Q. et al. (2017). Colorimetric biosensor for detection of cancer biomarker by Au nanoparticle-decorated Bi_2Se_3 nanosheets. *ACS Appl. Mater. Interfaces* 9 (8): 6931–6940.

77 Guo, C., Su, F., Song, Y. et al. (2017). Aptamer-templated silver nanoclusters embedded in zirconium metal-organic framework for bifunctional electrochemical and SPR aptasensors toward carcinoembryonic antigen. *Appl. Mater. Interfaces* 9 (47): 41188–41199. https://doi.org/10.1021/acsami.7b14952.

78 Uh, M., Kim, J.S., Park, J.H. et al. (2017). Fabrication of localized surface plasmon resonance sensor based on optical fiber and micro fluidic channel. *J. Nanosci. Nanotechnol.* 17 (2): 1083–1091. https://doi.org/10.1166/jnn.2017.12771.

79 Hahn, J., Kim, E., You, Y., and Choi, Y.J. (2019). Colorimetric switchable linker-based bioassay for ultrasensitive detection of prostate-specific antigen as a cancer biomarker. *Analyst* 144 (14): 4439–4446.

80 Mollasalehi, H. and Shajari, E. (2021). A colorimetric nano-biosensor for simultaneous detection of prevalent cancers using unamplified cell-free ribonucleic acid biomarkers. *Bioorg. Chem.* 107: 104605.

81 Chao, C.T.C., Kooh, M.R.R., Chau, Y.F.C., and Thotagamuge, R. (2022). Susceptible plasmonic photonic crystal fiber sensor with elliptical air holes and external-flat gold-coated surface. *Photonics* 9: 916. https://doi.org/10.3390/photonics9120916.

82 Miao, X., Zhu, Z., Jia, H. et al. (2020). Colorimetric detection of cancer biomarker based on enzyme enrichment and pH sensing. *Sens. Actuators, B* 320: 128435.

83 Teng, Y., Shi, J., and Pong, P.W.T. (2019). Sensitive and specific colorimetric detection of cancer cells based on folate-conjugated gold-iron-oxide composite nanoparticles. *ACS Appl. Nano Mater.* 2 (11): 7421–7431.

84 Xia, N., Deng, D., Wang, Y. et al. (2018). Gold nanoparticle-based colorimetric method for the detection of prostate-specific antigen. *Int. J. Nanomed.* 13: 2521–2530. https://doi.org/10.2147/IJN.S154046.

85 Prasad, K.S., Abugalyon, Y., Li, C. et al. (2020). A new method to amplify colorimetric signals of paper-based nanobiosensors for simple and sensitive pancreatic cancer biomarker detection. *Analyst* 145 (15): 5113–5117.

86 Bordbar, M.M., Samadinia, H., Sheini, A. et al. (2022). A colorimetric electronic tongue based on bi-functionalized AuNPs for fingerprint detection of cancer markers. *Sens. Actuators, B* 368 (February): 132170. [Online]. https://doi.org/10.1016/j.snb.2022.132170.

87 Nawrot, W., Drzozga, K., Baluta, S. et al. (2018). A fluorescent biosensors for detection vital body fluids' agents. *Sensors* 18 (8): 1–21. https://doi.org/10.3390/s18082357.

88 Yu, Y., Yang, Y., Ding, J. et al. (2018). Design of a biocompatible and ratiometric fluorescent probe for the capture, detection, release, and reculture of rare number CTCs. *Anal. Chem.* 90 (22): 13290–13298. https://doi.org/10.1021/acs.analchem.8b02625.

89 Tan, J., Lai, Z., Zhong, L. et al. (2018). A graphene oxide-based fluorescent aptasensor for the turn-on detection of CCFR-CEM. *Nanoscale Res. Lett.* 13: 66.

90 Wu, M., Chen, Z., Xie, Q. et al. (2021). One-step quantification of salivary exosomes based on combined aptamer recognition and quantum dot signal amplification. *Biosens. Bioelectron.* 171: 112733. https://doi.org/10.1016/j.bios.2020.112733.

91 Lai, Z., Tan, J., Wan, R. et al. (2017). An activatable aptamer-based fluorescence probe for the detection of HepG2 cells. *Oncol. Rep.* 37: 2688–2694.

92 Zhao, L., Cheng, M., Liu, G. et al. (2018). A fluorescent biosensor based on molybdenum disulfi de nanosheets and protein aptamer for sensitive detection of carcinoembryonic antigen. *Sens. Actuators, B* 273: 185–190.

93 Cui, F., Ji, J., Sun, J. et al. (2019). A novel magnetic fluorescent biosensor based on graphene quantum dots for rapid, efficient, and sensitive separation and detection of circulating tumor cells. *Anal. Bioanal.Chem.* 411 (5): 985–995. https://doi.org/10.1007/s00216-018-1501-0.

94 Kalkal, A., Pradhan, R., Kadian, S. et al. (2020). Biofunctionalized graphene quantum dots based fluorescent biosensor toward efficient detection of small cell lung cancer. *ACS Appl. Bio Mater.* 3 (8): 4922–4932. https://doi.org/10.1021/acsabm.0c00427.

95 Ding, J., Xu, W., Tan, J. et al. (2022). Fluorescence detection of cancer stem cell markers using a sensitive nano-aptamer sensor. *Front. Chem.* 10: 1–9.

96 Loyez, M., Hassan, E.M., Lobry, M. et al. (2020). Rapid detection of circulating breast cancer cells using a multiresonant optical fiber aptasensor with plasmonic amplification. *ACS Sens.* 5 (2): 454–463. https://doi.org/10.1021/acssensors.9b02155.

97 Sun, D., Fu, Y., and Yang, Y. (2020). Label-free detection of breast cancer biomarker using silica microfiber interferometry. *Opt. Commun.* 463: 125375. https://doi.org/10.1016/j.optcom.2020.125375.

98 Liang, L., Jin, L., Ran, Y. et al. (2017). Interferometric detection of microRNAs using a capillary optofluidic sensor. *Sens. Actuators, B* 242: 999–1006. https://doi.org/10.1016/j.snb.2016.09.153.

99 Carneiro, M.C.C.G., Sousa-Castillo, A., Correa-Duarte, M.A., and Sales, M.G.F. (2019). Dual biorecognition by combining molecularly-imprinted polymer and antibody in SERS detection. Application to carcinoembryonic antigen. *Biosens. Bioelectron.* 146: 111761.

100 Fan, M. et al. (2021). 'On-off' SERS sensor triggered by IDO for non-interference and ultrasensitive quantitative detection of IDO. *Sens. Actuators, B* 344: 130166.

101 Muhammad, M., Shao, C.s., and Huang, Q. (2021). Aptamer-functionalized Au nanoparticles array as the effective SERS biosensor for label-free detection of interleukin-6 in serum. *Sens. Actuators, B* 334 (February): 129607. https://doi.org/10.1016/j.snb.2021.129607.

102 Maier, S.A. (2007). *Plasmonics: Fundamentals and Applications*, 1e. New York: Springer.

103 Shin, H., Jeong, H., Park, J. et al. (2018). Correlation between cancerous exosomes and protein markers based on surface-enhanced Raman spectroscopy (SERS) and principal component analysis (PCA). *ACS Sens.* 3 (12): 2637–2643. https://doi.org/10.1021/acssensors.8b01047.

104 Ning, C.F., Wang, L., Tian, Y.F. et al. (2020). Multiple and sensitive SERS detection of cancer-related exosomes based on gold-silver bimetallic nanotrepangs. *Analyst* 145 (7): 2795–2804. https://doi.org/10.1039/c9an02180a.

105 Butt, M.A., Kaźmierczak, A., Kazanskiy, N.L., and Khonina, S.N. (2021). Metal-insulator-metal waveguide-based racetrack integrated circular cavity for refractive index sensing application. *Electronics* 10 (12): 1–12. https://doi.org/10.3390/electronics10121419.

106 Ben Salah, H., Hocini, A., Bahri, H., and Melouki, N. (2021). High sensitivity plasmonic sensor based on metal–insulator–metal waveguide coupled with a notched hexagonal Ring resonator and a stub. *ECS J. Solid State Sci. Technol.* 10 (8): 081001. https://doi.org/10.1149/2162-8777/ac1805.

107 Khani, S. and Hayati, M. (2022). Optical biosensors using plasmonic and photonic crystal band-gap structures for the detection of basal cell cancer. *Sci. Rep.* 12 (1): 1–19. https://doi.org/10.1038/s41598-022-09213-w.

108 Liang, Z., Khawar, M.B., Liang, J., and Sun, H. (2021). Bio-conjugated quantum dots for cancer research: detection and imaging. *Front. Oncol.* 11 (October): 1–14. https://doi.org/10.3389/fonc.2021.749970.

Index

Biosensors: Nanomaterials, Approaches, and Performance-Enhancement Strategies, First Edition. Baljinder Kaur, Santosh Kumar, and Brajesh Kumar Kaushik.

Published 2025 by John Wiley & Sons, Inc.
Companion website: www.wiley.com/go/kaur

t

v

w

z

IEEE Press Series on Sensors

Series Editor: Vladimir Lumelsky, Professor Emeritus, Mechanical Engineering, University of Wisconsin-Madison

Sensing phenomena and sensing technology is perhaps the most common thread that connects just about all areas of technology, including technology with medical and biological sciences. Until the year 2000, IEEE had no journal or transactions or a society or council devoted to the topic of sensors. It is thus no surprise that the *IEEE Sensors Journal* launched by the newly minted IEEE Sensors Council in 2000 (with this Series Editor as founding Editor-in-Chief) turned out to be so successful, both in quantity (from 460 to 10,000 pages a year in the span 2001–2016) and quality (today one of the very top in the field). The very existence of the *Journal*, its owner, IEEE Sensors Council, and its flagship IEEE Sensors Conference, have stimulated research efforts in the sensing field around the world. The same philosophy that made this happen is brought to bear with this book series.

Magnetic Sensors for Biomedical Applications
Hadi Heidari and Vahid Nabaei

Smart Sensors for Environmental and Medical Applications
Hamida Hallil and Hadi Heidari

Whole-Angle MEMS Gyroscopes: Challenges and Opportunities
Doruk Senkal and Andrei M. Shkel

Optical Fibre Sensors: Fundamentals for Development of Optimized Devices
Ignacio Del Villar and Ignacio R. Matias

Pedestrian Inertial Navigation with Self-Contained Aiding
Yusheng Wang and Andrei M. Shkel

Sensing Technologies for Real Time Monitoring of Water Quality
Libu Manjakkal, Leandro Lorenzelli, and Magnus Willander

Solid-State Sensors
Ambarish Paul, Mitradip Bhattacharjee, and Ravinder Dahiya

Biosensors: Nanomaterials, Approaches, and Performance-Enhancement Strategies
Baljinder Kaur, Santosh Kumar, and Brajesh Kumar Kaushik

Printed and bound by CPI Group (UK) Ltd, Croydon, CR0 4YY
17/09/2026
14964332-0002